Osteopathic Athletic Health Care

JOIN US ON THE INTERNET VIA WWW, GOPHER, FTP OR EMAIL:

WWW: http://www.thomson.com
GOPHER: gopher.thomson.com
FTP: ftp.thomson.com   A service of I(T)P
EMAIL: findit@kiosk.thomson.com

Osteopathic Athletic Health Care

Principles and practice

W. Llewellyn McKone DO

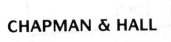

CHAPMAN & HALL

London · Weinheim · New York · Tokyo · Melbourne · Madras

Published by Chapman & Hall, 2–6 Boundary Row, London SE1 8HN, UK

Chapman & Hall, 2–6 Boundary Row, London SE1 8HN, UK

Chapman & Hall GmbH, Pappelallee 3, 69469 Weinheim, Germany

Chapman & Hall USA, 115 Fifth Avenue, New York, NY 10003, USA

Chapman & Hall Japan, ITP-Japan, Kyowa Building, 3F,
2–2–1 Hirakawacho, Chiyoda-ku, Tokyo 102, Japan

Chapman & Hall Australia, 102 Dodds Street, South Melbourne,
Victoria 3205, Australia

Chapman & Hall India, R. Seshadri, 32 Second Main Road, CIT East,
Madras 600 035, India

First edition 1997

© 1997 W. Llewellyn McKone

Typeset in 10½/12pt Times by Photoprint, Torquay, Devon

Printed in Great Britain by The Alden Press, Oxford

ISBN 0 412 59090 5

A catalogue record for this book is available from the British Library

Library of Congress Catalog Card Number: 96-86087

∞ Printed on permanent acid-free text paper, manufactured in
accordance with ANSI/NISO Z39.48–1992 and ANSI/NISO Z39.48–1984
(Permanence of Paper).

DEDICATION
TO DAD

Mum, Vivienne, Ernest, Claire, James,
Benjamin, Julian, Katharina and Maximillian
for putting up with me

Acknowledgements

I would like to say thank you to the following people.

Donald R. Alagiah (World Health Organization), George Anderson (Los Angeles Raiders Football Club), Jim Anderson (Los Angeles Rams Football Club), Mayfield Armstrong (London Monarchs, Nichols State University), Dot Blake (Royal London Hospital, Department of Sports Medicine), British College of Naturopathy and Osteopathy (BCNO), British School of Osteopathy (BSO), Dr P. Choi (Nottingham University Department of Psychology), Dr Martin Collins (BSO), Peter Colvin, DO, Jonathan Curtis-Lake, DO (BSO) Otho Davis (Philadelphia Eagles Football Club and National Athletic Trainers' Association), Andrea van Dongan (Landestheatre, Altenburg, Germany), Ian Eaves (Medisport Int.), Dr Brian English, Alice Fung (library, BCNO), Garret Giemont (Los Angeles Rams Football Club), the late Bill Granholm (National Football League), John Gustaad (Sports Pages), Haringey Rugby Football Club, Billy Hicks (Dallas Cowboys Football Club and London Monarchs Football Club), Peter Higgs (*Mail on Sunday*), Elliot Hill, Mrs N. Iacovou, Mr Andrew Jackson, Colin Jarman, Professor Keith Johnson (Genetics), Leo Jordan (good conversation), Alain Lebret, DO, Sir Norman Lindop, Professor Brian Kneale (Royal College of Art), Kent Rams Football Club, the late K. Keuls DO, Norm Killion (Wisconsin), Mr John King (Royal London Hospital, Department of Sports Medicine), Robin Kirk, DO, John LeGear (Timothy Communications, USA), John McKone, London Monarchs Football Club, Robert (Bobby) Alles King (for making me read), Ken Locker (Dallas Cowboys), Mr Simon Moyes, Dr Carlos Oliveros (Gym Nuevo Estilo, Fuengirola, Spain), Dr John Nixon, Tony Owens and family, Rozanne Oggoian (Chicago College of Osteopathic Medicine), Dr Ashwin Patel, William Podmore (BSO library), Stephen Sandler, DO, the Starting Gate Public House, Kenneth Underhill and family, Richard Weatherall (*The Times* and the *Independent*), Chris Willis (Willis Medical, Dallas, Texas), David Worton (computer man) and all my students and patients.

Contents

Introduction

Schools concentrate too much on knowledge and not enough on insite.

Jostein Gaarder, philosopher, Bergen

The problems of the world cannot possibly be solved by sceptics or cynics whose horizons are limited by the obvious realities. We need men who can dream of things that never were.

John F. Kennedy, Dublin, Ireland, 28 June 1963

It is only when practitioners realize what they are dealing with that they can even begin to understand how to begin to help. This book was compiled and written with the intention of starting the ball rolling, and is a general overview of as much as possible. Practitioners from other disciplines have asked me to direct the book at their professions, so that I may achieve a greater readership. This is impossible: I am an osteopath. Due to the scope of sports medicine, especially in the field of osteopathy, this book is by no means complete. I may have omitted some basic concepts but they can be found elsewhere as the reader searches the references. What I have included is some basic concepts that I feel need driving home.

The book is directed at my students, who always moan at me about not knowing where they can find information on applying osteopathic concepts, principles and practice in the field of sports medicine. Here is some of that information, so now they have no excuses! The book is aimed at giving a general explanation of over 100 years of findings by some of the most respected men and women in the field of health care. The order of the chapters and sections is a personal preference. Chapter 2 is a melting pot of basics that may seem disjointed, but it seemed the only way to put together areas that are always paramount in my mind. In Chapter 3 I have attempted to present in-the-field topics. It includes understanding of physiological responses to trauma, first aid and subsequent stabilization. Chapter 4 covers the principles of dysfunction, or how things can begin to go wrong. It may seem strange that I have included skin infections at the end of this chapter; the reason for this is that it is important osteopathically to consider the skin as part of the other systems, and its 'dysfunction' may be related to an expression of another system's dysfunction. Chapter 5 covers the approach of the osteopath to the patient. In Chapter 6 I have tried to bring all the previous information together. I have presented this regionally in an attempt to make it more applicable in practice. Chapter 7 is a brief look at other approaches to the athlete, in both exercise and treatment.

Few of the ideas in this book are originally my own. Many of the references from books and papers are out of print and I had to search in the library at the British School of Osteopathy, British College of Naturopathy and Osteopathy, and the British Science Library in the Aldwych, London.

I hope to bring to the forefront the fact that osteopathy has had the beginnings of a workable system for a long time, but has been too busy dealing with the mass of musculoskeletal sprains and strains, and became distracted from looking at the base of the triangle representing the beginnings of dysfunction leading to illness. No book can give you all the information, no book can teach you how to think in a certain way. It is important that this book is used as a springboard towards further searching for the answers to questions. There is no right or wrong way to treat a presenting condition, and if the practitioner does not continually read and investigate then he or she becomes an instrument, not a thinking, analytical and feeling human being.

I have chosen sports medicine as the stage on which to present the information, principles and concepts first developed by Andrew Taylor Still and furthered by Denslow, Burns, Sutherland and Korr, to name but a few. These doctors realized the importance of the musculoskeletal system in the maintenance of health. This massive system heals quickly when injured, and nature has designed it in such a way that large sections can be lost without a threat to life. Why? Because it is the 'primary machinery' in the expression and achievements in everyday life. Due to this powerful ability for self-regulation and adjustment, allopathic practitioners have chosen to reduce its importance from general health to a postgraduate speciality, missing the fact that this system influences neuroendocrine/immune responses and homeostasis.

Why sports medicine? We need a yardstick by which to measure the concepts of well-being and health. This sports medicine yardstick allows me to take the patient as far as he or she wishes to go. If I have no original concept of exercise, nutrition and applied psychology, where will I direct my patients on their quest for good health? But a word of warning: like any system the quest is cyclic; you may end up where you began.

After years of travelling and lecturing around the world, it has become more and more apparent to me that the concept of osteopathic medicine has more of a complete approach to health maintenance than any other system. Restrictions on the ability to carry out these concepts change from country to country. This came home to me even more so in the closed environment of full-time professional sport. Application of osteopathic concepts would not only have returned the players to the field more quickly, but would also save thousands of dollars. Unfortunately, the orthodox system of sports medicine practice is far bigger than that of osteopathy. If every sporting body and athlete turned to osteopathy for help tomorrow morning, osteopaths would be in trouble. Many osteopaths want to be as good as the doctors and physiotherapists and adopt some of their techniques and machines. What we are left with is a system that is itself practised in a fragmented nature on both sides of the water. The other unfortunate situation is that we have to deal with a dynamic, psycho-physiological, socio-economic, manipulating variable, the human being.

There are no rules to the practice of osteopathic medicine, just principles. Rigid rules and procedures are a weakness in any system. This does not mean that 'osteopathy means different things to different practitioners', as I have heard a few times. This is not a how-to-do-it book, but a combination of the results of applying osteopathic principles and my experience. The concepts and practical approaches are a thought process towards preventing, or a presenting situation. It is important that the practitioner asks the right questions if he or she expects to receive the right answer. The ability of the osteopath to help a patient with any condition is based on the practitioner's application and continuing education. If a practitioner wants a practice with only low back pain or musculoskeletal trauma patients then that is what you will spend the rest of your practising days treating. It is important that sports medicine is not practised full time as this tends to place the practitioner in a false sense of security.

The layout of the book is that of presenting the facts, and the application of this information to situations encountered both on the field and in the office. This is a mosaic of osteopathy. Students of osteopathic sports medicine will understand very quickly what is being said. To bring this home to you it may be felt that certain ideas and information have been repeated. Contrary to popular belief this is not to pad out the book, but to make sure that the concepts and principles are pressed home. I hope that students will use this book to continue to search for facts that will fit into the individual puzzles, which are their patients. The very least that I hope to achieve is that, when the reader has read this book, he or she will be motivated to argue with me. And to all those of you who are not osteopaths, I do hope you understand the overview between these pages.

> [Then] the *science* of osteopathy is not merely the punching in a certain segment or cracking of the bones, but it is the keeping of a *balance* – by the touch – between the sympathetic and the cerebrospinal system! *That* is real osteopathy!
> Edgar Cayce's *Wisdom for the New Age: Keys to Health,*
> *The Promise and Challenge of Holism.*

When osteopaths, doctors, physiotherapists or anyone with a basic knowledge of science or medicine meets me they will probably tell you that I have an annoying habit of opening book after book, showing them information that is not new and confirms osteopathic principles. This book is a written version of this habit. It is was not written to prove anybody wrong or right, but to touch on the subjects and skills that are important in ostepathic sports medicine. I hope you enjoy reading this book, my first attempt.

I was brought up on osteopathy; my uncle, Llewellyn McKone, was an osteopath. In addition to this I was looked after from childhood by the osteopath Kenneth Underhill. As a child I was always fascinated how Mr Underhill could remove the signs and symptoms of another uncle's 30 year debilitating migraine in just one treatment. There had to be a principle on which he worked.

Science changes constantly. I remember how disappointed I was when I started my chemistry A level at school. I had just become used to the concept that atoms had rings around them, then they moved the goal posts by telling me that they are in fact clouds. Just when you think you are happy and comfortable, somebody comes along and changes things. It has happened to me before and no doubt it will happen again. Fortunately, the principles of osteopathy cannot change.

History of osteopathy $\boxed{1}$

To ask a doctor's opinion of osteopathy is equivalent to going to
Satan for information about Christianity

Mark Twain

In 1874 Andrew Taylor Still, MD (1828–1917) suggested a hypothesis that
addressed preventive medicine. His supposition was simply that the body
contained within itself healing substances and means of combating disease.
The discoveries of immunology have substantiated this hypothesis rather
than supplanted it. Still was a frontier doctor who developed in the
crucible of turbulent times and was motivated by a personal tragedy. Like
his more sophisticated and 'acceptable' medical colleagues and pre-
decessors, Still was dissatisfied with the status quo of medicine. He was
one of the first in his time to point out that if one studied the attributes of
health one might be better able to understand the handicaps and processes
of disease. In Hoag, Cole and Bradford's publication, *Osteopathic
Medicine*, it is written that during Still's time in medical history, the
practice of medicine was for the most part in confusion. In the post-Civil
War period, 'Cnidian practice' was especially rampant, named after one
of the ancient schools of Greek medicine at Cnidus (Knidos). Meerloo
(1964) describes it as follows:

> In ancient Greece we find this controversy (between the two
> schools of medicine) expressed in the antinomy between the two
> dominant medical schools, the one on the Isle of Kos, the other
> from the town of Knidos. The school of Kos emphasized that there
> was only the individual sick man to be treated, man in all his
> varieties of misery. Knidos emphasized disease, viewing it as
> an intruder from the outside that had to be chased away. Kos
> emphasized the study of individual health, Knidos studied its
> antimony, the dis-ease; disease, pain, and suffering. Through the
> ages we find more important; the diseased, the sick man in his
> individual singularity, or the disease, the separate, morbid entity
> subservient to general rules of pathology.

The confusion could perhaps be excused; the disgrace lay in the
deliberate rejection of logic and reason, in favour of the indiscriminate
and ever-increasing application of 'remedies' that seemed to be killing
more people than they cured. Still was a reformer. He wanted to initiate a

medical reform within medicine, but was rebuffed by his own medical colleagues. Encouraged by liberal-minded physicians and patients coming from all over the world for his services, Still continued his medical reform as an independent movement within the world of medicine. He developed a medical philosophy which, upon its rejection by orthodox medicine, became the philosophy of osteopathic medicine. This philosophy is distinctive and distinguishable, original in its implementation but otherwise deriving in a direct line from the ancient Hippocratic school.

Because Still was opposed to the standard practice of dosing every patient with the useless, often disastrous medications of his day, many labelled him, and still do, a 'drugless practitioner'. The fact was that there were certain drugs that he recognized in therapy.

Since allopathic medicine was still the dominant therapeutics system, Still knew he must train his students well for the competition they would face when setting up practice. This goal would require special physical facilities such as a large building with enough space for classes, clinical services and, hopefully, a laboratory and dissection programme (Still, 1991). On 10 May 1892, Dr Still received a charter from the Missouri state capital granting him the right to teach the science of osteopathy. On 14 May 1892, the certificate of incorporation was filed in the office of the secretary of state. The purpose and object of the school (American School of Osteopathy, ASO) was

> To improve our systems of surgery, midwifery and treatment of diseases in which the adjustment of the bones is the leading feature of this school of pathology. Also to instruct and qualify students that they may lawfully practice the science of osteopathy as taught and practised by A.T. Still.
>
> (Chila, 1990)

Even before osteopathy caught the attention of national magazines, fellow Missourian Mark Twain – a free-thinking spirit in his own right – testified on behalf of the osteopaths in the New York State Legislature in 1901. Twain's aversion to the medical profession had begun in 1896, when his daughter Susy died of spinal meningitis. More outspoken than Still (who lost three children to that disease), Twain declared that the physicians had assassinated Susy. When another daughter, Jean, developed epilepsy during the late 1890s, the Twains sought treatment for her at Jonas Henrik Kellgren's Swedish Institute in Sanna, Sweden. As the whole family received Kellgren's drugless treatments, Twain became enthusiastic about Kellgren's system and more disgusted with traditional medicine. Intrigued by the similarity of Kellgren's theories to osteopathy, Twain began to search for a good osteopath who could provide treatments for Jean so they could return to America. It seems that Twain even had the young man in charge of Kellgren's Institute come to America to attend Still's American School of Osteopathy (Trowbridge, 1991).

Following the establishment of the first school at Kirksville, other osteopathic colleges rapidly sprang into existence from coast to coast. At one time there were 37 colleges. Many of these were private institutions which had been started solely for profit, and some were nothing but correspondence courses or 'diploma mills'. The damage they did the profession still lingers today in the misconceptions which were built into the public's mind by inadequately trained physicians who were not worthy of being doctors of osteopathy (DOs). Osteopathy was not a drugless therapy or a glorified massage. The famous 1910 Flexner Report on medical education divided the colleges into two groups: the scientific, or traditional, and the sectarian which included the osteopathic, eclectic, homeopathic and physiomedical schools. Flexner did not classify the chiropractic and the mechano-therapists as medical sects, but claimed they only masqueraded as such. Flexner criticized the osteopathic colleges for accepting applicants without high school diplomas, and found the number of faculties inadequate. The report also stated that the education received at many of the orthodox medical colleges was inadequate, and recommended that only 31 of 155 colleges be allowed to remain in operation. During the next decade over half the medical schools were closed. Flexner's report was responsible for upgrading both allopathic and osteopathic institutions. In 1915, the osteopathic colleges increased their course of study to four years, and in 1916 required a high school diploma for entrance (Walter, 1981). Another type of manipulative therapy was emerging at this time, a method which in some ways was derived from the osteopathic principles established and taught at ASO. In 1896, David D. Palmer visited Dr Still. He stayed around for several weeks, and it is reported he visited with students and looked over the clinic before he returned to Davenport, Iowa, where he had been practising as a 'magnetic healer'. Two years later he opened a school in which he taught his own type of manipulative therapy called chiropractic. For the first several years Palmer's school had only a few students: in 1902 only 15 students were enrolled; a few years later, only a dozen or so more. Not until 1906, when Palmer's son B.J. took over the operation of the Davenport school, did the chiropractic movement experience any expansion. B.J. understood the value of advertising and under his aggressive leadership the chiropractic college grew considerably in strength (Still, 1991).

Table 1.1 shows that, by 1916–17, the osteopathic colleges gave a course equal to that of medical colleges whose graduates were accepted without question by all state-examining boards. The approved standard for an osteopathic education is 4 years, of at least 8 months each, spent in a recognized college of osteopathy after graduation from a high school or its equivalent.

By 1924, 38 states had legally recognized osteopathy. An organization was founded in 1897 to establish professional standards of practice. That organization later became the American Osteopathic Association whose constitution reads: 'The objects of this association shall be to promote the public health, to maintain and improve high standards of medical education in osteopathic colleges' (Walter, 1981). In an affidavit dated 4 April 1940, Dr Charles E. Still stated

That he personally witnessed his father, the said Andrew Taylor Still, personally perform a large number of surgical operations and administer anaesthetics and narcotics in connection therewith, all of which the said Andrew Taylor Still believed to be and expressed to be an integral part of the practice of Osteopathy.

(Siehl, 1984)

In World War I the doctors of osteopathy met opposition to volunteering their services. This happened again during World War II. As the MDs left home to join the services, the DOs closed the gaps in health care throughout the United States. By proving their ability to provide excellent medical service to the civilian population, they gained respect, acceptance and many new friends for their profession (Walter, 1981). Modern osteopathic physicians are sometimes embarrassed by the recorded

Table 1.1 Comparative courses in medicine and osteopathy (Compiled from catalogues of 1916–17). Average hours in each subject and the average totals at the following six leading medical colleges: Johns Hopkins, University of Pennsylvania, Cornell, Harvard University, University of California and University of Illinois; the following six osteopathic colleges: American School, Chicago College, College of Osteopathic Physicians and Surgeons, Des Moines Still College, Massachusetts College and Philadelphia College

	Medical colleges		Osteopathic colleges
Fundamental subjects			
Histology	171		188
Anatomy	489		696
Physiology	329		279
Embryology	72		52
Chemistry	284		288
Pathology	405		342
Bacteriology	157		154
Diagnosis	146		201
Hygiene	66		119
Gynaecology	131		135
Genito-urinary	42		48
Surgery	549		489
Obstetrics	196		172
Jurisprudence	13		25
Eye, ear, nose and throat	187		154
Paediatrics	123		60
Dermatology	41		50
Orthopaedics	71		62
Psychiatry	160		155
Syptomatology	531		653
Total	4163		4322
Therapeutic subjects			
Pharmacology	119		—
Materia medica	33		—
Therapeutics	90	Technique	454
Action and effects of drugs	—		51
Electives etc.	109		458
Total	4490		5285

statements and admonitions from that earlier time. In this tranquillized, antibiotic, hormone-energized and sometimes sterile age, it is easier and more comfortable to take advantage of the miracle drugs – for how could a miracle be exaggerated? – and forget warnings like these:

> One of the first duties of the physician is to educate the masses not to take medicine . . . Man has an inborn craving for medicine. Heroic dosing for several generations has given his tissue a thirst for drugs. The desire to take medicine is one feature which distinguishes man, the animal from his fellow creatures.
>
> (Bean, 1961)

These statements were not made by Still but by one of his distinguished contemporaries, Sir William Osler.

Early in the 1950s, the American Medical Association (AMA) appointed a committee to investigate the osteopathic colleges. The committee report stated that there were no significant differences between allopathic and osteopathic educational programmes. The report was rejected by the House of Delegates. Again, in 1954, another committee looked into the matter. They recommended that the 'cultist' label be dropped, that MDs be allowed to teach in osteopathic schools and that inter-professional relations be instigated. However, long years of bias could not be overcome and, again, it was rejected by the AMA House of Delegates (Walter, 1981).

As we know Dr Still first announced osteopathy in 1874, but it was not until 1897 that one of the first definitions was recorded:

> Osteopathy is that science which consists of such exact, exhaustive and verifiable knowledge of the structure and function of the mechanism, anatomical, physiological and psychological, including the chemistry and physics of its known elements, as has made discoverable certain organic laws and remedial resources, within the body itself, by which nature under the scientific treatment peculiar to osteopathic practice, apart from all ordinary methods of extraneous artificial or medicinal stimulation, and in harmonious accord with its own mechanical principles, molecular activities, and metabolic processes, may recover from displacements, disorganisations, derangements, and consequent disease, and regain its normal equilibrium of form and function in health and strength.
>
> (A.T. Still, 1897)

Dr Still put great emphasis on a working knowledge of general and regional anatomy. Believe it or not, when he first developed his philosophy he did not even mention manipulation (Siehl, 1984).

Donald Siehl, DO wrote a paper titled 'Andrew Taylor Still Memorial Lecture: The Osteopathic Difference – Is it Only Manipulation?', which was presented at the 1983 Annual Convention and Seminar of the American Osteopathic Association held in New Orleans in October of that year, which gave details of osteopathic principles. These were originally written by Dr George Laughlin in 1924 under the title 'The Scope of Osteopathy'. Siehl quoted from this latter article the following:

The underlying principle of Osteopathy is, we all know, a very simple but truthful proposition – that is, disease is produced and maintained by mechanical causes and physical causes; that when the body is out of repair, when it is mechanically wrong, there will be disturbance of function which is disease, and that in the main is the fundamental of Osteopathy; that is the underlying principle, but Osteopathy is more than that. When it comes to the treatment of diseases it includes more than the application of that principle. Osteopathy started with and grew upon that principle. Osteopathy has developed today so that it has outgrown its swaddling clothes . . .

There is no question that there are many cases where spinal lesions exist that do not respond to other forms of treatment but do respond to osteopathic treatment. But we must not hope to confine our practice to this class who cannot be helped by other methods – but we must prepare ourselves to engage successfully in practice in competition with practitioners of other systems. In my opinion the scope of Osteopathy is unlimited – that is if we have the right kind of osteopathic physicians. If you have a narrow view of osteopathy, your scope is that much. If you have a wide liberal view and sufficient knowledge of Osteopathy, your scope of application is just that broad. Now as an example. An osteopathic practitioner should be prepared to engage in general practice. He should be prepared to engage to a certain degree in surgical practice. I do not mean that every osteopathic physician should be a surgeon. It is impossible. It is not necessary, but every osteopathic physician should have a knowledge of surgery, and if he engages in general practice he should be able to do such minor surgery that comes within the scope of general practice. An osteopathic physician should engage in obstetrics. What did the charter say when the original school was founded? Did it say I propose to treat only cases of deformity? No. 'That osteopathy is a system to improve general practice, surgery and obstetrics.' And that is what the first charter said and that is what all college charters should read today.

Just a few words more in regard to the relation of surgery to osteopathy. I maintain that practitioners should make no differentiation between surgery and osteopathy. Surgery is osteopathy; that is if we make it osteopathy. Surgery is part of the osteopathic system. The practice of medicine does not mean that the practice is confined solely to the administration of drugs. Take the average successful medical practitioner. Is his work confined to doping people with drugs? It may be in some cases, but not with the better qualified practitioner. Surgery is a part of the practice of medicine. Hydrotherapy is a part of the practice of medicine. Public health is a part of the practice of medicine. All these things are in common with the practice of medicine and osteopathy. They are part of the osteopathic system. The point I am trying to make is that one should not confine his osteopathic practice to adjusting the spinal lesion, as good and useful as that is. If you will practice all these things your method of practice of osteopathy is a broad method and you will make osteopathy a system that is practical and useful. We must use common sense in the treatment of disease. We must be in favour of progress and growth . . .

Just a word or two in regard to the thing that differentiates osteopathy from the other systems of practice. What is the difference between osteopathy and medicine as we generally understand these terms? Here is a man who practices osteopathy in the sense I have outlined – does a general practice. Here is a man who practices medicine – both practices are fairly successful. What is the difference? They do a lot of things in common; they both practice obstetrics; both give advice with regard to diet; there is no difference there. They both practice to some extent minor surgery. There is no difference there. Here is the difference: The man who practices osteopathy looks upon diseases – acute and chronic – as being produced at least to some extent by something mechanically wrong with the human body which affects the nerve and blood supply to the organs that are diseased. With this mental conception of disease he immediately has his form of treatment outlined and takes hold of the body and adjusts the spine for the purpose of improving innervation and blood supply. We know the nerves control everything. On the other hand, here is the man who practices medicine. He does not pay any attention to the physical side. He does not think in osteopathic terms. He thinks in terms of medicine. If the patient has pain, he gives him something to relieve the pain. If the patient has diarrhoea he gives him something to check the diarrhoea. If the patient is constipated, he gives him something to make his bowels move. He treats symptomatically. The difference is that we believe disease is produced and maintained by spinal abnormalities. By helping nature to cure diseases, we find it useful to make spinal adjustments – normalising the spine to regulate the nerve and blood supply. So every osteopathic physician should look upon osteopathy as a system that will apply to all diseases and should prepare himself to handle all cases that come to him for treatment.

Dr Siehl goes on to say:

what is the osteopathic component? You and I are asked that question many times. The osteopathic component is much more than osteopathic manipulative treatment or musculoskeletal diagnosis. Osteopathic manipulative treatment is valuable for more than just musculoskeletal disease. Osteopathic medicine is more than manipulative treatment and structural diagnosis. The osteopathic cardiologist who may not use manipulative treatement still approaches the patient differently. He has the osteopathic concept in the back of his mind and he ends up treating the patient differently than the allopathic physician. He considers the whole individual and the specific and overall effect of the problems he has found in various areas.

Illness is a disparity between the neuromuscular system and the visceral system in many instances and this forms a cycle which must be broken into in order to adequately treat the problem. We cannot always normalise all tissues and have to be content with partial treatment or partial normalisation and this is why in many instances regular osteopathic manipulative treatment is needed and why in many instances we have to assist the manipulative aspect of treatment with other measures such as medications, diet and nutrition, rest and physiotherapy modalities.

EUROPEAN OSTEOPATHY

The main connection between osteopathy on either side of the Atlantic is John Martin Littlejohn (1865–1947). Littlejohn was a native of Glasgow, Scotland. His education covered areas of the arts, theology, Oriental languages, political economy and physiology and anatomy (Berchtold, 1975). Littlejohn received a PhD from Columbia University in 1894, although most of his previous qualifications were from the University of Glasgow. It was while he was serving as President for Amity College at College Spings, Iowa (1894–8) that his health began to suffer, particularly his throat and neck. He found his way to Kirksville, and had several treatments from Dr Still. He was so impressed that he became a student at the ASO (receiving his DO in 1900), and soon after was appointed Dean of the Faculty and Professor of Physiology. Together with his brothers James and John, he founded the American College of Osteopathic Medicine (1900), later to be called the Chicago College of Osteopathic Medicine. A paper that introduced osteopathy to Britain was read at the Society of Science and Arts in London around this time. This led to the first osteopath to practice in Britain, Dr F.J. Horn, in 1902. After this, several American osteopaths travelled across the Atlantic to settle in Scotland (Dr Willard Walker) and Ireland (Drs Jay Dunham and Harvey Foote).

Littlejohn put greater emphasis on physiology than Still, who emphasized anatomy. Many osteopaths rejected the use of drugs, anaesthetics and antiseptics at the time. Littlejohn preferred to use these agents in moderate amounts. It is ironic that today British osteopaths are more faithful to the original principles than their American colleagues. As early as 1903 Horn and Littlejohn discussed the forming of a British school. In 1913 Littlejohn left America for London and in 1915 started the British School of Osteopathy (BSO), later to be incorporated in 1917. Under British law, anyone could practice osteopathy, chiropractic or naturopathy (nature cure, diet). As early as the 1920s the osteopaths were formulating a register to protect the public from untrained osteopaths. In 1925 a petition to establish a government-sanctioned registry for osteopaths was rejected by the Minister of Health, and again in 1931, 1933 and

1934. The circumstances under which these were turned down were very dubious.

The year 1978 saw the establishment of the London College of Osteopathic Medicine (LCOM), which enrolls practising physicians from around the world on a short course in an attempt to teach osteopathic manipulative therapy. The British Naturopathic and Osteopathic Association (BNOA), initially a naturopathic group which over time added spinal manipulation, operates from the British College of Naturopathy and Osteopathy, which is in Frazer House, Hampstead, London. The Maidstone Osteopathic Clinic and Institute of Applied Technique was founded in 1954 in Maidstone, Kent, by John Wernham and T. Edward Hall, both originally students of the BSO.

French and Belgian training requires that students are at least qualified physiotherapists (who are trained practitioners independent of the medics, unlike in Britain where physiotherapists work under medical supervision). Slowly the Continental European physiotherapists are developing an osteopathic attitude. In 1951 the Ecole Francaise d'Ostéopathie was established in Paris.

REFERENCES

Bean, W.B. (ed.) (1961) *Sir William Osler: Aphorisms from His Bedside Teachings and Writings*, Charles C. Thomas, Springfield, IL.

Berchtold, T.A. (1975) *To Teach, To Heal, To Serve: The Story of the Chicago College of Osteopathic Medicine*, Chicago College of Osteopathic Medicine, Chicago.

Chila, A.G. (1990) The beginning of osteopathic medicine. Andrew Taylor Still Memorial Address. *The DO*. October. pp. 68–79.

Hoag, J.M., Cole, W.V. and Bradford, S.G. (1969) *Osteopathic Medicine*, McGraw Hill, New York.

Meerloo, J.A.M. (1964) *Ilness and Cure: Studies on the Philosophy of Medicine and Mental Health*, Grune & Stratton, New York.

Siehl, D. (1984) Andrew Taylor Still Memorial Lecture: The osteopathic difference – is it only manipulation? *Journal of the American Osteopathic Association*, **83**(5), 47–51.

Still, C.E. Jr (1991) *Frontier Doctor Medical Pioneer. The Life and Times of A.T. Still and his Family*, Thomas Jefferson University Press at Northeast Missouri State University, Kirksville, MI.

Trowbridge, C. (1991) *Andrew Taylor Still: 1828–1917*, Thomas Jefferson University Press at North Missouri State University, Kirksville, MI.

Walter, G.A. (1981) *Osteopathic Medicine: Past and Present*, Kirksville College of Osteopathic Medicine, Kirksville, MI.

2 | Principles

BASIC AND APPLIED ANATOMY AND PHYSIOLOGY

Introduction

As I mentioned in the Introduction, this chapter may seem not to have an overall objective, but it introduces ideas and topics that I consider important. These topics are presented in a basic format that may seem logical to some readers, and strange and out of context to others. All these topics in their various depths are vital in the forming of an overall understanding of osteopathic athletic health care. Details may change after this book is written, but the principles will still be the same, as you will see in later chapters.

Energy

Before we can really begin to understand the concepts of body function it is necessary to review the elements of energy systems used by the body. These systems are important for a clearer interpretation of how and what can go wrong. Placing humans correctly in the bioenergetic cycle leads to a broader concept of their needs; these include nutritional changes, drug interactions, fluids and training techniques which may influence the energy systems to such a degree as to disrupt any treatment programme, advice you may give, and ultimately the prognosis for the athlete.

Sources of energy

The main source of energy is the sun. Energy released from the sun loses mass as expressed by Einstein's formula: $E = mc^2$. The energy reaches the earth at a rate of 2×10^{13} kilocalories per second. This released energy is stored in chemical, electrical, mechanical and thermal forms. As we now know this solar energy is in fact nuclear energy. Besides heat there is also light energy. Light energy is used by plants in a process known as **photosynthesis**. This process combines molecules to form basic food structures such as glucose, cellulose, proteins and fats from carbon (CO_2) and water (H_2O). As humans we are not able to perform this function, so we are to a large extent dependent on plants and other animals for our food (energy) source and indirectly dependent on the sun. When we have eaten this food it can then be broken down, in the presence of oxygen (O_2), to the original CO_2 and H_2O, releasing energy. This process is known as **respiration**.

This **biological energy cycle** is not a one way system; it does not begin with the sole purpose of supplying humans with energy so they can run, jump, swim etc. This cycle is continually in a state of flux with no beginning or end. It is a delicate cycle that, like any biological system, has the capability to adapt, but this adaptive capability is not endless.

So, we now know where the energy comes from. We now have to be able to understand how this energy is used to allow us to perform work, i.e. muscular contraction. Energy released from the process of respiration is not directly used to allow the muscles to contract; it is used to make a compound present in muscle cells. This compound is known as **adenosine triphosphate** or ATP. It is the repeated breakdown and re-formation of this compound that provides the energy for muscular contraction.

As you can probably work out from the name, adenosine triphosphate consists of one complex compound called adenosine and three simpler phosphate groups. The bonds between the adenosine complex and the phosphate groups are of a high energy type. When one of these bonds is broken (hydrolysation), energy (E) is released with the production of between 7000 and 12 000 calories. As a result we are left with the complex adenosine compound attached to two phosphate molecules, which is known as **adenosine diphosphate** (ADP), and a free phosphate molecule (Pi). Further breakdown of the ADP molecule would yield an adenosine monophosphate (AMP) molecule and one molecule of phosphate (Pi).

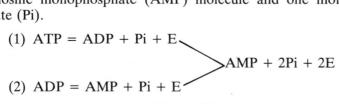

(1) ATP = ADP + Pi + E

$$\qquad\qquad\qquad\qquad\qquad\searrow \text{AMP} + 2\text{Pi} + 2\text{E}$$

(2) ADP = AMP + Pi + E

We can see that the reactions of (1) and (2) yield one molecule of AMP with two phosphate molecules and two units of energy.

ATP is supplied to the muscle in three basic ways. The first is through the ATP–phosphocreatine (PC) system. Breakdown of PC needs to occur for the ATP to be available. The **lactic acid system** (anaerobic) and the **oxygen system** (aerobic) are two more sources of ATP as a consequence of the breakdown of foodstuffs. These are also known as the chemical and metabolic pathways, respectively.

The ATP–PC system

PC is stored in muscle tissue and when the phosphate group is removed, energy is released. The result is creatine and free phosphate. ATP is thus re-formed from the re-forming of ADP and Pi using the energy liberated from the breakdown of PC which is stored in the muscle cells. PC is re-formed from Pi and creatine from the energy released by the breakdown of ATP. The ATP–PC system is used in situations where power is needed in a few seconds, for example footballers, sprinters and shot putters. It is a rapid system that does not use a series of reactions or oxygen from the air.

Anaerobic and aerobic pathways

The anaerobic (lactic acid) pathway, discovered by Gustav Embden and Otto Meyerhof and also known as the Embden–Meyerhof cycle, does not require oxygen, uses only carbohydrates (glycogen and glucose) as fuel, and produces relatively few ATP molecules. In this system food groups are broken down incompletely to lactic acid.

The aerobic (oxygen system) pathway requires oxygen, uses all three food groups (fats, carbohydrates and proteins) as fuel, and results in a relatively large amount of ATP. In this system the result of the aerobic process is CO_2 and H_2O. With oxygen, a glucose molecule is completely broken down to CO_2 and H_2O with production of 38 molecules of ATP.

Within the oxygen system is the **Krebs' cycle**, named after its discoverer, Sir Hans Krebs, who was awarded the Nobel Prize in 1953. Other names for this cycle are the **tricarboxylic acid** (TCA) and the **citric acid cycle**. This cycle occurs in the mitochondria in cells (e.g. skeletal muscle) under aerobic conditions. Two main chemical reactions occur in the Krebs' cycle; they are the production of CO_2 and the removal of electrons (oxidation). The CO_2 is excreted via ventilation. The electrons are removed as a hydrogen atom containing a positive charge (proton) and a negative charge (electron):

$$H \quad \rightarrow \quad H^+ \quad + \quad e^-$$

hydrogen atom   hydrogen ion   electron

At the end of this cycle, H_2O from the Krebs' cycle is combined with the oxygen that we breathe. The series of reactions in mitochondria that results in this combination is known as the **electron transport system** or **respiratory chain**.

Anaerobic and aerobic conditions in rest and exercise

Lactic acid is formed continuously, during rest as well as submaximal exercise. Additionally, lactic acid is formed in contracting muscles under fully aerobic conditions. Further, lactic acid is an indirect product of carbohydrate digestion and is a means of shuttling oxidizable substrate and gluconeogenic and glycogenic precursors between cells, tissues and organs (Brooks, 1987).

What needs to be considered is the foodstuffs metabolized, the roles played by each pathway and the accumulation and clearance of lactic acid in the blood.

At rest our aerobic system is the main pathway involved. This is because at rest the aerobic pathway can supply all cells with sufficient oxygen, and ATP is sufficient to supply all energy requirements. But, it must also be recognized that: (1) lactic acid (although an anaerobic product) can be formed under fully aerobic conditions (e.g. at rest as an indirect product of digestion in the glucose paradox or as part of the Cori cycle mechanism); (2) lactic acid is actively and continuously formed during sustained, submaximal exercise; and (3) lactic acid formed during exercise can be removed during exercise (Brooks, 1987). The constant amount of lactic acid present in the blood is approximately 10 mg/100 ml of blood.

During exercise both the anaerobic and aerobic systems contribute to the production of ATP, but the amount each contributes depends on the type of exercise undertaken. The main types of exercise are: (1) that performed with maximum exertion for a short distance/time; (2) that performed with submaximal effort for a long distance/time; and (3) combinations of the two. Examples of exercise with maximum exertion for short distances/times include running 100 or 200 m, lifting heavy weights and push-ups. The predominant pathway is anaerobic with the major fuel being glucose; some fat is also used but the protein contribution is negligible. However, it should be understood that the aerobic pathway is not completely switched off. Energy is supplied by the ATP–PC and lactic acid system (anaerobic) and cannot be supplied by the aerobic system alone.

Everybody has a limitation to their aerobic pathway in supplying adequate ATP. There are two main reasons for this limitation: (1) we all have a maximum rate at which we can consume oxygen; and (2) the increase of oxygen consumption to a higher level takes a few minutes. Trained athletes have aerobic capacities of approximately 3 and 5 l O_2/min for females and males, respectively; untrained females and males have a maximum capacity of around 2.2 and 3.2 l/min, respectively. At all these capacities there is nowhere near enough O_2 consumed to supply all the ATP required, for example, in the 100 m sprint which could demand around 45–60 l/min.

To reach a level where the amount of oxygen consumed meets the ATP requirements takes a few minutes. It is this delay in the biochemical process of rate of supply and demand that leads to what has been termed the **oxygen deficit**. To continue the exercise of high intensity when the oxygen consumption level is not supplying enough energy, the ATP–PC and lactic acid systems come into play. During this oxygen deficit these two systems supply most of the ATP required to continue.

The result of this quick supply of energy is an equally rapid accumulation of lactic acid in the blood and muscles. This accumulation interferes with muscular contraction, leading to **fatigue**. The major effect of training is on lactate metabolic clearance rate (MCR) (MCR = rate of lactate turnover/[lactate]) (Brooks, 1987). So, the ability to clear the metabolic products of activity is a major prerequisite of athletic ability.

In the case of submaximal effort for a long distance or time, e.g. more than 5 min, we primarily use glucose and fats. If the activity continues for longer than about 1 h there is a shift from glucose as the main energy source to fats. This is due to exhaustion of the glycogen stores. The aerobic pathway is the major source of ATP, with the ATP–PC and lactic acid systems being the supplier at the begining of the exercise until the O_2

plateaus out and there is a steady supply. There is also enough oxygen supplied at this time to pay back the oxygen deficit incurred at the begining of the activity.

As we have seen above, fatigue may be due to lactic acid accumulation during anaerobic activity, but this is not the only factor. Factors causing fatigue during aerobic activity include low blood glucose levels due to the depletion of liver and muscle glycogen stores, dehydration, loss of electrolytes, an elevation of body temperature, repeated minor trauma, contractions etc. These are major contributory factors in injury and illness of the athlete.

In the prevention of injuries it is important to remember that coaching or training should follow the energy system demands of the activity as closely as possible. Therefore, understanding the anaerobic/aerobic needs of the activity will allow formulation of a training programme to achieve the best from athletes. Think of the activities on an energy demand basis. The wrong type of training schedule may expose your athletes to fatigue too early, increasing the risk of injury.

Body type, body fat, body fluids, electrolytes and their distribution

Teddy Bear
A bear, however hard he tries,
Grows tubby without exercise.
Our teddy bear is short and fat,
Which is not to be wondered at;
He gets what exercise he can
By falling off the ottoman.
But generally seems to lack
The energy to clamber back.

Now tubbiness is just the thing
Which gets a fellow wondering;
And Teddy worried lots about
The fact that he was rather stout,
He thought: 'If only I were thin!
But how does anyone begin?'
He thought: 'It really isn't fair
To grudge me exercise and air.'
A.A. Milne

Body type

Body type is also known as body build or **somatotype**. There are three basic forms of body type:

1. **endomorph** – round, undefined, soft body, short neck, predominance of abdomen over thorax.
2. **mesomorph** – square body, slender waist, muscular, rugged, well-defined, broad shoulders, strong wrists, fingers and ankles.

3. **ectomorph** – small boned, thin, long muscles, long thin neck, little muscularity, abdomen and thorax are flat and continuous from an anterior–posterior plane.

These three body types are known as the Sheldon somatotypes. They are extremes, the usual athlete being a combination. For example, female gymnasts are usually ecto-mesomorphs, and basketball players are often endo-mesomorphs. Certain body types seem to be sports specific. The process of fitting a body type to a suitable activity or specialist position within a sport is known as **body composition profiling**. The body composition profile of athletes permits a detailed analysis of the body's major structural components – i.e. muscle mass, fat and bone (Katch and Katch, 1984). However, body type is not always an indication of athletic ability.

Endomorphs have less heat tolerance than the other two groups, while mesomorphs have a tendency towards malignant hyperthermia. Also known as malignant hyperpyrexia, this is a rare muscle disorder in which the body temperature rises rapidly, acidosis ensues, and the heart rhythm becomes irregular; the disease sometimes results in death (Hunter *et al.*, 1987).

Body fat

There are two types of body fat. **Essential fat** is stored in the marrow as well as in the heart, lungs, kidneys and lipid-rich tissues of the central nervous system (important when considering the trophic or nutritional function of nerve tissue). It is essential for normal physiological function. Female essential fat includes sex-specific or sex-characteristic fat. The other type is **storage fat**, which is the major fat of the body and is a nutritional reserve under the skin as well as a protective layer for the internal organs.

Since body fat (BF) cells do not contain ATP, fat is less metabolically active than lean body mass (LBM). LBM (muscle mass) is increased by exercise, while body fat is reduced.

Dietary fats in the blood tend to be cleared within a couple of hours of eating, by the liver and other body tissues. The liver is important because it not only uses fat as a fuel, but converts lipids from chylomicrons (globules) into other blood lipid products such as lipoproteins.

There is a higher percentage of fat in the female body. Boys rapidly gain muscle mass and loss about 3–5% of body fat between the ages of 12 and 17, whereas girls gain some lean body mass as well as fat (Mellion *et al.*, 1990).

The threshold body fat value in a young woman is between 16% and 18%. Below this she may well temporarily stop menstruating. This amenorrhoea may be associated with a degree of osteoporosis, or calcium loss from bones, which may in turn be associated with stress fractures. Therefore teenage and young sportswomen should not allow their body fat to get too low (Sharp, 1986).

Many people believe that to lose fat as part of a training programme, exercise must be performed at low intensity. This is not true, as anyone who watches a 10 km run, marathon, triathlon or other endurance sports event will recognize (Puhl and Clark, 1992).

Obesity can be defined as follows.

> Obesity is an excess of body fat frequently resulting in a significant impairment of health. The excess fat accumulation is associated with increased fat cell size; in individuals with extreme obesity, fat cell numbers are also increased. Although the aetiologic mechanisms underlying obesity require further clarification, the net effect of such mechanisms leads to an imbalance between energy intake and expenditure. Both genetic and environmental factors are likely to be involved in the pathogenesis of obesity. These include excess caloric intake, decreased physical activity, and metabolic and endocrine abnormalities. Hence, a number of subtypes of obesity exist.
>
> National Institutes of Health, 1985

The methods used to measure body fat/obesity are often sophisticated and expensive. Three simple methods for a general approach are recommended.

1. Estimation of relative weight:
   relative weight = body weight/midpoint of medium frame desirable weight
2. Body mass index:
   body mass index = body weight (kg)/height (m²)

It should be remembered that the weight of an individual may not be an indication of their obesity, as weight includes lean body mass. Overweight does not necessarily mean too much fat.

3. Skinfold measurements:

Here, we are attempting to directly measure the fat tissue. Although it is not the most precise method, it is a cheap and convenient way to get a rough estimation. Measurements for body fat of male athletes are taken from:

1. triceps: back of the upper arm over the triceps, midway on the upper arm; the skinfold is lifted parallel with the axis of the arm pendant;
2. subscapula: below the tip of right scapula; the skinfold is lifted along the long axis of the body;
3. abdomen: about 5 cm lateral from the umbilicus avoiding the abdominal crease; the skinfold is lifted on the axis with the umbilicus (Buskirk, 1974).

Body fluids

Water accounts for between 45% and 80% of body weight. This varies between sex, age and body type. The average 75 kg male is made up of about 45 l of water. Two-thirds of this is intracellular fluid. The remaining 15 l is extracellular fluid and is divided between the interstitial fluid (10 l) and the vascular compartment (5 l). There is a fourth transcellular compartment, which includes cerebrospinal, synovial, pleural and pericardial fluids, including the water in the gastrointestinal tract.

Water loss

Normal water loss figures are approximately as follows: gastrointestinal tract, 200 ml/day; respiratory tract, 400 ml/day; skin, 500 ml/day; kidneys, 1500 ml/day = 2600 ml/day. An intake of water to equal this loss could be as follows: as fluid, 1300 ml; as water in food, 1000 ml; water liberated during oxidation in cells, 300 ml = 2600 ml/day.

Water loss increases considerably as the individual begins to exercise heavily. Glycogen is the fuel primarily used during exercise. Approximately 2.7 g of water is combined with each gram of glycogen. Glycogen gives up the water during combustion. This is why if you ingest a high carbohydrate meal it is important to also consume water. Glycogen combines with the water to become an energy-producing compound.

Body salts and proteins

The combination of body salts differs between compartments. In intracellular fluid the main ions are potassium and phosphate. The fluid outside the cells, i.e. extracelluar fluid, contains mainly sodium, chloride and bicarbonate ions. Due to the permeability of the capillary walls to salt, there is a similar salt concentration in blood and interstitial fluid.

Protein content differs in these compartments. Interstitial fluid is predominantly protein free, because capillaries are practically impermeable to the macromolecular proteins. Proteins are present mainly in the venous side of the capillary bed, mainly as albumin. These cause an 'oncotic pressure', drawing fluid towards the venous capillary bed.

All three main compartments are separated by membranes of varying permeability. This means that water can distribute itself under different conditions. The composition of intracellular, extracellular and transcellular fluids is given in Tables 2.1 and 2.2.

Control of fluids

The excretion or retention of sodium and water from the renal system is the basic regulatory mechanism that is used to control the circulating

Table 2.1 Composition of transcellular fluids (mmol/l)

	Plasma	Saliva	Gastric juice	Bile fluid	Pancreatic fluid	Ileal fluid	Colonic fluid	Sweat
Na	140	20–80	20–100	150	120	140	140	6
K	4	10–20	5–10	5–10	5–10	5	5	8
Cl	102	20–40	120–160	40–80	10–60	105	85	39
HCO_3	27	0–60	0	80–120	40	40	60	16

Source: *Surgery* (1994), **12** (4).

Table 2.2 Composition of intracellular and extracellular fluids (mmol/l)

	Intracellular fluid	Extracellular fluid	
		Plasma/serum	Interstitial fluid
Cations			
Na	10	140[a]	14
K	160	4	4
Others	14	2	2
Anions			
Cl	3	102	117[b]
HCO_3	10	27	27
PO_4 and others	106	1.0	1.0
Protein	65	16	0
Total[c]	368	292	302

[a] Note that ions in plasma are usually expressed as mmol/l plasma. However, these ions are distributed in plasma H_2O, which forms only 93% of plasma and hence the concentration of ions in plasma H_2O is higher (Na concentration in plasma H_2O is 153 mmol/l). If the amount of solids (proteins and lipids) is grossly elevated, as in hyperlipidaemia or hyperproteinaemia, the concentration of Na when expressed per litre of plasma may be artificially low (pseudohyponatraemia) without changes in Na concentration in plasma H_2O.
[b] The difference in the composition of interstitial fluids and plasma is due to the effect of proteins, which are negatively charged.
[c] The higher total ion concentration in intracellular compared with extracellular fluid (368 vs 302) is caused by the presence of higher concentrations of non-diffusible anions (e.g. protein and organic PO_4).
Source: *Surgery* (1994), **12** (4).

blood volume. Increasing the reabsorption of salt, associated with water retention, expands the vascular and interstitial compartments.

Myofascioskeletal system

> Rewarding as the visceral emphasis has been through the centuries, it is important to keep in mind, however, that human activity – behaviour of the person – is not a composite of visceral functions, such as peristalsis, secretion, digestion, vasomotion, and glomerular filtration. Human activity is the continually changing composite of the activities of striated muscles, most of them pulling on bony levers, their contractions and relaxations orchestrated by the central nervous system, in response to external and internal stimuli and to volition.
>
> Irvin M. Korr, PhD

Osteopathic principles tell us that the myofascioskeletal system (MFS) is the system that produces the most metabolic waste and uses the most energy. This system does conform to the laws of nature, physics and mathematics, but our reliance on these physical sciences as methods of investigation and explanation takes us further away from what is literally in our hands. The MFS should not be looked at as a system who's primary and only objective is that of movement. This could not be further from the truth. If it is only thought of in this capacity then an understanding not only of what can go wrong with this system, but also the effects it has on the entire organism, will be further away from the osteopath. The MFS should be regarded as a sensory system that responds biomechanically. In its maturation through an individual's life, the stress of postural adaptation and an upright, or orthograde, stance takes its toll on the sensitivity and as a consequence the response of this system.

Structure of muscle

Whole muscle is held together by various components of connective tissue. Wrapped around this whole muscle is connective tissue called the **epimysium**. Bundles of muscle fibres, known as **fasciculi**, are held together by **perimysium** which makes up the bulk of whole muscle. Around each muscle fibre is the **endomysium** and within this is the muscle cell membrane, the **sarcolemma**, which is not connective tissue. Within this cell membrane is a protoplasm called **sarcoplasm**.

The microstructure of the muscle fibre under the light microscope reveals a striped or striated appearance. The sarcolemma is formed from sarcoplasm, a viscous, reddish fluid, in which are found the mitochondria and nuclei. In addition to this are myoglobin, ATP, fat, glycogen, phosphocreatine (which is a reservoir of high-potential phosphyl groups (Stryer, 1981)) and hundreds of threadlike protein strands, **myofibrils**. It is these myofibrils that are composed of alternating black and white areas. The dark areas are called A bands and the light areas are called I bands. When light passes through A bands its velocity is not equal in all directions, i.e. it is **anisotropic**, whereas light passing through the I band emerges the same in all directions, i.e. it is **isotropic**. In between these light I bands is a dark line called the Z line (from *Zwischen*, meaning 'between' in German).

Around the myofibrils is a network system of tubules called the **sarcoplasmic reticulum**. The sarcoplasmic reticulum consists of longitudinal tubules which are parallel to the myofibrils and run into outer cisterns or vesicles at the end of each longitudinal tubule section. Each longitudinal tubule section is repeated along the length of the myofibril, and separated by transverse tubules, the T system or T-tubules. The T-tubule and the two outer cisterns as a complex are known as a triad.

The A and I bands consist of two different protein filaments, the thinner one called **actin** and the thicker one **myosin**. The actin filaments consist of globular molecules linked together forming a double helix, to which are attached two proteins, **tropomyosin** and **troponin**. The tropomyosin filament is a long thin structure wrapped around the actin molecules which end in spherical molecules which are the troponin proteins. Myosin has tiny projections of protein, extending towards the actin filaments. These myosin projections are called **cross-bridges**. Actin filaments make up the entirety of the I band and are not continuous within one sarcomere, that is the distance between two Z lines. These filaments are attached in the Z line zone at each end of the sarcomere, partly extending into the A band zone. The A band contains a small amount of actin filaments even though its main composition is myosin. A zone in the middle of the A band that is free of actin filaments is known as the H zone.

Sliding filament theory

The interdigitation of the actin and myosin filaments has led to the 'sliding filament' theory. In this action the length of the actin and myosin filaments does not change; they slide over each other shortening the I band but not changing the A band, and resulting in disappearance of the H zone. A chemical bond forms between the myosin cross-bridges and selected sites at the actin filaments resulting in a protein complex, **actomyosin**. In its simplest form, when actomyosin is extracted from muscle and ATP is added, the muscle contracts. The events that take place in the process of muscular contraction can be broken down into five broad phases: (1) rest; (2) excitation–coupling; (3) contraction (shortening and tension development); (4) recharging; and (5) relaxation.

Rest
At rest the cross-bridges of the myosin filaments point towards the actin filaments. The ATP molecule at the end of the cross-bridge is not active and the complex is called an **'uncharged' ATP cross-bridge complex**. Within the cisterns (outer vesicles) of the sarcoplasmic reticulum, calcium (Ca^{2+}), vital in the contraction process, is stored in large quantities. While it is stored it is not free. Under these conditions the troponin of the actin filament inhibits the myosin cross-bridge from binding with actin, i.e. actin and myosin are uncoupled.

Excitation–coupling
As we know, nerve impulses at the end plate release acetylcholine onto the sarcolemma spreading the impulses via the T-tubules. This releases the store of Ca^{2+} from the cisterns which then attach to the troponin molecules on the filaments of actin. The 'uncharged' ATP cross-bridge complex becomes 'charged' causing an attraction of the actin and myosin proteins. This forms the actomyosin complex.

Contraction
The formation of this actomyosin complex leads to the activation of an enzyme component of the myosin head called **ATPase**. This enzyme breaks down ATP to ADP and Pi, releasing energy, causing the actin filament to slide over the myosin filament toward the centre of the sarcomere. This leads to shortening of the muscle.

Recharging
Recharging takes place on the myosin cross-bridge by breaking the bond in the actin and myosin complex. It is the resynthesis of ATP that reloads the myosin cross-bridge, breaking the active site on the actin filament. After breaking the bond and the resynthesis of ATP, the cross-bridge site

is ready for recycling. When ATP is not available then the cross-bridge does not break, e.g. rigor mortis in death.

Relaxation

Relaxation begins once the neural input to the muscle stops. There is an unbinding of Ca^{2+} from troponin. The Ca^{2+} is actively pumped back into storage in the sarcoplasmic reticulum cisterns. As a result of this pumping back into the cistern the actin filament is 'turned off', the complex broken, ATPase activity stops, and no more ATP is broken down. Elastic recoil allows the muscle to return to its relaxed (tonic) state.

Muscle spindles and Golgi tendon organs

Much has been written over the past century about the muscle spindles and Golgi tendon organs. Osteopaths are fed on understanding these mechanisms to the point that many of us do not know who said what any more. So, to clarify the situation I will briefly review previous works.

Golgi tendon organs are contraction-sensitive mechanoreceptors of mammalian skeletal muscles innervated by fast-conducting Ib afferent fibres. Control of posture and movement requires permanent monitoring of muscle length and tension, which is provided in mammalian muscles by two kinds of mechanoreceptors, spindles and tendon organs, which are sensitive to changes in muscles' length and tension, respectively (Jami, 1992). Anatomically, it is clear that the spindles are arranged parallel to the extrafusal muscle fibres and are thus suited to sensing length changes of the muscle. The tendon organs, on the other hand, are located in series with the muscle fibres and are thus suited to detecting force generated by the muscle fibres. Spindles have been known for some time to be sensitive to very small perturbations in muscle length, producing a reflex activation, or shortening, of the muscle being stretched. In contrast, tendon organs were thought to respond only to high levels of force and to provide protection against the development of too much force by inhibiting the muscle (i.e. muscle of origin of the reflex) (Howell *et al.*, 1986).

Muscle spindles are found in large numbers in most striated muscles of mammals. These sensory receptors signal information about muscle length to the central nervous system, information that is used in the control of muscle contraction and in the perception of body position. It is an elaborate sense organ, sensitive to dynamic and static changes in muscle length, and is controlled by efferent neurons from the central nervous system. The sensory endings are mostly located at or near the equatorial region. The largest sensory axon to the spindle, the Ia (primary afferent) axon, has extensive annular terminations on all the intrafusal fibres of the spindle in their nucleated regions (the primary ending). The smaller group II axons terminate in 'flower spray' endings disposed principally on the nuclear chain and bag 2 (the secondary ending). Most spindles have only one sensory region (simple spindle); some have more than one sensory region (tandem spindles). The muscle spindle was shown to be a sense organ by Sherrington in 1894. The primary ending arises from the large Ia sensory axon that divides repeatedly as it approaches the intrafusal muscle bundle. The parent Ia axon has a diameter of 12–20 µm in its course from dorsal root to muscle. Of the two branches produced at its division on approaching the spindle, one often goes exclusively to terminals on the bag 1 fibre while the other innervates the bag 2 and chain fibres. The secondary ending has its terminations on the bag 2 and chain fibres and occasionally a few on the bag 1 fibre. Although some of its terminations have an annular form, many do not encircle the intrafusal fibres to the extent seen in primary endings. The overall appearance is more patchy, as suggested by Ruffini's description of the secondary ending as flower spray. Whereas the primary ending is distributed over the nucleated region of the intrafusal fibres, the secondary terminals overlie regions of the fibres more completely occupied by sarcomeres, which are presumably more contractile (Hunt, 1990).

The term 'tension' (i.e. the constrained condition resulting from elongation of an elastic body) is used in physiological studies to designate the force that has to be opposed to a muscle to maintain it at a given length. When a non-contracting muscle is extended it develops, by virtue of its elastic properties, a 'passive tension'. By analogy, the term 'active tension' is often used to designate the force developed by contraction. Both active and passive tensions are usually measured with transducers (strain gauges) and are expressed in 'gram' units rather than newtons, dynes or gram-force.

Given the mechanical properties of muscle tissue, length and tension are physically inseparable parameters, but while spindles monitor muscle length rather than tension, assessment of muscle tension rather than length is considered to be the task of tendon organs (also called musculotendinous end organ, Golgi organ or tendon spindle). However, tendon organs are not equally sensitive to passive and active tensions. In recent years the most important advance in our knowledge of tendon organs was the demonstration that contraction is their adequate stimulus and that an individual receptor can monitor the activity of a single unit.

Commonly accepted ideas that have to be revised represent the tendon organ as a stretch receptor with a high threshold and a low dynamic sensitivity. In fact, muscle stretch does not consistently or significantly activate tendon organs, whereas contraction does. Moreover, tendon organs display a very low threshold and an appreciable dynamic sensitivity when tested with their adequate stimulus: they can signal very small and rapid changes in contractile force. This is likely to have functional consequences that are not yet fully appreciated. It should also be realized that, notwithstanding their denomination, tendon organs are not located within tendons. As originally reported by Golgi, they are mostly found at points of attachment of muscle fibres to tendinous tissue, including deep intramuscular tendons or aponeuroses.

Recent studies have shown that there is no 'private' pathway for Ib input at the segmental level, since a variety of peripheral and central inputs converge on the interneurons mediating autogenic inhibition.

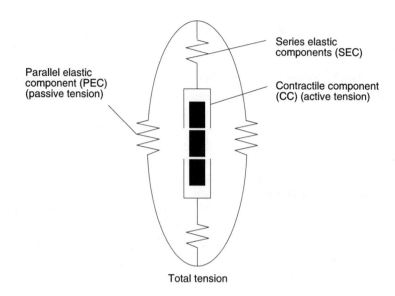

Parallel elastic
component (PEC)
(passive tension)

Series elastic
components (SEC)

Contractile component
(CC) (active tension)

Total tension

Fig. 2.1   Model of the functional components of striated muscle.

Information from tendon organs is co-processed with information from other receptors and dispatched, as from a turntable, via different 'alternative pathways' selected by descending motor commands. The fact that inputs from tendon organs reach the cerebral cortex suggests that they contribute to conscious sensations, allowing assessment of the force developed in a voluntary contraction. It is difficult to disentangle the relative contributions of spindles, tendon organs and other muscle receptors, but it seems likely that all these contributions are co-processed at the highest level, as in the spinal cord, in light of centrally generated information derived from motor commands (Jami, 1992).

Isometric and isotonic contractions

Contractions of muscles occur in one of three ways: (1) shortening of the distance between fixed points at bones and/or fascia (isotonic); (2) increasing tension within the muscles without shortening (isometric); and (3) combinations of these two. A simple model of the muscle (Fig. 2.1) shows how these types of contraction work. This model is important in understanding the treatment protocols later in the book. The model shows a contractile component attached in series to elastic tissue called the series elastic component and a parallel elastic component.

Fascia

It was not until the latter part of the 19th century that connective tissue was studied in detail. Around 1890, chemists and physicists became interested in its composition. Prior to this A.T. Still conceived his new method for the treatment of disease, with connective tissues playing a central role in the new concept. Connective tissue proper may be subdivided into three descriptive types: loose or areolar, in which the fibres form a loose network, the interspaces (areolar) of which are filled with semi-fluid, amorphous ground substance; dense (fibrous) connective tissue, which is characterized by a great many more closely packed fibres with correspondingly less matrix; and special connective tissues, which represent modifications of the loose variety and comprise the adipose, pigment and haemopoietic tissues.

The structural role of connective tissue for intervisceral support and as a binding for every cell of the body is well known. As a bed for all vessels and nerves, connective tissue serves a mechanical and important physiological role. One of its most important functions is as a manufacturing centre for intercellular substances, blood and lymph cells, heparin and antibodies. The significance of the reactivity of this tissue in the prevention and control of noxious forces in the body, by antibody production and phagocytic cell activity, together with its role in the inflammatory reaction and in the prevention of spread of infection, cannot be overestimated.

Finally, the osteopathic physician appreciates the value of connective tissue in synchronizing motion between muscles, viscera, vessels and nerves, but little factual information is available on this (Snyder, 1956).

Contractility of connective tissue persists throughout life, but elasticity decreases with age. The contractile phase not only persists but supersedes all other qualities of fascia.

Fascial attachments have a tendency to shorten after a period of great activity followed by a period of inactivity. With increasing age the ligaments become thicker and tighter. Although the arc of forward bending is not expected to be very marked in the elderly person, the arc should not be limited at around 20–40 years of age, as is so frequently seen.

That part of treatment in which the fascia is important must take advantage of the properties and functions of fascia (Cathie, 1974).

1. It is provided with sensory nerve endings.
2. Its outstanding properties are contractility and elasticity.
3. It gives extensive attachment to muscles.
4. It helps regulate circulation especially that of the venous and lymphatic systems.
5. It both gives support and is a stabilizer, helping maintain balance; the balance is suggestive of motion.
6. It assists in the production of motion, the control of motion, and interrelation of motion of related parts.
7. In many of the conditions resulting in deformities of a chronic nature, i.e. the degenerative diseases characteristic of the ageing process, fascial change will precede changes in cartilage and bone.
8. Fascial contraction and thickening predispose to chronic passive congestion.

9. Chronic passive congestion precedes the abnormal production of fibrous tissue. It is followed by an increase in the hydrogen ion concentration of articular and periarticular structures.
10. Many fascial specializations have special postural functions. In these, definite stress bands can be demonstrated.
11. Sudden stress on fascial membranes will often be accompanied by a burning type of pain.
12. Fascia (connective tissue) is the arena for inflammation.
13. Infections and fluid often track along fascial planes.
14. The dura mater is a connective specialization surrounding the central nervous system. In the skull it is attached to the bone. Changes in its tension and structure are important in the production of headache, and many disturbances of the brain.

Motion

Faulty mechanics can hasten some of the ageing process.

(Kraus, 1947)

The musculoskeletal system may be viewed as a complex system of levers, pulleys and joints functioning interdependently under the motive power of inertial forces and forces supplied by the contractile properties of muscle. This link system approach to the human body permits us to characterize motion, and limits to motion, under normal and pathologic influence, and to understand the effects that local dysfunctions produce for the rest of the body. Frequently, we fall into the trap of assuming that muscle is the single motive force acting on the musculoskeletal system. Indeed, it is a major force, but a variety of inertial forces are also highly influential (Wells *et al.*, 1980).

Movement is an interlinked system in all animal motion. This interrelationship of the link system is vital to the understanding of both normal function and dysfunction. Observing normal action is best done with the trained human eye, as the observer is able to discriminate between what is good and what is bad within the context of the athlete. Osteopathic manipulative therapy can then be prescribed on the basis of the interaction of this link system approach, taking into consideration lesion patterns, which are three-dimensional, as well as an area of more simple adaptations.

Posture, sacral base and the short leg

Throughout the training of an osteopath the concept of postural analysis and its associated factors, sacral base and the short leg, are continually being taught and referred to. Posture is an easy component to blame for the problems of your athlete patient, similar to telling your patient they are overweight.

The normal posture is a dynamic and static physical balance within the system that interacts to the best of its ability with the person's internal and external environments. If everybody was bent double due to an increase in gravitational pull then this would be the normal posture. Changes to posture are generally thought to be due to the effects of gravity, short leg, sacral plane dysfunctions, muscle, fascia and joint problems etc. This is only partly true. Although these tissues are affected in various ways, it is the effect of what has happened elsewhere that we are seeing in a large majority of cases. These include genetic, infective, traumatic, gastrointestinal, genitourinary and cardiorespiratory dysfunctions (metabolic, nutritional, traumatic etc.), and the accumulative adaptive processes of the nervous, endocrine and immunological systems.

This means that the patient's posture has developed the way that it has owing to the individual's life, and is a form of organic history, with gravity the only constant between all of us. Measuring or analysing the individual's posture can be performed by various methods, from observation to the most advanced forms of computer-based analysis. It is still believed by many that dynamic analysis while running on a treadmill and videotaping the athlete is an adequate way of analysing the lower extremity dynamic postural function. Any postural assessment is meaningless without also taking a full history. Attempts at postural correction should be individualized and not generalized. Generalizations will naturally give us an overview of the problem, but the most difficult people to help are those who do not fit into the mould. Methods of helping athletes, as with general health, should involve the use of nutrition, osteopathic manipulative therapy, exercises, medication, psychology etc. It is not a case of just making somebody stand up straight. Many athletes will have developed a certain posture over years of training for a particular reason. Just because it looks different from everybody else does not mean that it is wrong. What you should be asking is, is it functional for the needs of the individual? Does it work?

The word 'posture' has a variety of meanings, depending on the context. The definition in *Webster's New International Dictionary* is: 'Relative arrangement of the different parts of the body; the position or bearing of the body as a whole, whether characteristic or assumed for a special purpose'. For the purpose of this book we shall define posture as the total reaction of the body to fundamental forces, chiefly that of gravity, whatever the position of the body. The word 'reaction' as used here means the total reaction of the body and not that of the musculoskeletal system only.

With this definition before us, let us propound a question as to the significance of posture, and by an examination of osteopathic fundamentals, answer that question clearly and definitely. The question would be something like this: 'Is posture a significant factor in the cause and treatment of disease?' To rationalize, we may say that since, in the osteopathic concept, we link pathological evidence with osteopathic lesions, if posture can be demonstrated as producing or maintaining osteopathic lesions, then surely it is a basic factor in the cause of disease. If this is true, then conversely, we must consider posture in any therapeutic regimen (Nelson, 1948).

Optimal postural balance exists when there is perfect distribution of the body mass around the centre of gravity, with compressive forces on spinal discs balanced by ligamentous tension. In this state, the muscles have normal tone and are not required to contract actively in order to support the body mass. This latter point is clinically significant since the muscles are required to contract to maintain postural balance.

The base of support can be considered from several perspectives. In the standing position, the feet are the base of support for the whole body, and the sacrum is the base of support for the spinal column. If the patient is observed from the back or front, he is considered to have symmetric right and left halves (which is not the case); ideally, a vertical plumb line should exactly bisect the cranium and spine and fall at a point equidistant between the patient's feet, dividing him into equal halves. If the patient is viewed from the side, a vertical plumb line should pass through the external auditory meatus, shoulder, hip and lateral malleolus.

An anatomical short leg has the potential for causing disturbances of postural balance. 'Anatomical short leg' is variation in leg length as measured between the floor and top of the femur with the patient standing. There are many causes of anatomic short leg; however, the effect on postural balance tends to be the same for all. The resultant asymmetry causes strain at some point in the body; specifically, certain muscles must contract in order to maintain balance.

Approaches to the short leg problem

Short leg and its associated problems may be viewed differently by different observers. However, these points of view fit into three general categories. The first two emphasize structure, while the third emphasizes function (Kapler, 1982).

Leg length discrepancy
The first point of view considers the short leg as an isolated entity. The objective of examination would be to measure leg length, using whatever methodology is available. Treatment is based on the general assumption that because of short leg problems, treatment (lifts, shoe modifications, surgery) should correct leg length inequality, and that should solve the problem. However, those who take this view are looking only at leg length differences and are observing only part of the total problem. Correcting the leg length difference could help the patient, but could also cause additional problems or exacerbate existing ones.

Sacral base declination
Some physicians prefer to consider the plane of the sacral base and assume that this plane must be horizontal in order for proper postural balance to occur. Examination is carried out to detect sacral base levelling or unlevelling (sometimes called sacral base declination).

Those who measure and observe sacral base declination take into account the fact that the sacral base plane is not always the same as the plane between the tops of the two femurs. There may be several reasons for this: there may be anatomical asymmetry between the two halves of the pelvis; there may be inequality of sacral halves with one side of the sacrum being larger than the other. In addition, the sacrum is movable between the two halves of the pelvis. Motions of the sacroiliac joint include flexion–extension, rotation and sidebending. Although sidebending is usually accompanied by rotation, it is the sidebending motion of the sacroiliac joint which changes the sacral base plane. Chronic sacroiliac somatic dysfunction will result in a positional change of the sacrum, with sacral base declination. Although it certainly tends to occur with problems of short leg and postural imbalance, it can also occur when leg length is equal.

Postural balance
A third approach to the short leg problem is to evaluate the patient's postural balance. The fundamental question is this: where is the sacrum (base of support for the spine) in relation to the midline, viewed either from the front or the back, or from the side? Examination is directed at observing not only differences in leg length and sacral base levels, but also sacral position in relation to the right or left of midline (anteroposterior or posteroanterior), sacral position anterior or posterior to the midline (lateral), distribution of body mass in relation to the midline, body asymmetry, motion change and tissue texture change resulting from disturbances of postural balance. It must consider the interrelationship of structure and function; to consider only structural relationships without considering function is a departure from osteopathic philosophy.

Postural balance and motion patterns (1982). R.E. Kapler, DO, FAAO.

The above extracts are from the series of papers published by the American Academy of Osteopathy: Postural Balance and Imbalance: Clinical and theoretical significance of posture and imbalance (1983).

Central and peripheral nervous systems

> During thirty years of a challenging and absorbing general practice, I observed that certain somatic and visceral symptom complexes and pain patterns respond satisfactorily only to osteopathic manipulative medicine. I also frequently observed that patients treated for neuromusculoskeletal problems reported concurrent improvement in visceral functions. These phenomena occurred too frequently to be dismissed as incidental.
>
> (Isaacson, 1980)

It is the integration of the nervous system through normal, unconscious, reflex activity that is of major interest to the osteopath, and more importantly the communication between the somatic and visceral components, their communications within themselves and especially what can be done when they are disturbed.

Autonomic nervous system

This system is divided into the sympathetic and parasympathetic systems. Although to some extent the two divisions have opposite effects, they share an objective of homeostasis. They are not fighting or 'antagonizing' each other. It must also be remembered that there are no rigid barriers between this nervous system and the central or peripheral divisions, or between the autonomic system and the endocrine system. In general, however, there is a quantitative as well as qualitative difference between the two subdivisions: sympathetic effects tend to be rather diffuse, whereas parasympathetic effects tend to be specific (Hoag *et al.*, 1969).

Reflex activities

Wilbur V. Cole, the Associate Professor of Anatomy at the Kansas City College of Osteopathy and Surgery, describes the various reflex activities as follows (Hoag *et al.*, 1969).

Certain basic reflex patterns have been substantiated as the basis for more complex reactions observed in a disease process. These reflexes have a potential for altering either psychic or somatic responses, and when the pattern of reflex activity is altered to some non-definable degree, disease is the result. It is for the basic purpose of understanding that the reflexes are separated and described as units as: (1) somatosomatic; (2) somatovisceral; (3) viscerosomatic; and (4) viscerovisceral.

Somatosomatic
'Somatic' is used here in its broadest sense, including head, trunk, walls of the body cavity and the appendages. Both receptors and effectors are present in somatic structures. In other words, this reflex may affect any portion of the body. The stimulus evoking a somatosomatic reflex may be a variation in temperature, mechanical stress, chemical irritation or environmental or structural stress. The major criterion, which holds for all reflex activity, is that the stimulus should be above threshold level, or else that the threshold of the reflex circuit be low enough that activation can be induced by that particular stimulus. This reflex pattern has a direct application to the problem of muscle alterations in the paravertebral region, as noted by the osteopathic physician. When conditions are such that the stimulus elicits and abnormally prolongs a muscle contraction in this area, the tissues become a secondary source of irritation with the potential of disturbing homeostatic balance. If the individual's inherent resistance cannot compensate for the imbalance, clinically recognizable symptoms are the result. It is possible that this state of muscle shortening may be classified as a physiological contracture.

Somatovisceral
Here the reflex receptor is located in a somatic structure and the effector in a visceral structure. The central synapse in the spinal cord is between the afferent neurone and the mediolateral cells of the grey matter of the

spinal cord which give rise to the sympathetic outflow of the thoracic and lumbar regions. Similar reflexes take place in the parasympathetic division of the autonomic system and follow the same general plan: the neurologic structures involved are parasympathetic cranial nerves and the outflow of the sacral region of the spine. In the normal individual, the somatosomatic and somatovisceral reflexes function in a correlative manner in both health and disease. The object of manipulative therapy is to re-establish adequate function of both somatosomatic and somatovisceral reflexes and their interrelationships.

Viscerosomatic
Otherwise known as visceromotor, viscerotrophic or viscerosensory reflex. These variants in the name emphasize one or another of the elements in the viscerosomatic reflex. The stimulus may result in a motor response that is limited to somatic structures, but this is not always the case. Trophic alterations in the skin may result from a chronic reduction in the peripheral blood supply, and these can be recognized by gross observation, but the restrictive term viscerotrophic offers no advantages over viscerosomatic. In this reflex the stimulus is visceral, originating in an autonomic afferent neurone which has its central connection between the anterior horn cells or cranial nerve or both, and the sacral spinal cord (parasympathetic), again with cells giving origin to voluntary efferent fibres. The reflex indicates that either functional or organic visceral disturbances are present which affect somatic structures, usually on a chronic basis rather than an acute one. In connection with pain in the back, it has been suggested that careful study of such patterns in relation to recurrent and chronic diseases of the abdomen might indicate the proper diagnosis or at least suggest the proper line of investigation. It is stressed that pain in the back is a common symptom of many diseases and should not be regarded solely as a local symptom. Visceral diseases should be ruled out by history and examination before a diagnosis of postural back pain is suggested. Not all back pains are due to visceral disease; they may signify inherent factors within the spinal complex.

It is a common situation that patients with visceroptosis are told they have to tighten up their abdomen by doing exercises. One reason they suffer from back problems is due to viscerosomatic irritation that has been caused by shortening of the paravertebral structures that can no longer support the patient's posture. If visceroptosis were the only cause, then all abdominally large patients would have back pain; they do not.

Viscerovisceral
This is primarily an autonomic mechanism that cannot be divorced from those described above or from other influences expressed through autonomic activity. Any evaluation of the autonomic nervous system predicted on a dichotomy, with the sympathetic division on one hand and the parasympathetic on the other, is useful only from the standpoint of description: physiologically it would be a failure. Here, the stimulus arises from a viscus and is transmitted by the afferent sympathetic neurone to

the spinal cord where it synapses with the mediolateral autonomic motor cells. Efferent neurones transmit the impulses to segmentally related visceral structures. It should be remembered that although there is no anatomically distinct visceral–afferent system divided into sympathetic and parasympathetic components, such a system, or such afferent fibres, do exist and do play a highly significant role in body function. A simple example would be the visceral afferent fibres arising from the carotid sinus.

Immune/neuroendocrine system

It is important that sports physicians understand that the immune/neuro-endocrine system has a common circuitry and is an integrated bidirectional system. Acute stress has been known to precipitate the presentation of epidemics like flu, for example in the Japanese earthquake of January 1995. Exercise precipitates an immune/neuroendocrine response under normal circumstances. Taken to extremes, the ability to adapt to demand breaks down and the athlete becomes susceptible to infections.

The human body is intended by nature to be immune to infection and disease. If natural immunity is lacking it may be acquired; if it is lost, it may be restored; if it is present, it may be safeguarded and reinforced. All of these may be provided by osteopathic treatment (Hazzard, 1938).

Metal'nikov and Chorine (1926) showed that, similar to many other physiological responses, immune reactions could be conditioned. The conclusion from these studies was that the central nervous system is involved in immune responses. More recently, these studies have been refined, confirmed and extended by Ader and Cohen (1981). With the integration of the neurosciences and endocrinology and the development of the concept of stress came a possible explanation for one means by which the immune system might be regulated by the central nervous system. This explanation in part resided in Selye's (1936) observation of thymic involution during stress. Of course, the thymus is now recognized as an important organ for the maturation of lymphocytes, and adrenal glucocorticoids that are released during stress can have profound immunological consequences. Today, although we recognize that the situation is not so simple as to involve only glucocorticoids, there are few who question that the neuroendocrine system can control immunological functions. A less well accepted but perhaps more important recent advance in neuroimmunoendocrinology is the recognition that the immune system can regulate neuroendocrine functions. Observations related to this latter concept have begun to provide a biochemical basis for what we now understand is bidirectional, rather than unidirectional, communication between the immune and neuroendocrine systems (Bla-lock, 1989).

By 1966, through an extensive analysis of dominant immunological concepts, Szentivanyi (1989) came to the following conclusion.

1. The significance of the pharmacological mediators of immune responses in normal physiology is that they are the chemical organizers of central and peripheral autonomic action.
2. This suggests the inseparability of the immune response system from the neuroendocrine system.
3. Such inseparability indicates the *de facto* existence of immune/neuroendocrine circuits and the necessity for a bidirectional flow of information between the two systems.
4. One must distinguish between the concept of autoregulation as one that primarily revolves around one effector molecule of immunity, the antibody, and satisfies the requirements of antibody diversity and specificity, in contrast to the more complex requirements of immune homeostasis.
5. In contrast to autoregulation that is always self-contained, homeostatic control is always beyond the constraints of one single cell or tissue system.
6. Thus, immune homeostasis must represent a far more sophisticated level of control than autoregulation, and is based on immune/neuroendocrine circuits.
7. While the many similarities between the immune and nervous systems are fully realized, the immune system has an additional level of complexity over that of the nervous system. Although the nervous system, with its spectacular masses of much-revealing and well-defined projection patterns, is well moored in the body in a static web of axons, dendrites and synapses, the elements of the immune system are in a continuously mobile phase incessantly scouring over and percolating through the body tissues, returning through an intricate system of lymphatic channels, and then blending again in the blood. This dynamism is relieved only by scattered concentrations called lymphoid organs. These circumstances would appear to indicate that the functional plasticity of the immune system is far greater than that of the nervous system, and, consequently, its regulation must require a more complex and sophisticated level of control. For these reasons, I have raised the question in the above mentioned text in 1966 whether the immune system is more 'intelligent' than the brain (Szentivanyi, 1989). Currently, animal models are demonstrating that understanding of this mechanism is at an early stage. The sympathetic nervous system seems to inhibit antigen processing/presentation and, indirectly, T helper responses (Van Buskirk, 1990; Heilig *et al.*, 1993).

Nociceptors also have the potential for direct and indirect influence on the immune system. They may affect the immune system indirectly through the sympathetic nervous system. The thymus, spleen, lymph nodes and other lymphoid tissues are innervated by autonomic postganglionic neurones that appear to modulate the T-independent B cell antibody response (Bulloch and Moore, 1981; Miles *et al.*, 1981; Williams *et al.*, 1981; Bullock, 1985). Robuck discussed in 1915 the place of bony lesions in lowering immunity, and included with this discussion some phases of the pathology of the lesion (Burns, 1933).

Adaptations to exercise

Adaptations to exercise are important to the osteopath, not just due to the physiological changes, but also the palpatory changes. Physiological changes due to various stages of training can be looked at under the following headings.

Submaximal

Following submaximal exercise, there is no change or a slight decrease in VO_2 with a decrease in lactic acid production and an increase in the number and size of the mitochondria. There can be a decrease or no change in cardiac output. Stroke volume is increased, resulting in an increase in cardiac hypertrophy and an increase in myocardial contractility. The heart rate decreases with a decreased sympathetic drive. There is a decreased blood flow per kg of muscle and an increased extraction of oxygen by the muscles.

Maximal

Following maximal exercise, VO_2 is increased, with an increase in both total blood volume and the muscles' ability to extract oxygen. This is accompanied by increased lactic acid production with enzyme activities. Cardiac output, stroke volume and myocardial contractility will continue to increase. As with submaximal drive, there is an increase in heart volume and a resultant decrease in sympathetic drive. The changes in blood flow volume will level out with no real difference per kg of working muscle.

At rest

Most osteopaths will see their patients at rest. Adaptations of the athlete seen at rest include a cardiac hypertrophy that is the result of marathon or endurance training leading to an increased ventricular capacity, and sprint or non-endurance athletes presenting with increased myocardial thickness. There will be decreased heart rate and increased vagal tone as a consequence of parasympathetic inhibition.

Integration of these systems

There are no rigid barriers between the above division of the nervous system (autonomic nervous system) and the central or peripheral divisions, or between the autonomic system and the endocrine system. Though each of these systems may act independently, there are frequent examples of obligatory interdependence (e.g. the action of the hypothalamus in promoting gastric secretion by vagal activity), and circumstances in which one system will elicit a response in the other (e.g. the increase in sympathetic and adrenal activity in the presence of strong emotion) (Hoag *et al.*, 1969).

The field of neuroimmunomodulation encompasses all of the interactions between the central nervous system and the immune system. In essence, the nervous system layers the functions of the immune system via the neural, hormonal and paracrine actions. Neural and humoral influences from the immune system feed back to the CNS to modulate its influences. This is a subject which was in its infancy until the last 5–10 years; there has recently been an explosive increase in our knowledge of these interactions.

The nervous system controls the immune system by release of hypothalamic peptides which alter the secretion of anterior pituitary hormones. These circulate through the blood and act on the immune cells, either directly or through their own target gland secretions to either increase or decrease immune responses. In addition, there is direct innervation of immune cells which can lead to alterations in their function in response to immune challenge. In response to host challenge the cells of the immune system release a variety of cytokines that circulate to the brain to alter temperature regulation, sleep, food intake and other vegetative functions. The cytokines alter efferent output to the immune cells and release of hypothalamic peptides to alter secretion of pituitary hormones. In addition to acting on the CNS via the circulation, various neurones and glial elements can also produce cytokines and thus directly affect the nervous system. Furthermore, circulating cytokines act directly on the pituitary to alter secretion of its hormones. Cytokines are also produced in the pituitary gland to exert direct effects on the output of pituitary hormones (McCann, 1994).

Soon after the emergence of physiology as a distinct discipline, Claude Bernard tested the concept of *vis medicatrix naturae* (the healing influence of nature) in experiments which demonstrated glycogen storage in the liver, along with what he called 'internal secretion' of glucose into the hepatic vein. He also pointed out the peripheral vasomotor neural control mechanisms, which later were recognized as part of the temperature-regulating system. On the basis of such findings he concluded that all the body's vital mechanisms 'have only one object, that of preserving constant the conditions of life'. The human body is an optimum-seeking physiological system (Hoag *et al.*, 1969). (Fig. 2.2). The body must be interpreted as a cybernetic or servomechanism, that is self-regulating.

In the 1972 *American Academy of Osteopathy Year Book*, George Malcolm McCole, DO, in his chapter on 'Historic and Philosophic Foundations of the Osteopathic Concept', describes the overall system and the role of the osteopath as follows:

Oscillation in control systems

In an excellent chapter on the 'Internal Environment and the Physiology of Its Control', Guyton (1961) outlines the characteristics of physiological

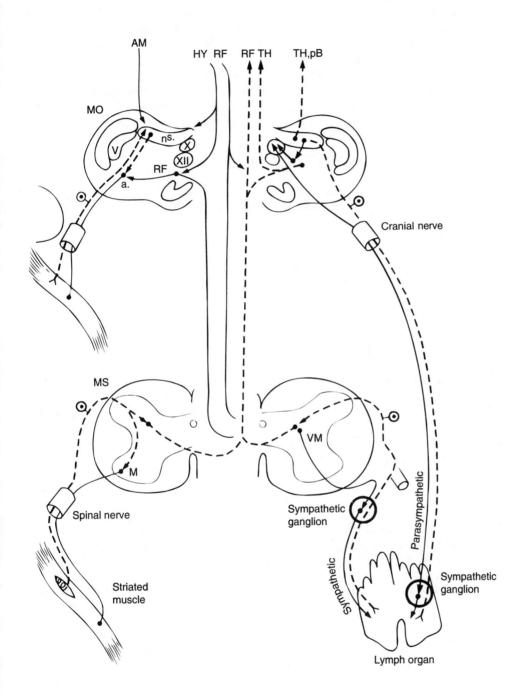

Fig. 2.2 Immune–somatic connection. V, sensitive nucleus of trigeminal nerve; X, nucleus of dorsalis nervi vagi; XII, nucleus of nervi hypoglossi; MS, spinal cord; ns, nucleus solitarius; M, spinal motor neurone; AM, amygdalar nuclei; a, nucleus ambiguus; RF, reticular formation; HY, hypothalamus; MO, medulla oblongata; TH, thymus; VM, visceral motor neurone; pB, nucleus parabrachialis.

control systems. He points out that oscillation – normal and desirable in many living systems – depends on two traits of the servomechanism: delay and amplification. Delay must be appreciable, between receptor excitation and response; and amplification must produce overshoot in the response.

In the reflex type of control system familiar to us in biology and medicine, delay and strong amplification almost always are present. Oscillation of the homeostatic 'constant' concerned therefore is expected. Oscillation is necessary for control, and control regulates (limits) oscillation.

Driving, damped and waxing oscillations

Guyton (1961) describes three types of control system oscillation: driving, damped and waxing (runaway). Of these, the driving type is more or less normal, as in blood pressure curves or in the alternation between endometrial hyperplasia and menstrual slough.

Damped oscillation may be normal for some physiological control systems (e.g. tendon reflexes). Damping, on the other hand, may be decidedly abnormal – as in failure of respiration due to loss of sensitivity of the respiratory centres. In abnormal damping it may be necessary to supply additional stimulus periodically, as (in example just given) by thumping the chest wall.

Waxing oscillation results when the amplification factor is exaggerated (as in the conclusive response of the strychninized animal); or when the sensitivity of detector elements is increased (e.g. the grotesque arterial pressure fluctuation caused by excessive bleeding). Waxing oscillation results also when damping factors are decreased. An example is the familiar pendulum-type (clonic) tendon reflex response when the cerebellum, basal ganglia or other extrapyramidal control (damping) system has been impaired.

The physician as servosystem engineer

The physician must understand these patterns of control, in order to achieve maximum insight into the condition of his patient – and in order to intervene *pro re nata*. According to the ancient and still valid doctrine of 'first, do no harm', the physician intervenes minimally. He serves nature. But in terms of 'controls engineering', the physician may and must intervene as indicated.

1. To decrease the amplification factor, as by relieving structural aberrations which cause hyperexcitability and irradiation in brain and spinal cord systems. Among the familiar methods by which amplification factors can be decreased are sedative drugs, local anaesthetic agents and selective manipulation. Less familiar perhaps is the administration of an agent (physical or chemical) to increase blood flow; ischaemia irritates (before it destroys), helping to initiate and perpetuate lesions of all types. When ischaemia yields to appropriate therapy, amplification often is decreased.

2. To increase damping, as by improving the flow of blood to a part; by otherwise warming the region; by helping the patient to gain insight into his condition so that his inherent damping systems may have full play; or by systemic retraining of reflex sets, as in the rehabilitation of the cerebral palsied, or residually damaged anterior poliomyelitis patient.

Occasionally a condition may call for increase of amplification or decrease in damping, but such occasions are relatively infrequent.

Osteopaths are servosystem engineers.

Circadian rhythm

It was not until I began work with the World League of American Football London Monarchs that the concept of international flight and crossing backwards and forwards across time zones and the effect of circadian rhythm upset really meant anything to me. Having to travel east and west through time zones of more than 5 hours sometimes every weekend for up to 3–4 weeks had some strange effects on players and staff.

Every practitioner knows that different people have different oscillatory patterns over a 24 hour period. This is an aspect of sports medicine that is not taken into account in many sports-related injuries, training sessions, events and reaction to osteopathic manipulative therapy. A basic understanding of the cyclic variation in body systems is necessary to understand these physiological rhythms that naturally occur in sleep–wake cycle, pulse rate, ventilation, arterial pressure, diuresis and excretion of electrolytes (Winget *et al.*, 1985). For example, the athlete has a lower body temperature in the morning and higher temperature in the evening.

What is circadian rhythm? It has been described as a system that comprises specialized photoreceptors and circadian (Latin *circa dies*, 'about 24 hours') oscillators whose complex mutual interactions are integral to daily patterns of brain function and, in many species, to the seasonal control of reproductive and metabolic phenomena (Cassone, 1990). It is the internal daily and seasonally tuned body clock, that adjusts physiology and metabolism for the short- and long-term benefit of the organism.

What is of interest here is the effect on athletic performance. If as we understand the circadian rhythm mediates physiology etc. in an oscillatory pattern over a 24 h period, then training and competing at certain times will not only be an advantage, but would allow to plan and have the edge, if possible. When arriving in another country, overcoming the effects of jet lag to allow you to get back on schedule is paramount. Most parameters influential for athletic performance, such as grip strength, maximal ventilation, oxygen consumption and tolerance to an all-out effort, are closely related to the body temperature curve, which peaks in the late afternoon (Winget *et al.*, 1985; Minors *et al.*, 1986). The direction of travel and the number of time zones crossed are two major factors

influencing the duration and magnitude of depressed athletic performance. When travel is in a westward direction, the length of the day is
extended and the body's circadian system must undergo a phase delay
(lengthen). This is a natural direction for the body to adjust. It has been
shown that humans, isolated from all environmental and light cues,
display internal rhythms of about 25 hours. In contrast, with travel in an
eastward direction the length of the day is shortened and the circadian
system must undergo a phase advance (shorten) to resynchronize. With
the body demonstrating a natural tendency toward a period of longer than
24 hours, it is more difficult for the body to adjust itself to advances in
daily rhythms. Thus, adjustment to eastward travel is more difficult. It has
been suggested that at least three time zones must be crossed before the
deleterious effects of jet lag are evident (Jehue *et al.*, 1993). The problem
is how to reset the time difference. Eichner (1988) uses the principle of
zeitgeber (German for 'time giver'). Humans, with a 25 hour free running
period, adapt to a 24 hour day by resetting their biological clock each day.
To reset the clock, we must perceive an indicator of environmental time –
a *zeitgeber*. Temperature and other physical measures that vary diurnally
are potential *zeitgebers*. It is speculated that social contacts and the timing
of meals may also be *zeitgebers* for humans.

Several components of this system have been identified. First, the
hypothalamic suprachiasmatic nucleus (SCN) is a crucial component in all
amniote species studied. Second, the pineal gland, which synthesizes and
secretes the indoleamine hormone melatonin rhythmically such that
melatonin levels are highest at night, appears to vary from species to
species in its importance for circadian organization. Third, in all mammals
photoreceptors within the ocular retinae, which project directly to the
SCN via the retinohypothalamic tract (RHT), are the sole source of visual
input controlling the circadian phase and period of rhythms generated by
the circadian system (Cassone, 1990). There is growing evidence that
human circadian organization is profoundly melatonin-sensitive. As mentioned above, the hormone melatonin (N-acetyl-5-methoxytryptamine) is
secreted during the darkness hours. The pineal gland and the retina are
the primary sites of melatonin production. While the role of the pineal is
well established, the mammalian retina is just begining to be appreciated
as an independent site of melatonin synthesis (Wiechmann, 1986; Nowak
et al., 1989; Olcese and Møller, 1989). Because environmental light
inhibits melatonin synthesis by direct action on the retina and indirect
action on the pinealocytes via the SCN pathway, a classical (and physiological but non-selective) way to regulate the melatonin system has been
to alter the animal's photoperiod by changing the time and/or duration of
the light stimulus.

Melatonin is synthesized in photoreceptors of the retina and in the
pinealocytes of the pineal gland and then secreted locally (retina) or into
the bloodstream (pineal). It acts on specific high-affinity receptors in the
retina, CNS and pituitary which regulate a variety of physiological and
behavioural effects. Melatonin is metabolized by separate degenerative
pathways in the brain and liver. The system is active during the dark

phase of the daily cycle with nightly peaks seen in the activity of *N*-acetyltransferase (NAT), the rate-limiting enzyme for melatonin synthesis, and in the levels of melatonin (in retina, pineal, cerebrospinal fluid and plasma) and urinary 6-hydroxymelatonin, the liver metabolite of melatonin. The darkness is permissive in that the circadian rhythm of melatonin production is actually driven by an endogenous clock in the SCN of the hypothalamus (and possibly also in the retina). Information from the SCN is conveyed via a multisynaptic pathway [retinohypothalamic tract→SCN→paraventricular hypothalamus→medial forebrain bundle→mediolateral nuclei of upper thoracic spinal cord→superior cervical ganglion-→sympathetic nerves (nervi conarii)] that terminates with sympathetic input to the pineal gland. The system is dramatically inhibited by environmental light, the external cue that synchronizes the melatonin rhythm to the prevailing day/night cycle and allows the organism to maintain precise 24 hour rhythms and stay in tune with the time of day and season (Krause and Dubocovich, 1990).

Questionnaire: Are You a Lark or an Owl?

Circle the number that follows the response you selected for each of the following questions.

1. **If you were free to plan your day, when would you get up and when would you go to bed?**

Get up (a.m.)		Go to bed (p.m.)	
5 to 6:30	5	8 to 9	5
6:31 to 7:45	4	9:01 to 10:15	4
7:46 to 9:45	3	10:16 to 12:30	3
9:46 to 11	2	12:31 to 1:45	2
11:01 to 12 noon	1	1:46 to 3	1

2. **If you have to get up at a specific time, how dependent are you on the alarm clock to wake you up?**

Not at all dependent	4
Slightly dependent	3
Fairly dependent	2
Very dependent	1

3. **How easy is getting up in the morning?**

Not at all easy	1
Not very easy	2
Fairly easy	3
Very easy	4

4. **During the first half hour after waking up:**

How alert are you?		How tired are you?	
Not at all	1	Very tired	1
Slightly	1	Fairly tired	2

Fairly	3	Fairly refreshed	3
Very	4	Very refreshed	4

How's your appetite?

Very poor	1
Fairly poor	2
Fairly good	3
Very good	4

5. **When you have no commitments the next day, when do you go to bed compared with your usual bedtime?**

Seldom or never later	4
Less than 1 hour later	3
1 to 2 hours later	2
More than 2 hours later	1

6. **Some friends want you to exercise hard with them. How would you perform:**

From 7 to 8 a.m.?		**From 10 to 11 p.m.?**	
Quite well	4	Quite well	1
Reasonably well	3	Reasonably well	2
Poorly	2	Poorly	3
Very poorly	1	Very poorly	4

7. **When in the evening are you tired and ready for bed?**

8 to 9 p.m.	5
9:01 to 10:15 p.m.	4
10:16 p.m. to 12:45 a.m.	3
12:46 to 2 a.m.	2
2:01 to 3 a.m.	1

8. **When would you be at your peak for:**

A gruelling two hour quiz?		**Two hours of exhausting physical work?**	
8 to 10 a.m.	6	8 to 10 a.m.	4
11 a.m. to 1 p.m.	4	11 a.m. to 1 p.m.	3
3 to 5 p.m.	2	3 to 5 p.m.	2
7 to 9 p.m.	0	7 to 9 p.m.	1

9. **You've gone to bed several hours later than usual, but you can wake up when you wish to. What is the most likely to happen?**

You'll wake up at the usual time and not fall back asleep	4
You'll wake up at the usual time and doze thereafter	3
You'll wake up at the usual time but fall back asleep	2
You'll wake up later than usual	1

10. One morning you must be on watch from 4 to 6 a.m. You have no commitments the rest of the day. Which of the following would you do?

Would you not go to bed until watch was over	1
Would you take a nap before watch and sleep after	2
Would you take a good sleep before watch and nap after	3
Would you take all sleep before watch	4

Score (total points) _____

To learn what type you are, find your score on the scale below.

Score	Type
14–23	Owl (evening type)
24–31	Almost an owl
32–44	Neither (intermediate type)
45–52	Almost a lark
53–65	Lark (morning type)

(Source: Eichner, 1988.)

FUNDAMENTALS OF OSTEOPATHY

> The physician must . . . have two special objects in view with regard to disease, namely, to do good and to do no harm. The art consists of three things, the disease, the patient and the physician. The physician is the servant of the art, and the patient must combat the disease along with the physician.
>
> Hippocrates

While the fundamentals of osteopathy are quite straightforward, putting these principles into practice is a challenge. There have been slight alterations over the years in the application of these principles, with changes in social, disease (viral epidemics) and global political trends. Here, we look at the laying down of these principles by some of the leading men and women in osteopathic medicine. Even though the underlying current is still the same, it is important to look at the many interpretations of these principles. It is also important to compare and contrast them, understanding why they are 'pulling the same way' even though they are all 'holding different ropes'. This is one of the sections in any book that students tend to bypass. Many of you who are students, and some practitioners for that matter, will ignore this chapter, and instead attempt to seek out answers to questions you have about the treatment of presenting conditions and situations that you have or will find yourself in. However, a knowledge of the fundamentals of osteopathy is essential to good practice.

In 1899, Dr Still wrote that 'osteopathic medicine was a recently discovered, unknown sea and that its practitioners were only acquainted with its shoretide. It is my object to teach principles and not rules.' He went on to say in the same year in *Philosophy of Osteopathy*: 'I do not instruct the student to punch or pull a certain bone, nerve, or muscle for a certain disease, but by a knowledge of the normal and abnormal, I hope to give a specific knowledge for all diseases.' He further stated that it was a desire to 'give to the world a start in a philosophy that may be a guide in the future'. In passing, it is interesting to note that, contrary to common belief, Dr Still was aware of and recommended the use of all diagnostic or treatment methods that would benefit his patients. An announcement in his 1899 book reads:

> . . . the A.T. STILL INFIRMARY is full prepared to receive and handle the most difficult cases requiring the highest order of skilled surgery, and it is not necessary to send such cases to the city hospitals in the East for even the most difficult and delicate operations . . . Cases requiring careful and delicate surgery, the removal of fibrinoid tumours, and in fact any operation of whatever nature will receive the best and most scientific treatment and care in this situation. The management has now secured a powerful and perfect Roentgen or x-ray apparatus which will be used in connection with this department, in the examination of difficult cases.

Without principles of approach the practitioner will look for absolute trends, i.e. every lateral elbow strain is 'tennis elbow', every infrapatella discomfort is 'jumper's knee'. There are no rules.

It does not matter what speciality you are involved in, osteopathic principles are applicable in any field. If the practitioner is not applying them, then he or she is letting the patient down.

> Cardiologists and other specialists need to look beyond 'the organ', 'the system', and 'the disease'. They need to think about the body as a unit, as a whole.
> I. Philip Reese, DO, a board-certified cardiologist and internist,
> Fort Worth, Texas (Sprovieri, 1992).

Definitions of osteopathy

Here are four definitions taken from *Osteopathic Principles in Disease* by Carter Harrison Downing, MD, DO.

> Osteopathy is that science which consists of such exact, exhaustive and verifiable knowledge of the structures and functions of the human mechanism, anatomical, physiological, and psychological, including the chemistry and physics of its known elements as has made discoverable certain organic laws and remedial resources, within the body itself, by which nature, under the scientific treatment peculiar to osteopathic practice, apart from all ordinary methods of extraneous, artificial, or mechanical principles, molecular activity, and metabolic processes, may recover from displacements, disorganisations, derangements, and consequent disease, and regain its normal equilibrium of form and function in health and strength.
> Mason W. Pressly, AB, PhD, DO

Osteopathy is that science of healing which emphasises, (a) the diagnosis of disease by physical methods with a view to discovering not the symptoms but the causes of diseases, in connection with misplacements of tissue, obstruction of the fluids and interference with the forces of the organism; (b) the treatment of diseases by scientific manipulations in connection with which the operating physician mechanically uses and applies the inherent resources of the organism to overcome disease and establish health, either by removing or correcting mechanical disorders, and thus permitting nature to recuperate the diseased part, or by producing and establishing antitoxic and antiseptic conditions to counter toxic and septic conditions of the organism or its parts; (c) the application of mechanical and operative surgery in setting fractured or dislocated bones, repairing lacerations and removing abnormal tissue growths or tissue elements when these become dangerous to the organic life.

J. Martin Littlejohn, LLD, MD, DO
(the founder of The British School of Osteopathy)

Osteopathy is that science or system of healing which, using every means of diagnosis, with a view to discovering, not only the symptoms, but the causes of diseases, seeks, by scientific manipulations of the human body, and other physical means, the correcting and removing of all abnormalities in the physical relations of the cells, tissues and organs of the body, particularly the correcting of misplacements of organs or parts, the relaxing of contracting tissues, the removing of obstructions to the movements of fluids, the removing of interferences with the transmission of nerve impulses, the neutralising and removing of septic or foreign substances from the body; thereby restoring normal physiological processes, through the re-establishment of normal chemical and vital relations of the cells, tissues, and organs of the body, and resulting in restoration of health, through the automatic stimulation and free operation of the inherent resistant and remedial forces within the body itself.

C.M. Turner Hulett, DO

Osteopathy is a philosophy, an art, and a science of medicine founding its system of therapeutics on all fundamental, physical, chemical, and biologic sciences, basing its treatment of all abnormal conditions of the body on the natural laws and vital principles governing life; namely the adjustment of all these vital forces of the body, whether physical, chemical or mental, in so far as we have knowledge thereof.

C.H. Downing, MD, DO

In 1961 Angus Gordon Cathie, DO, put forward his theme, 'The Pyramid of the Osteopathic Armamentarium'. This is a very important interpretation as it gives one of the clearest layouts of the principles and allows for some direction and structure for the student. Here is an extract from the *American Academy of Osteopathy 1974 Year Book*, titled 'Osteopathic Principles':

> Permit me to rather briefly refer to the structure of the Pyramid of Osteopathic Armamentarium or schematic representation of the relationship of the major sciences incorporated into the study of man and osteopathic principles. It has as its base Anatomy, Physiology, and Pathology. Resting upon this base is a block representing Biophysics upon which is superimposed one representing Biochemistry. Next comes a block representing Hydrodynamics, then Thermodynamics, and finally Logic. These blocks are surmounted by one representing Application of the subject's name, and at the apex, is one representing Results. Above the apex of the pyramid is an arch having three divisions. The first division represents integration, the second interplay, and the third homeostasis. The value of such schema lies in the truth it calls to mind. Here we are brought face to face with the major sciences operating in man to make him what he is and that we are responsible for the reasons we behave like humans. We are reminded that they are interrelated and interdependent; that there is a continuous yet ever changing interplay between them that is essential if the homeostatic mechanism of the body is to be maintained. Thus we may obtain a glimpse of the wide variety of biophysical and biochemical combinations that account for an expansive range of variations many of which contribute to the organism. The only danger in the use of such a schematic representation is that of oversimplification. To me it portrays a scientific starting point in the study of man in the comprehension and application of osteopathic principles. It points to the importance of the somatic component of disease.
>
> Osteopathic principles are then the scientific application of basic sciences in the study and care of man. It also recognises the importance of the relationship existing between body, mind, and spirit. From its inception this profession has recognized these truths and has endeavoured to promote a reasonable approach to the study of health and disease. Behind each physical sign and symptom there lies an anatomicophysiological basis which, if comprehended, permits one to understand the reason for the appearance of these manifestations of disease.
>
> From what has been said about the scientific basis of osteopathy it is possible to consider the following conclusions to which I refer as, 'Values that Remain and Endure'.
>
> 1. All changes recognized in the body are related, directly or indirectly to the sciences named in the Pyramid of the Osteopathy Armamentarium.
> 2. If all changes found are directly or indirectly related to the sciences named, detection of these changes is more readily

accomplished by a knowledge of these sciences as they relate to the human body.

3. The osteopathic concept, philosophy, and principles are based upon these truths or scientific facts.
4. The study of physical man is primarily the application of biophysical and biochemical principles. (The term 'physical man' is used in contradistinction to 'spiritual man'.)
5. The structure and function of the musculoskeletal system is related primarily to biophysics. The state of nutrition of these tissues is related primarily to biochemistry.
6. Problems of hydrodynamics and thermodynamics are the result of biophysical and biochemical activity.
7. Change in tissue density is, from a functional point of view, related especially to biophysics.
8. The somatic component of disease is definitely related to biophysical change. Biophysical changes may be produced by biochemical change. The interrelation becomes obvious.
9. The application of these sciences to the animate is more difficult than their application to the inanimate.
10. The interrelationship existing between these sciences, as seen in the human body, is complicated by the state of character of the neuroendocrine system. (Sometimes the state or character of the neuroendocrine system is referred to as one's 'Autonomic Personality.')
11. The intricate mechanism responds or reacts biophysically and biochemically to external and internal stimuli. The type and intensity of the reaction varies greatly among individual members of the same species.
12. These observations lead us to recognize the individuality of man.
13. The interrelationship existing between the various systems of the body is such that the condition of one is reflected in the others. The unitary concept of man is thus scientifically correct.

The osteopathic profession was the first to make use of this course of investigation and to develop from it an adequate examination of the somatic component of disease. It was the first to develop a system of therapy based on these principles although history cites earlier physical methods of the treatment of disease.

To disregard the scientific approach to the study of man is, I believe, potentially dangerous. We must first identify the elements to be organized and must attempt to intelligently interpret the concepts, weigh the values, and improve our skill.

Angus Gordon Cathie (1902–70)

The future of the osteopathic profession cannot be predicted with certainty. The fundamental principles which underlie osteopathic practice are of course permanent and will endure under whatever name they are practised. The osteopathic profession must maintain its independence until the principles which it represents receive universal recognition by the therapeutic world. The fear is sometimes expressed that osteopathy will be absorbed by medicine. This cannot be so, since osteopathy is a part of medicine and consists of a set of principles which are true. As long as the profession of osteopathy maintains its own institutions and abides by its principles it will maintain its identity. When the principles of osteopathy are identical with the principles of medical practice, the profession of osteopathy would have fulfilled its mission. The question as to whether the healing art will adopt the name osteopathy is a minor matter. The history of the osteopathic profession at any such time will speak for itself, and the contribution of Andrew Taylor Still will be recognized for its true worth (Page, 1927).

The structure–function relationship

Too often biologists simply cannot bring themselves to make a sufficiently serious study of the structural aspects of their problems. Yet there can be no reason to assume that, while Nature uses methods of infinite subtlety in her chemistry and her control mechanisms, her structural approach should be a crude one (Gordon, 1987).

The structure–function relationship is one of the most basic of biological concepts. From insects to mammals, structure denotes an ability to function in a certain way and function is limited or controlled by structure. Changes in the structure–function relationship can be influenced by the interaction of the external and internal environments or combinations of both. Functional changes in the athlete can range from immediate to gradual, via the neuroendocrine system. Demands on the make up of the body, visceral and somatic, need time to change structurally in the face of changing functional demands. Sometimes this is easy; other times it is nearly impossible. The functional demands may include changes in psychological, mechanical, emotional, intellectual or nutritional aspects. Any factors that change the functional interaction of the individual with his or her environment will lead to some kind of structural change.

This interrelationship can also be reduced to a cellular level, and was documented as early as 1855 by the German scientist Rudolph Virchow. He wrote: 'All diseases are in the last analysis reducible to disturbances, either active or passive, of large or small groups of living units, whose functional capacity is altered in accordance with the state of their molecular composition and is thus dependent on physical and chemical changes of their contents.'

Essential to the application of a unifying philosophy of medicine, as expressed in the basic physiological principles of osteopathic medicine, is recognition of the inseparability of anatomy (structure), physiology (function) and pathology (disease or aberrant structure–function). It is this basic theme around which occurs the greatest opportunity to initiate further advances in medical practice (Hoag *et al.*, 1969).

Martin D. Young, DO, wrote in *Laws of Structure and Function*:

Let us cite a simple example. We have a normal body with a normally functioning digestion. There is introduced into that digestive tract a combination of food chemistry that is decidedly incompatible which the normal digestion cannot handle and we say the digestion is upset. Mind you, the structure is in a perfectly normal state. The stomach does the best it can and passes it on to the intestines and the colon. Disturbance and irritation to the lining and glands of the digestive tract and to the circulation to these structures and to the nerves which supply them is inaugurated. Continued abuse results in definite changes in those organs and a perverted function. Those changed structures can only express the perverted function for which they were in no way responsible.

The nervous irritation thus set up is transferred by metastasis to the spinal segment corresponding, causing irritation to, and consequent contraction of, the supporting tissues of that joint and a spinal lesion ensues. The spinal lesion is not the cause in this case. The perverted function determined all of these structural changes and determined what they should become. So much so that now the digestive tract cannot perform its normal function of digestion with the simplest diet, for a reversal has taken place and the perverted structure becomes the expressor (or if you prefer the term, governor, though by compulsion) of the perverted function.

To say that the structure–function relationship between the musculoskeletal system and the other body systems is important is an understatement. The importance of the musculoskeletal system in the hierarchy and interrelationship of the body systems was recently emphasized in relation to hypokinetic disease. It was pointed out that the role of striated musculature was far more important than that of assisting locomotion. Activity of striated muscle affects bone structure and body posture; it influences circulatory and metabolic function and endocrine balance; it mediates the expression of emotions and nervous responses (Hoag *et al.*, 1969).

On a gross level, the palpation skills of the osteopath are suited to reading the structural changes in human tissue which are then interpreted as functional disorders. These biophysical quality changes lead to biochemical functional expressions in immediate or distant organs.

The osteopathic lesion

Yes, more definitions. Definitions are always a good place to start, to reduce the risk of confusion.

The following are extracts from George W. Northup, DO, who wrote in Hoag *et al.* (1969) on the subject of osteopathic lesions.

The term osteopathic lesion is traditional, deriving from the time when the disturbance in joint function and relationships was the most obvious feature, and the contributing factors were little understood. Objective definition and impeccable classification are certainly desirable attributes. However, it may also be pointed out that if medical fact were dependent on correct definitions, we would indeed be in trouble. As far as the requisites for definition are concerned, it should be noted that the word itself is derived from the Latin *definire*, meaning 'to set limits or to describe'.

It is possible, however, to describe observations made through the years concerning osteopathic lesions and their importance in the structure–function of biomechanical man. The importance of these lesions is enhanced by the unavoidable conclusion that both their local and remote effects occur through the unifying and communicating channels of the neuroendocrine and circulatory systems. Therefore, the osteopathic lesion can no longer be considered merely a mechanical disorder; it must be viewed as one intimately connected with the biological structure–function of the total body economy. Its definition and significance must be assessed in relation to the total body state in the individual under consideration.

Osteopathic lesions are biological processes observed in the musculoskeletal system. They cause both subjective and objective signs and symptoms, which may appear in the area of the lesion itself, or in segmentally related but remote portions of the musculo-skeletal system, or as disturbed function in other body systems. This triad of cause and effect comprises the common disorders occurring in the musculoskeletal system. Their influence, channelled through the neuroendocrine and circulatory systems, makes these biomechanical lesions potentially capable of affecting every tissue of the body. This concept has been greatly illuminated by the systems analysis techniques of modern research.

Emphasis is placed on the idea of impairment of response, which is a purely qualitative concept. There is no single, universally typical response to any given inciting factor. The disease state can occur only if the homeostasis of the body tissues becomes altered, and such alteration can progress to almost any degree. Homeostatic balances and disturbances are regulated at the cellular level; therefore, cytopathologic changes mark the beginning of altered function, which may increase considerably before symptoms appear that the clinician recognizes as disease.

The foregoing concepts and definitions are recognized in the official statement of principles issued by the American Osteo-pathic Association (1963). In addition to the factors mentioned above, this document cites the view that the musculoskeletal system plays a prominent role in homeostasis and therefore in total body health, exerting a twofold influence: it is an especially vulnerable site for the origin of stressful factors which may disturb equilibrium, and it offers a physiologic approach to diagnosis and the application of therapy. Faults in joint motion are especially likely to instigate excessive reflex activity, because of the rich sensory innervation from articulations. Impulses arising at any of such initiating stations may produce changes at the synaptic junction which in turn modify the total integrating functions and systems of the body.

Lesions similar to those described by osteopathic physicians have also been noted and described by others. The following description includes observations and hypotheses similar to those made by osteopathic physicians for almost a hundred years:

> Entrapment neuropathy . . . is a region of localized injury and inflammation in a peripheral nerve that is caused by mechanical irritation from some impinging anatomical neighbour. It may occur at the point at which a nerve goes through a fibrous or osseofibrous tunnel or at which the nerve changes its course over a fibrous or muscular band. Although external force may have been applied directly to the region, in many cases there is no discernible relationship of the condition to external trauma.

Entrapment neuropathy, then, on the basis of this description, denotes the non-specific neurological lesion which is often described, particularly if an articulation is involved, as an osteopathic lesion. An important difference is that the osteopathic physician would not necessarily expect the lesion to be associated with local signs of trauma, and in the absence of such signs he would search for contributing factors elsewhere in the nervous and musculoskeletal systems.

It is important to note, in this connection, that failure in response is not taken to indicate irreversibility of the lesion. The osteopathic lesion is a dynamic disturbance and when manipulative therapy is impossible or ineffective it is understood that the disorder has advanced beyond the lesion stage.

This osteopathic lesion concept is best described as a working model. You will encounter again and again research papers that discuss and make conclusions without realizing the total concept of their interpretations. Denslow and Hassett (1944) were the first physiologists working in the osteopathic field to have papers published in the *Journal of Neurophysiology*, under the title 'The central excitatory state associated with postural abnormalities'. After this terms like 'lesion reflex', 'lesion areas', 'irritable focus', 'final common path' and 'central excitatory state' started to appear in scientific journals.

Taking a big jump to recent publications, there seems to be poor continuity of terminology, and repeating of fundamentals. On a positive point, such papers have indirectly reinforced those theories of principles in practice laid down at the turn of the century. A good example of this is the work by Woolf and Walters (1991), who discuss concepts of 'central and peripheral sensitization' in post-traumatic situations. We shall look at this in more detail later.

The neural basis for the osteopathic lesion

In the December 1947 edition of the *Journal of the American Osteopathic Association*, a paper was published with the title 'The neural basis for the osteopathic lesion', written by Irvin M. Korr. To this day, as a result of his experiments, this concept still holds true. Admittedly, there have been further discoveries in the field of physiology since 1947, but the concept and the findings of Korr still hold. Here, I will use Korr's work as the basis for this section, mixing it with references to other papers and findings.

The four main principles in osteopathy appear to be:

1. Joints and their supports are subject to anatomical and functional derangements.
2. These derangements have distant as well as local effects.
3. They are related, directly or indirectly, as well as having pathological influences.
4. Their local and distant effects are influenced favourably by manipulation.

The osteopathic lesion (joint derangements, in single and multiple presentations) has many aspects which are partly revealed in the local and distant effects referred to in 2 above. Included among these are:

1. Hyperaesthesia, especially of the muscles and vertebrae.
2. Hyperirritability, reflected in altered muscular contraction.
3. Changes in tissue texture of muscle, connective tissue and skin.
4. Changes in local circulation and in the exchange between blood and tissues.
5. Altered visceral and other autonomic functions.

Within the nervous system, in the phenomena of excitation and inhibition of nerve cells, and in synaptic and myoneural transmission, lie the answers to some of the most important theoretical and practical osteopathic problems.

The activity and condition of the tissues and organs are directly influenced, through excitation and inhibition, by the efferent nerves which emerge from the central nervous system and which conduct impulses to these tissues and organs (Fig. 2.3). For example:

Muscle:
- anterior horn cells (motor neurones) – muscular contraction;
- lateral horn cells (sympathetic preganglion neurones through post-ganglionic neurones) – vasomotor activity.

Skin:
- lateral horn cells – vasomotor activity;
- lateral horn cells – sweat gland secretion;
- lateral horn cells – piloerection.

Viscera:
- lateral horn cells – smooth muscle contraction.
- lateral horn cells – glandular secretion.
- lateral horn cells – vasomotor activity.

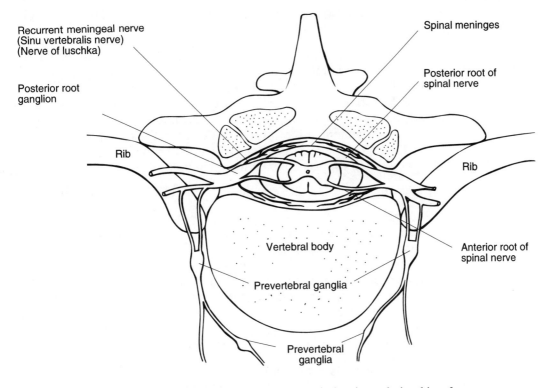

Fig. 2.3 Cross section of thoracic spine and spinal cord showing relationship of nerves to bony anatomy.

The activity of these organs and cells is directly determined by the activity of their motor nerves. The amount of contraction (tension produced or degree of shortening) at any moment is in proportion to the number of motor neurones which are conducting impulses at that moment and the average number of impulses per second which each is conducting to the muscle. It is important to emphasize, however, that not all the effects of overactivity or underactivity of the efferent neurones are direct and immediate. Thus, a muscle's overactivity, over a long period of time, may result in fibrosis and major chemical and metabolic changes, while under-activity may result in atrophy.

Overactivity of sympathetic fibres which control arterioles may result in local anoxaemia, inflammation, altered capillary permeability, oedema etc. Imbalance in the efferent neurones controlling the smooth mus-culature of the gastrointestinal tract may result in flaccidity or spasm with serious effects on digestion and absorption and, therefore, on the entire body economy. Overactivity or underactivity of the neurones controlling glands may result in disastrous shifts in acid–base, fluid and electrolyte balance and in such conditions as peptic ulcers. If the gland happens to be one of the endocrines, the effects may be especially serious and extensive.

Korr went on to ask three main questions, with efferent neurone activity in mind.

1. What factors control activity, i.e. the number of impulses, in the efferent nerve fibres?
2. How does structural abnormality, i.e. the osteopathic lesion, play upon these factors to produce overactivity or underactivity of these fibres and, therefore, of the organs which they innervate?
3. How does manipulative therapy play upon these factors to restore balance and cause regression of signs and symptoms? This I will discuss in the section on principles of manipulation.

The following models of factors controlling efferent activity were proposed.

1. The principle of reciprocity states that through the network of interneurones (also known as internuncial neurones, intercalated neurones and connector neurones), which is situated within the central nervous system, every neurone potentially influences, and is influenced by, almost every other neurone in the body.
2. The principle of convergence states that many nerve fibres converge upon, and synapse with, each motor neurone. These presynaptic fibres convey impulses from a large variety of sources to the efferent neurone which, therefore, represents a final common path.

These were then presented in more detail.

1. Each anterior horn cell receives impulses from a large number of sources through the presynaptic fibres which converge upon and synapse with it. All the descending tracts in the spinal cord, conveying impulses from such sources as the cerebral cortex, red nucleus, medulla oblongata, vestibular nuclei, cerebellum, pons, superior colliculi and other higher centres, establish synaptic connections with the anterior horn cell for the mediation of voluntary motion, equilibrium, postural reflexes, visuospinal reflexes and others. The proprioceptors, stretch and tension receptors situated in the tendons and in the muscles themselves are a steady continuous source of impulses. Afferent fibres from the viscera may also play an important role. In fact, every afferent nerve fibre, whether it mediates touch, pain, pressure, temperature, sight or any other sense modality, exerts influence upon the final common path represented by the motor nerves.
2. Some of the converging fibres exert an excitatory influence, while others have an inhibitory influence on the same motor neurones.
3. The activity of the motor neurone at any moment, that is, the frequency with which it delivers impulses to the muscle fibres, represents a dynamic balance among all the excitatory and inhibitory influences being exerted by the many neurones which converge upon it. The proprioceptors and some of the higher centres, through their steady, tonic control, act as governors or buffers. The balance, however, is shifted from moment to moment in accordance with changes in the internal and external environment and in response to

volition. As previously stated, pathology results when the balance is shifted too far in one direction or the other (excitation or inhibition) for too long.

4. The collective action of the presynaptic nerve fibres upon the final common path is further reflected in the phenomena known to physiologists as **reinforcement** and **facilitation**. Before the anterior horn cell can discharge impulses into the muscle fibres, it must itself receive excitatory impulses simultaneously from a number of presynaptic fibres. Stated another way, before a given stimulus (e.g. to the skin) can produce a reflex muscular response, the anterior horn cell must first be 'warmed up' or 'put on edge' (facilitated) by impulses from other (excitatory) fibres which synapse with it. The efferent neurone must already be in a state of subthreshold or subliminal excitation. In other words, the various fibres converging upon a given group of motor neurones must cooperate (reinforce each other) in order to open the final common path leading to the muscle. In a whole nerve it has been demonstrated that a considerable portion of the nerve fibres must be in a state of subliminal excitation before any of them fire and cause muscular contraction.

5. This requirement serves as a margin of safety or an insulation, preventing muscles from responding to every impulse which reaches the anterior horn cell.

6. When a significant percentage of the anterior horn cells in a given segment of the spinal cord is maintained in a state of subliminal excitation, they require little additional stimulus to produce a reflex response. This is reflected in our frequent use of the terms 'on edge', 'jumpy' and 'tense', which imply motor aspects of psychic imbalance. In individuals thus characterized the anterior horn cells are maintained close to, or at, threshold, even during rest.

The osteopathic lesion and the factors controlling efferent activity

In answering the second question, Korr had to address another question. How do anatomical and functional derangements of the joints and their supports operate on these factors to produce seriously altered activity of the efferent neurones? In answering this question he presented research work which was in progress at that time at Kirksville College of Osteopathy and Surgery under the directorship of J.S. Denslow. The research revealed close relations between lesion mechanisms and certain well-established physiological principles.

In this original paper Korr goes on to give an overview of the experimentation; I will leave the reading of this section up to you. Needless to say, it is very interesting in its approach and rationale, and discusses reflex thresholds, sore spines, hyperirritable motor neurones, intersegmental spread of excitation, procaine studies, bilateral differences, rest activity and an interpretation of experiments.

In his interpretations he came to the following general conclusions.

1. An osteopathic lesion is associated with a segment of the spinal cord which has a low motor reflex threshold, i.e. it represents a hyper-excitable segment of the cord. At least in the lesioned segments studied by us it may be said that the balance has been shifted too far for too long toward the excitatory side.
2. The lowered reflex thresholds are demonstrable independently of the related spinous process. Even though changes in the palpable character-istics and in pain sensitivity of the spines are important diagnostic features, they are apparently secondary to other, more fundamental alterations in the cord. This aspect will be discussed later.
3. The lesion represents an anterior root at least some of whose motor neurones are maintained in a state in which they are relatively hyperexcitable to all impulses which reach them. In a severe lesion many of the motor neurones are so close to threshold, even when the subject is at rest and reclining comfortably, that it requires very few additional impulses from the neurones which synapse with them to trigger these motor neurones into overt activity. These additional impulses may come apparently from almost any source; the spinous process is but one such source.
4. The lesion, therefore, is to be conceived not as a radiating centre of irritation, spreading excitation to other segments, but rather as a segment upon which irritation is focused. It represents a place in the cord where barriers to motor neurone excitation have been lowered and which, therefore, channels impulses into muscles receiving motor innervation from that segment.

On the topic of the basis for segmental hyperexcitability and the source of the impulses, Korr continues:

> These anterior horn cells can be maintained in this facilitated state by continuous and excessive bombardment from some untiring source or sources. The sources which, in our opinion, most closely fulfil these qualifications are the proprioceptors, i.e., the stretch, tension, and pressure receptors in the muscles and connective tissues.
>
> First, postural, mechanical, and articular derangements unques-tionably cause increased fibre length or tension in the muscles and tendons on at least one side of the articulation in question. The proprioceptors are highly sensitive to changes in fibre length or tension.
>
> Secondly, they are the only adapting type or receptor. They keep firing impulses into the cord via the dorsal root fibres as long as they are under tension and at frequencies which are pro-portional to the tension. The higher the tension, the higher the afferent bombardment for as long as the tension is maintained.
>
> Third, the afferents from proprioceptors not only have segmental distribution, but they specifically influence the activity of the muscles to which they are most closely related or in which they are situated. This specifically extends not only to the muscles them-

selves, but to specific muscles' heads. It is thought that the muscles spindle cells reflexly influence only the muscle fibres in their immediate vicinity. In this way, highly localized, viscous cycles of irritation may be set up.

We therefore believe that these receptors play an important role in maintaining segmental hyperexcitability in areas of lesion. As a result of the constant barrage of impulses which they fire into the cord at their level, the anterior horn cells of the corresponding segment are maintained in a state of chronic facilitation – at a high level of subliminal excitation, even during rest.

Effects of chronic facilitation

In these segments, therefore, it may be said that the normal 'insulation' which keeps the efferent neurones from firing in response to every impinging impulse has become worn. Since under normal conditions of life, requiring constant adjustment to the external and internal environments, and motion and the maintenance of the erect posture, so many impulses from so many sources are constantly impinging on the motor neurones, in all segments of the spinal cord, those which are already facilitated, as in the lesioned segment, will inevitably be more active than the others. If maintained for sufficient periods of time this hypertonus would lead to textural, morphological, chemical and metabolic changes, i.e. sources of irritation.

These experimental studies demonstrated that closely and quantitatively correlated with lowered motor reflex thresholds are three other features of the lesion:

1. alteration in the texture of the tissue overlying the spinous process;
2. lowered pain threshold;
3. increased susceptibility to trauma.

From this it was concluded that neurones other than the anterior horn cells may also be facilitated and maintained in a state of hyperexcitability in the lesioned segment. This appeared to be true, at any rate, of certain preganglionic fibres of the sympathetic nervous system and of the spinothalamic fibres conveying pain sensation to the higher centres.

Characterization of the lesion

As a result of this experimentation, Korr was able to progress and characterize the osteopathic lesion on the basis of the information available at the time.

1. Normally, efferent neurones are kept from firing in response to every impulse that reaches them by the fact that a relatively high level of subliminal excitation – or facilitation – must be established by other impulses converging upon them before the firing point is reached. This requirement serves as a sort of insulation.

2. In the lesioned segment this insulation has been weakened. A large portion of the efferent neurones are kept near the firing point (facilitated), even under conditions of rest, by chronic afferent bombardment from segmentally related structures.
3. Proprioceptors are undoubtedly an important source of this bombardment, but any segmentally related structure may be such a source. A pathological viscus, or a cutaneous trigger spot, or any other inflamed or irritated structure which concentrates its afferents in one or a few dorsal roots may be responsible for more or less tonic facilitation. (The close relation of the osteopathic lesion to referred pain mechanisms is clear, but space does not permit a discussion of this most important aspect.)
4. The firing process in the facilitated efferent neurones may be completed by any impulses impinging on those neurones, whether the source of these impulses be the cerebral cortex, postural and equilibrium centres, bulbar centres, cutaneous receptors or others. Should this superimposed bombardment be sufficient and enduring, the facilitated neurones (and the organs they innervate) may be maintained in a continuous state of excessive activity.
5. The state of facilitation may extend to all neurones having their cell bodies in the segment of the cord related to the lesion, including the anterior horn cells, preganglionic fibres of the sympathetic nervous system and apparently the spinothalamic fibres.
6. Because a structural defect, an osteopathic lesion, sensitizes a segment to impulses from all sources, and for reasons previously given, the lesioned segment is to be considered not a radiating centre of irritation, but rather a neurological lens which focuses irritation upon that segment. Because of the lowered barriers in the lesioned segment, excitation is channelled into the nervous outflow from that segment.
7. It is a truism in neurophysiology that when something is excited, something functionally related is simultaneously inhibited. Although in our studies we have not yet directed attention to this aspect, it cannot be doubted that facilitation in the segment of lesion also extends to neurones exerting inhibitory influences upon other neurones or organs.

It may then be concluded that an osteopathic lesion represents a facilitated segment of the spinal cord maintained in that state by impulses of endogenous origin entering the corresponding dorsal root. All structures receiving efferent nerve fibres from that segment are, therefore, potentially exposed to excessive excitation or inhibition.

Homeostasis

The word 'homeostasis' was coined by Walter B. Cannon, the great Harvard physiologist, who had a clear grasp of its hierarchic implications. He wrote that homeostasis liberates the organism:

> from the necessity of paying routine attention to the management of the details of bare existence. Without homeostatic devices, we

should be in constant danger of disaster, unless we were always on the alert to correct voluntarily what normally is corrected automatically. With homeostatic devices, however that keep essential bodily processes steady, we as individuals are free from such slavery – free . . . to explore and understand the wonders of the world about us, to develop new ideas and interests, and to work and play, untrammelled by anxieties concerning our bodily affairs.

(in Koestler, 1967)

We all have a concept of homeostasis as being a keeping in balance internally and externally with changes. This concept is central to the osteopathic concept. To stay within this balance concept the body and its interaction with the environment has to be constantly changing. This is important to remember when treating patients. They are not the same patient they were at their last visit; there should never be a treatment plan that is identical to the last; and treatments should have objectives, not repeated procedures.

Heraclitus of Ephesus, born some 2500 years ago, expounded a philosophy that still imbues modern sociology and religion as well as the basic sciences. In nature, he said, the only constant is change; things that appear the same are actually undergoing constant transformation: 'Man is like a fountain, always the same form, but never the same water' (Hoag *et al.*, 1969).

Principles of osteopathic manipulative therapy

Living tissue to the hands of an osteopath is like Braille to a blind man.

Harold Hoover, DO

Tactile textures are complex three-dimensional structures. Moreover, in exploring tactile textures we can scan our finger pads over the surface, so that the effective stimulus has a temporal component as well. This complex spatio-temporal stimulus is filtered by the skin mechanics before exciting the populations of low threshold mechanoreceptors. In the human fingerpad there are four types of low threshold mechanoreceptor. Meissner and Pacinian corpuscles respond transiently, whereas Merkel complexes and Ruffini endings give sustained responses. The nerve fibres transmitting receptor responses to the spinal cord innervate the fingertip densely in the case of the Meissner and Merkel endings and sparsely in the case of the Ruffini and Pacinian endings. The roughness of the surface being explored is 'coded' in the activity of the four populations of primary afferents (Goodwin, 1993). Other receptors that must be considered are the polymodal nociceptors. These are free nerve endings (FNEs), called polymodal because they respond to more than one form of energy, i.e. either mechanical or thermal stimuli of a degree that produces or threatens to produce tissue damage. FNEs are terminals of A (thinly myelinated) or C (unmyelinated) fibres. They are present over the entire cutaneous surface where they subserve the modalities of pain and temperature (Kennedy and Wendelschafer-Crabb, 1993). The hand is used to acquire information about a number of different characteristics of an object – its surface features, including texture, contour and irregularities, its overall shape, size and weight, its consistency and its thermal properties. Sensing of these different properties of the object rapidly leads to its identification and unified perception as a specific object, such as a key, coin or piece of rubber; this is termed 'stereognosis' in the neurological literature (Sathian, 1989).

> The essential characteristic of life is motion whether it be of the single cell or the universe. When death occurs in a tissue, an organ, or an organism the inherent motility slowly comes to a standstill.
>
> Viola M. Frymann, DO, FAAO, MB, BS

During the course of an osteopathic education, training in manipulative therapy is started as soon as possible. This is a clinical skill that is vital to the osteopath in reaching an objective in caring for his or her patient. However, one skill that can be considered even more important than manipulation in osteopathy is palpation. On the art of palpation, I believe, hangs the success or failure of the osteopathic physician. Without palpation there is no 'reading' of the tissue. If you cannot read you cannot even begin to interpret the needs of the patient. Manipulation is not exclusive to osteopathy, but the level of palpation can rarely be challenged.

When students begin their osteopathic manipulative therapy (OMT) training they complain about not being able to feel the tissues. This is not the case; it is their interpretation of what they are feeling that has not developed. No analogies have yet been made and integrated into their central nervous system. Palpation is a psychomotor skill, where visualization and interpretation come together. It was shown by Beal (1989) that many papers advocated teaching palpation as a psychomotor skill. It was pointed out that other disciplines such as music and sports analysed the body's role in skilled activity, and that such things as a firm base of support, centring of body weight, corrected leverage, exact timing, smooth muscular action and moment-to-moment coordination are prime requisites for skilful palpatory technique.

The importance of the teaching of palpation and other manual skills as a psychomotor development should not be underestimated. Like the playing of sports, there are aims and objectives in a dynamic environment. Pure demonstration and copying of OMT is a poor method of teaching. An integrated approach with as much emphasis on theory (what, where, when, why etc.) is just as important as a practical workshop. Slow uptake of those learning palpation will be because they have very little perception/visualization. Tyrell (1963) wrote that in normal visual sense perception, the elements of sensing and perceiving are not separated. A red brick is seen as a patch of red. Recognition of the patch is called sensing. Perception is a mental act based on sensing and the acknowledged existence of a particular material in the environment. In perception we make an uncritical jump from knowledge that there is a coloured patch to the belief that there is a brick. However, an uncritical jump may be wrong and result in an illusion.

This uncritical jump is common in students of osteopathy. An illusion can result from the lack of applied anatomy. What you are feeling you may believe you are treating. An example of this is the palpation of the articular pillars of the cervical spine. You cannot feel them; what you are palpating is the soft tissue over them. The tension in soft tissue makes a contribution to the movement (or lack of movement) of the joints in the cervical spine, even on passive examination.

Myron Beal has made an unparalleled contribution to an understanding of OMT. Without this understanding it would be hard to research into combinations of techniques and the individual prescribing of OMT for each patient. Palpatory findings allow the osteopath to place OMT into its proper clinical context; it is not always necessary to manipulate.

Beal described palpation as the following:

> Palpation is a clinical skill used as a physical examination pro-
> cedure to assess the patient's general physical condition, including
> the musculoskeletal system. The examination process consists of
> an interaction between patient and examiner. An assessment of
> the results of this interaction as it pertains to an evaluation of the
> patient's musculoskeletal system requires an understanding of the
> role of both physician and patient.

He went on to attempt an analysis of the subjective elements of palpation, which he divided into three phases:

1. reception or sensing;
2. transmission of the sensory impulses to the brain;
3. interpretation or perception and analysis.

He felt that the reliability of palpatory findings is dependent on an understanding of the examination process and attention to the steps involved.

Developing palpation

Frymann (1963) reminds us that the human hand is equipped with instruments to perceive changes in temperature, surface texture and surface humidity, and to penetrate and detect successfully deeper tissue textures, turgescence, elasticity and irritability. The textile expert, for example, can distinguish a synthetic material from a natural one no matter how similar it may appear to the untrained eye and hand.

Let us consider first the various phases of general palpation and what may be discovered in each one.

1. A very light touch, even passing the hand 5 mm above the skin, provides information on the surface temperature. An acute lesion area will be unusually warm, while an area of long-standing chronic lesion

may be unusually cold compared with the skin in other areas. This is a good method of distinguishing a tear (warm) from an overcontraction (cold). Both will present as acute pain and swelling.

2. Light touch will also reveal the cutaneous humidity, and the sudorific or sebaceous activity of the skin.
3. The tone, elasticity and turgor of the skin may be noted by light pressure.
4. A slightly firmer approach brings the examiner into communication with the superficial muscles (and fascia) to determine their tone, turgor and metabolic state.
5. Penetrating more deeply, similar study of deeper muscle layers is possible.
6. The state of fascial sheaths and condensations may be noted.
7. In the abdomen similar palpation will provide information about the state of the organs within.
8. On deeper penetration, firm yet gentle contact is reached with bone.

Many physicians will see the techniques used by the osteopath as similar to if not the same as they use. But, as Frymann says, 'touch can never be analysed by the eye'. Palpation is the root investigation, after which the construction of techniques to be used begins. Without palpatory skills the practitioner cannot begin to know the direction to take. Technique is not a vague or chance accomplishment, it must be relentlessly and assiduously pursued until it becomes your own. It must be remembered that it is the interpretation of what you feel that is important not the fingers, soft or otherwise. Technique is rather a matter of the mind than the fingers. It is necessary to acquire mentally the power muscularly so to direct the limbs in their work that the purpose shall be accurately fulfilled.

As we have just read, palpation has additionally been described as a clinical skill used as a physical examination procedure to assess the patient's general physical condition, including the musculoskeletal system. This skill can be broken down into three steps:

1. reception or sensing;
2. transmission of sensory impulses;
3. interpretation.

Different degrees of touch reveal different sources of information. Touch can be grossly divided into light touch and deep touch. Light touch investigates:

- skin temperature
- skin moisture
- skin drag
- changes in contour
- roughness and smoothness
- tensile state of subcutaneous tissue and fluid content.

Deep touch investigates:

- changes in muscle contour
- turgidity

- elasticity
- compressibility
- irritability
- density
- tensile state
- status of ligament, bone and fascia.

Palpatory findings can lead to the following basic assessments.

1. Acute
    - increased temperature (tear)
    - decreased temperature (contracture/spasm)
    - change in tissue contour due to swelling
    - oedema
    - tenderness.
2. Chronic
    - decreased temperature
    - change in tissue contour due to fibrotic thickening
    - rigidity of the tissues
    - limitation in joint mobility.
3. Subacute
    - transitional stage between acute and chronic.

These findings may or may not alter under certain conditions. They have been more generally described as transient or stable conditions, as follows.

1. Transient
    - usually superficial tissues
    - readily change with patient position, with repeated examination or limited mobilization procedures.
2. Stable
    - usually chronic
    - remain constant in different patient positions and repeated examinations and are resistant to limited mobilization procedures.

The major basis for any system is terminology. The following are some descriptive terms in addition to acute/chronic and transient/stable: fixed/non-fixed, painful/non-painful, red/white, circumscribed/diffuse, pliable/tight, irritable/placid, turgid/dehydrated, superficial/deep, hot/cold, moist/dry, compressible/rigid, yielding/non-yielding, symmetrical/asymmetrical, soft/hard, thick/thin, rough/smooth, flaccid/firm, restricted/free, tense/relaxed (from Beal, 1980).

If we are to obtain the best results an intelligent and scientific evaluation has to be made. This is impossible until the condition of tissues in question has been determined. With the facts clearly in mind, it is then possible to select the type of therapy that will accomplish satisfactory results. The most scientific treatment requires an automicrophysiological approach to the problem, the manipulation being designed in accordance with the structure and condition of the part that is at fault. There should be a reason for any treatment. The routine, stereotyped procedure carried out with utter disregard for the tissues involved or for the condition of the tissues becomes nothing more than a type of gymnastic manoeuvre and may not accomplish the desired results. Indeed, it may be nothing more than a bold experiment carried out upon the vitality of the patient (Cathie, 1974).

Passive gross motion testing

Passive gross motion tests should be part of the physical examination, but usually they are not. They are initial impression tests, especially appropriate during the physical examination when the body systems are first screened. The somatic system, however, receives only a cursory examination if the full significance of its neuromusculoskeletal function is not recognized by the physician, and if the major goals in testing are limited to measurement of structural geometry and motion range. Skilled use of palpation, within a format of simple passive gross motion tests for asymmetry of regional response to motion, will evoke signs of somatic dysfunction as an early step in diagnosis of somatic components in a disease process. Positive findings of somatic dysfunction provide evidence of disturbed somatosomatic and viscerosomatic reflex activities. The physician's attention thus is drawn to postural problems and to critical regions within the somatic system where there are major segmental dysfunctions that should appear on the problem list for consideration in total patient management (Johnston, 1982).

Introduction to osteopathic manipulative skills

> The object of treatment ought to be to make the patient master of himself; the means to this end is the education of the will, or more exactly, of the reason . . . When we obey the simple suggestion of our feelings, when we let ourselves do what we want to do, we do not speak of will, although our volitions are concerned. We know very well that we are then slaves to our tastes and appetites, and we change up this easy-going morality to our motor impulses.
>
> (Roscoe, 1948)

Osteopathic techniques are initially taught as psychomotor procedures. Students are then taught to individualize their manipulative skills based on principles of application. This individualization is important as it will exploit the best assets of the individual practitioner. These assets include weight, height etc.

Effective OMT is based on a working knowledge of the applied medical disciplines, which include anatomy, physiology, pharmacology, neurology, gastroenterology, pathology etc. This helps not only in the application of various procedures but in the formulation of proper prescription of manipulation. This we shall look at in more detail later. Manipulative techniques are next to useless, as is pharmacological intervention, if the prescription is wrong. Of paramount importance is the need for an accurate diagnosis. This takes us back to the importance of the clinical assessment of palpation. Modification of techniques is based on the results of clinical examination and the needs of the athlete. Any student should be able to asses the athlete's manipulative needs in cases ranging from a twisted ankle to upper respiratory tract infection (Schmidt, 1982).

Conceptually, we should not remove the musculoskeletal system or the disturbed joint from the patient, treat it, and put it back (Kappler, 1981). Techniques are influenced by the needs of the patient and the local dysfunction. It should be remembered that OMT is a part of the clinical skills an osteopath uses in diagnosis and treatment; manipulation is not osteopathy, just as antibiotics are not medicine.

Here, we shall look at the basic principles of teaching osteopathic manipulative technique. These include an understanding of the following:

- the barrier concept/tissue tension
- direct procedures
- indirect procedures
- modifications
- localization
- fixation or locking
- operator position.

The barrier concept

An understanding of the barrier is vital as a basis for the safety of any OMT procedure. The information the student receives due to feedback will determine the criteria such as amount of force, direction and technique used. Naturally, in practising barrier engagement it is best to practise on healthy tissue and various body types. This will allow the student to detect dysfunctional tissue more easily.

Let us look at these two major types of barrier engagement: normal (functional) tissue and pathological (dysfunctional) tissue.

Normal (functional) tissue
An easy joint to perform this procedure on is the elbow. Here, we have the athlete (or volunteer) lying supine. Moving the joint through simple passive movements of flexion, extension, pronation and supination we will try and feel for the following:

- physiological barrier
- anatomical barrier
- neutral position.

Physiological barrier This is where you should be able to feel an alteration in the freedom of movement in the range through which you are taking the joint. The feedback you should be aware of is a tightening of tissue. Students should remember that when they do feel this tension, an experienced osteopath would have felt it a long time before. No pain should be felt.

Anatomical barrier Here, the structure of the athlete halts any further movement. At the point before you hit the full anatomical barrier the athlete will feel discomfort and/or pain. The build up of tissue tension is progressive and the type of tissue tension employment involved in the anatomical barrier will depend on the anatomical make-up of the joint and surrounding tissue.

Neutral position Theoretically, this is a position where, in a three-dimensional sense, there is no tissue tension. As we will see in indirect techniques this is a very important concept, and, like the other barriers, should be practised on different bodies and as many times as possible.

With all three positions it is important to feel not only for the range of motion but also for the quality of motion (Fig. 2.4).

Pathological (dysfunctional) tissue

The barrier concept can be applied to any tissue. Damaged tissue, including visceral tissue, should be used to experience limitation in range or distance of movement in various directions. In intra-abdominal and intra-thoracic injury or disease the myofascioskeletal system may reveal patterns of barriers that will lead to the prescription of OMT.

Direct procedures

These consist primarily of the use of movement of body tissue to engage resistance. As in the barrier concept, force application against tissue resistance is important as a diagnostic tool. This is especially important in direct action techniques, as the wrong feedback could lead to tissue damage, and would certainly be ineffective.

In direct action techniques, once the barrier has been engaged an activating force continues to be applied to initiate change in the function of the tissue. This change in function can be in the form of increasing circulation, ligament stretch etc.

Muscle energy technique

A direct technique that aims to reduce muscle hypertonia and reduce the gamma-gain. This is achieved by 'overloading' the afferent neural input to the spinal cord producing a reflex decrease in the efferent neural impulses maintaining the tone of the muscle. This is also referred to as proprioceptive neuromuscular facilitation (PNF). Muscle energy is basically applied by holding the limb in a position of ease and asking the athlete to gently move the limb in a prearranged direction while the osteopath resists the athlete's attempts at movement. The athlete is asked to hold this attempt at movement for 3–6 seconds. The predetermined direction is either to reduce the hypertonia in a muscle or combine movements for groups of

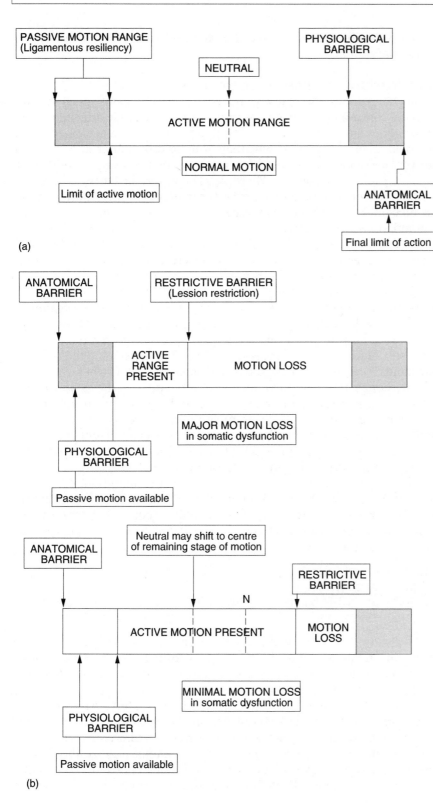

PASSIVE MOTION RANGE
(Ligamentous resiliency)

PHYSIOLOGICAL
BARRIER

NEUTRAL

ACTIVE MOTION RANGE

NORMAL MOTION

Limit of active motion

ANATOMICAL
BARRIER

Final limit of action

(a)

ANATOMICAL
BARRIER

RESTRICTIVE BARRIER
(Lesion restriction)

ACTIVE
RANGE
PRESENT

MOTION LOSS

MAJOR MOTION LOSS
in somatic dysfunction

PHYSIOLOGICAL
BARRIER

Passive motion available

Neutral may shift to centre
of remaining stage of motion

ANATOMICAL
BARRIER

N

RESTRICTIVE
BARRIER

ACTIVE MOTION PRESENT

MOTION
LOSS

MINIMAL MOTION LOSS
in somatic dysfunction

PHYSIOLOGICAL
BARRIER

Passive motion available

(b)

Fig. 2.4 Components of joint motion by physiological barrier (resistance) and anatomical barrier reached by bone and ligaments. (a) The presence of somatic dysfunction places a zone of restriction somewhere in the active range of motion. If the barrier is near one end of the range, it limits active motion to less than 50%. (b) When the zone of restriction is near the opposite end, it leaves more than 50% of active motion (Kimberly, 1980).

muscles. It can be used in normal stretching activities and in cases of pain due to hypertonia.

High velocity/low amplitude thrust technique

This technique has for many years been the subject of much debate, especially concerning its validity as part of the osteopathic armamentarium of techniques and when to use it. In osteopathic colleges it seemed that if you could 'click' or 'pop' a joint then you were far better at OMT than your fellow student. The reality in practice is that 'clicking' a joint on its own is a limited technique. There are, however, instances where one carefully chosen manoeuvre relieves the patient of pain, permanently. This mechanism is harmless when performed properly, and never results in an inflammatory reaction.

The centre of debate still revolves around the mechanism of the 'pop'. It must be remembered that myofascial structures move bones, and bones articulate around joints. There are many theories on this mechanism, ranging from Cyriax (1980), whose methods of manipulation were questionable at the best of times, and who stated that 'it is a fragment of [intra-articular] disc that moves', to my anatomy lecturer Professor R.W. Haines, who taught us that this was a decompression within the joint due to two soft, fluid-soaked surfaces separating. Try moistening the palms of your hands, pressing them together and them separating them.

Even though this compression may build up, it is the action of the nervous system through the resting tone and contracture of myofascial tissue that begins the compressive force process. This is not only due to purely neurophysical mechanics but, to an even greater extent in practice, there is a massive psychophysical influence. Therefore, a joint does not have to be damaged to be under compression.

With the experienced practitioner, safe thrust techniques are based on palpatory feedback. The practitioner 'searches' for restrictions within the joint. He or she 'listens' three-dimensionally, reducing the procedural mechanism of technique application. The thrust technique incorporates three main features:

1. localization of forces;
2. separation of joint surfaces;
3. motion toward a barrier, in the path indicated by the facet planes (Heilig, 1981).

The localization of forces is the key to specific thrust techniques, without which soft tissue will absorb the energy utilized to achieve a joint separation. This is most apparent in athletes who cannot relax. The practitioner who cannot localize forces will tend to use force. Localization of forces leads to a low amplitude procedure and safety. An example of inappropriate technique is a rebound thrust in which the force is directed away from the barrier and not into the barrier. An alternate term for this is 'exaggerated thrust'. Some chiropractic techniques utilize this type of technique, and perhaps it is for this reason that I choose to condemn it (Kappler, 1981). High velocity/low amplitude procedures are most effective when used on involuntary joints. The motions of these joints are accessory movements other than flexion, extension, rotation etc. that are not under our direct control. Again, this is in the majority of cases a qualitative 'joint play' (Heilig, 1981) that brings the athlete back to full function.

In the acute presentation the major contraindication is a haemarthrosis and/or inflammation. These tend to occur directly after a traumatic event. The use of a thrust technique after even the mildest acute joint injury should be discouraged, even if there is no significant joint patho's. The central nervous system has to calm down after a traumatic event. In areas such as the cervical spine, high velocity thrust after a minor joint disruption has been known to lead to exacerbation of symptoms and headache.

Soft tissue techniques
Objectives:

A. Cognitive.
   1. How to relax muscles.
   2. Indications.
   3. Precautions.

B. Skills.
   1. Evaluate change of tissue as you work on them.
   2. Specific techniques for relaxing muscles.
   3. Operator comfort in palpating.
      a. Working with tissues.
      b. Developing skilled hands.
   4. Affective?

The term 'soft tissue' is derived from a contrast between hard tissue (bone) and soft tissue (muscles, tendons, ligaments etc.). An alternative adjective is 'myofascial' soft tissue treatment. The usual objective of myofascial soft tissue techniques is to relax muscles and reduce fascial tension. However, it is important to realize that these techniques go even further, i.e. the treatment goes deeper than the muscle, down to the ligamentous or capsular tissue surrounding the joint or viscus, affecting whatever fascial plane may be between the skin and the affected joint or viscus. There is an increase in blood supply to the area with resultant processes of removal of toxins of function or disease, and changes in tissue chemistry such as increasing respiration and metabolism. It is maintained that the circulation of lymph with all its benefits is increased. Some practitioners use meaningless and purposeless gyrations or other ineffective manipulation, all of which require energy and do very little good (Keeler, 1948). Soft tissue techniques are not massage techniques.

Muscles can be relaxed using manual as well as pharmacological and physical approaches. In general, muscles can be relaxed by:

- slow longitudinal stretching
- lateral stretch
- deep careful kneading

It is possible to stretch or work muscles by moving the bony attachments, and the term 'articulatory treatment' is used when joints are moved through a range of motion. This type of treatment affects the muscles surrounding the joint(s).

Myofascial release technique
Direct myofascial release technique is a form of osteopathic manipulative technique which focuses on myofascial tissues (rather than joints). The operator contacts the tissues, engages a barrier by loading the tissue, and holds the position until release occurs by inherent forces. Release is a several-second phenomenon, not a sudden change.

Guidelines for myofascial soft tissue treatment

1. Apply the forces slowly.
2. Release forces slowly.
3. **Never** allow a muscle to snap back.
4. **Do not** allow fingers to slide over skin, as in massage.
5. **Do not** overstretch the skin.
6. Avoid excess force per unit area – spread forces out.
7. Avoid direct pressure over bony prominences.
8. The amount of force and distance used by the operator is gauged by the patient's tissue response. This demands a sensing approach.
9. The physician must perceive how the tissues are responding to the treatment, and adjust accordingly.
10. The usual response is for the muscles to relax. The skin may become warm. Continued treatment is associated with cutaneous vasodilatation (red skin) and ultimately the muscles will tighten.
11. Stop when the muscle relaxes; **do not overdose**; move to the next area.
12. Obtain feedback from your patient.

Paraspinal soft tissue treatment – lateral traction
The key is to contact the paraspinal muscle in the groove between the spinous process and the muscle, applying a firm pressure to the muscle mass and then pulling in a lateral direction. To avoid overstretching the skin, you may want to contact the skin over the muscle mass – move your fingers medially, without losing contact with the skin, then apply deeper pressure on the muscle and apply lateral traction.

Effective soft tissue technique employs the use of the entire body of the operator, not just the flexor muscles of the fingers, and you should not rub the skin as in massage.

Exercise Soft tissue technique for the cervical spine, patient supine.

1. Identify:
   (a) C1–C7 and review the palpable motions
   (b) trapezius muscle

    (c) scalene
    (d) sternocleidomastoid muscle
    (e) platysma muscle
    (f) thyroid cartilage
    (g) carotid pulses bilaterally
    (h) external jugular vein bilaterally.

2. Use one hand to stabilize the head by contact with the forehead. Have the fingertips of the other hand contact the paraspinal muscles in the mid-cervical region and apply a lateral force slowly to lengthen the muscles. When muscle relaxation occurs, release the lateral traction slowly to allow continued muscle relaxation. Concurrently applied rotation of the head will enhance muscle lengthening during this stretching technique.
3. Technique variation using traction (slow longitudinal stretching) along muscle fibres.

Thoracic technique
This is a procedure whereby the barrier or end point of joint motion is engaged repeatedly, i.e. the joint is carried through its entire range of motion in order to bring about an increase in freedom and range of motion.

Articulatory technique

1. Place the patient on the side, flex knees forward to stabilize.
2. Operator stands facing the patient.
3. Place pads of the fingers in the superior (the side up) paraspinal groove.
4. Apply a force towards operator and upward. This allows muscle to be stretched and ribs to be articulated.
5. Repeat several times, moving along entire thoracic spine.
6. Repeat for the other side.

Soft Tissue technique This is accomplished by direct manual treatment of the soft (non-bony) tissues themselves. The object of treatment usually is to relax ligamentous and muscular tissues or to promote an exchange of fluids. The following precautions should be observed.

- **Do not** permit fingers to slip over skin of muscle belly.
- **Do not** use excessive speed. Movements should be slow, rhythmic and steadily controlled.
- Pressure should be slowly applied and slowly released. **Do not** allow the tight muscle to snap back.
- Use the soft pads of the fingers and avoid gouging by the tips of the fingers or fingernails.
- Avoid direct pressure over a bony prominence.
- Avoid overdose of treatment. After relaxation, continued treatment will cause the muscle to become boggy and ultimately to spasm.

1. With patient prone, identify the erector spinae mass. Standing at the patient's side, reach across the midline and apply the heel of one hand against the medial aspect of the erector spinae mass, fingers pointing away from you. Direct firm pressure downward and laterally, increasing the pressure until the muscles are stretched (bowstring) and felt to yield somewhat. Slowly release the pressure. Repeat the procedure several times along the length of the muscle.
2. Apply the heel of one hand on to the soft tissue, medial to the blade of the scapula. Apply firm pressure distributed over the entire heel area. Gently apply a traction force slightly anterior and outward and return slowly. It is important to appreciate the muscle and soft tissue tone and resistance to your efforts as you work.
3. Repeat the above technique using the demonstrated alternative method of using fingertips rather than the heel of the hand. Which is more comfortable for the operator, and for the patient?

Lumbar treatment procedures
When applying soft tissue techniques remember:

- apply and release tissue forces slowly;
- do not apply pressure to bony prominences;
- do not allow skin or muscles to slip under fingers;
- be careful not to pinch muscles or skin between fingers;
- soft tissue should relax muscles, do not make them boggy and oedematous;
- always apply techniques to both sides.

Soft tissue treatment for erector spinae

1. Patient prone, head turned toward one side. Stand at patient's side.
2. Place your thenar eminence, thumbs or heel of hand in the paraspinal muscle group on the side opposite you.
3. Apply force slowly in an anterolateral direction (downward and outward).
4. Stop applying force when a barrier is reached (limit of muscle stretching or patient's tolerance).
5. Hold this position until you feel muscle relaxation.
6. Release force slowly.
7. Compare this side with the other side.
8. Treat the other side.

Deep articulation

1. Place patient on side. Stand behind patient.
2. Patient's upper arm should hang off the table.
3. Flex patient's legs for stability.
4. Place your hands on the paraspinal muscle (side up) at the thoracolumbar junction with your fingers wrapping gently over the patient's flank.
5. Slowly apply force toward the table and anteriorly. Release slowly.

6. This technique increases sidebending and extension. It facilitates range of motion.

Deep articulation

1. With patient prone, stand to the right side of your patient.
2. Place your right hand on the paraspinal musculature at the thoracolumbar junction.
3. Grasp the patient's left hip at approximately the anterior superior iliac spine.
4. Use your right hand as a holding force.
5. Lift the pelvis slowly and roll it towards you.
6. The object is to localize forces with your right hand, which stretches the soft tissues and extends the vertebral column.
7. Hold until muscles relax. Release slowly.

Indirect procedures

Strain/counterstrain
To effect release of a tender point, the part of the body being used as 'the handle' is carried into extension, sidebending and rotation away from the point of tenderness on the posterior aspect of the body, or the head (for example) is moved into flexion, sidebending and rotation towards the tender point if on the anterior aspect of the body, correcting and fine tuning as directed by the monitoring digit at the tender point (Woolbright, 1991).

Facilitated positional release
The object of facilitated positional release is to place the tissue or region into a 'neutral' position. By 'shortening' tissue in the lesioned area this allows the extrafusal muscle fibres (muscle spindle-gamma loop) to lengthen to their normal relaxed state. The response to this treatment is in the muscle tissue. The joint motion will normalize if its mobility was impaired by muscle hypertonicity. If joint motion asymmetry is caused by other factors such as meniscoid or synovial impingement or degenerative arthritis, then mobility will remain restricted (Schiowitz, 1990).

Modifications

These include adapting the OMT to the patient in their environment on a gross level. For example, the patient may have a physical disability, or you may not have the facilities at your disposal. The practitioner's height, weight and level of skill, and the age, sex and psychology of the athlete are important considerations. This means that it is important for the osteopath to remove him or herself from the clinically stable treatment room to develop the infinite range of adaptations that are theoretically possible. On a more local level, modifications of the particular OMT techniques are again affected by the parameters of age, sex, injury and illness presentation. Your OMT modifications should be dictated by the needs of the athlete.

Localization

This is the ability both to concentrate the application of forces in barrier engagement and to focus forces in an attempt not to engage a barrier. Both rely, to a great extent, on perception of what is felt.

Fixation or locking

This is a concept of barrier engagement that allows the osteopath to visualize and palpate both physiological and/or anatomical limitation of a range of passive motion.

Visualization

This is a three-dimensional 'in the mind's eye' representation of the anatomy and physiology, and its change in structure as a consequence of being palpated and manipulated while being moved through a space by the osteopath.

Contraindications

The contraindications to OMT can be either absolute or relative, based on technique applied, intensity of the application, and the areas it is applied to. There are areas where the application of OMT will remove restrictions to healing, e.g. fractures, but only if applied to areas around or away from the injury site, as we shall see. Therefore, the list of contraindications is a guide and every patient should be treated individually. As much information as possible should be obtained, to reduce the chances of making an uninformed judgement which could be detrimental to the patient or even fatal.

The main contraindications to OMT are as follows (General Council and Register of Osteopaths, 1993):

- primary bone tumours;
- sarcomas;
- metastases;
- fractures;
- recent trauma without X-ray;
- local infectious conditions (e.g. osteomyelitis);
- acute inflammatory conditions (e.g. acute osteoarthritis, rheumatoid arthritis, ankylosing spondylitis);
- aneurysms;
- severe osteophytosis;
- any condition that will introduce ligamentous instability;
- increased pain or radicular symptoms on positioning;

- angiomas;
- active growth disorders (e.g. Sheuermann's disease);
- pregnancy in the 8th to 12th weeks;
- haemophilia;
- thrombocytopenia;
- active phase of MS, myalgia encephalomyelitis, AIDS;
- prodromal symptoms (e.g. migraine, epilepsy, viral infections);
- gross morphological congenital abnormalities (e.g. cervical ribs);
- metabolic conditions (e.g. osteoporosis, Paget's, Cushing's, osteo-genesis imperfecta);
- prolapsed intervertebral disc;
- arterial insufficiency;
- nerve or spinal cord compression manifesting neurological deficit;
- transient ischaemic attacks;
- patients on long-term medication (e.g. anticoagulants, steroids).

Introduction to craniosacral techniques

Objectives:

1. Review of cranial landmarks.
2. Learn the vault hold.
3. Learn the fronto-occipital hold.
4. Palpate the craniosacral rhythm at the cranium.
5. Palpate the craniosacral rhythm at the sacrum.
6. Perform the lumbosacral decompression technique with the use of the craniosacral rhythm.

Cranial landmarks

Locate, identify and note the significance of each of the following landmarks.

1. Head and neck: posterior and posterolateral:
   (a) Inion (external occipital protuberance), junction of the skin of the scalp and neck.
   (b) Mastoid process.
   (c) Superior nuchal line (runs from the inion base of the mastoid process).
   (d) Zygomatic arch, zygoma (trace from mastoid process to the body of the zygoma; forms the prominence of the lateral facial area).
   (e) External acoustic meatus.
   (f) Angle of mandible.
   (g) Transverse process of atlas (Cl) (midway on a line from the tip of the mastoid process to the angle of the mandible). Place your index fingers (bilaterally) on this point (first with patient supine, then with him sitting); note all changes in the relationship to these three points of reference (tip of the mastoid process, transverse

process of the atlas, and angle of the mandible) in forward bending, backward bending and sidebending, and sidebending rotation.

2. Face: anterior and anterolateral:
    (a) Temporomandibular joint (anterior to external acoustic meatus; below zygomatic arch).
        (i) Palpate bilaterally as follows:
            • mouth closed;
            • mouth open;
            • during opening and closing of mouth (joint in motion), note all deviation in motion; note all restriction or hyper-mobility.
        (ii) Have patient retract lips to show teeth; observe irregularity of mandibular motion during depression and elevation; test again with fingers placed to test motion at articulation by palpation.
    (b) Masseter muscle. Useful test for motor portion of mandibular division of the trigeminal nerve (VIII): place palmar surface of fingertips below the zygomatic arch; have the patient clench his teeth; normally the muscle should become prominent.
    (c) Facial muscles. Test facial nerve (VII), motor: have patient smile; observe action of facial muscles; compare bilaterally and be sure to observe the angles of the mouth.
    (d) Facial artery. May elicit a pulse approximately 1 cm in front of the anterior border of the masseter muscle.
    (e) Frontozygomatic suture. Handy reference to ascertain location of the pterion (which is approximately 35 mm posterior and 11 mm above this suture); pterion is a point at the junction of the frontal, parietal, temporal and great wing of the sphenoid bone; useful in examination and surgical diagnosis; at pterion is great wing of sphenoid, anterior branch of the middle mengeal artery, middle cerebral artery and insula.
    (f) Nasion and nasal bone. Note lower borders of nasal bones; never exert undue pressure here while treating.
    (g) Supraorbital foramen. Ophthalmic division of the trigeminal nerve (VI).
    (h) Infraorbital foramen.
    (i) Mental foramen. Mandibular division of the trigeminal nerve (VII).
    (j) Note that 7, 8 and 9 fall in a vertical line; pressure will indicate if sensorium is intact, i.e. all three divisions of the trigeminal nerve.
    (k) Symphysis menti.
    (l) Glabella. Smooth area on frontal bone between the superciliary arches.

3. Neck:
    (a) Sternocleidomastoid muscle (outline muscle).
    (b) Supraclavicular space.
    (c) Anterior cervical arches (important in diagnosis, surgery and treatment).
        (i) Lower border of mandible.

(ii) Hyoid bone.
(iii) Thyroid cartilage.
(iv) Cricoid cartilage.
(v) Jugular notch (episternal fossa).

Some basic techniques

Vault hold
The vault hold is used to assess the general motion of the bones of the cranium. It is used in treatment to normalize the motion in both the cranial base and vault. It is also used to isolate specific restrictions within the cranial mechanism.

The patient should be in a supine position, comfortable and relaxed. The patient should remove glasses, non-fixed dental appliances and bulky objects in pockets. The practitioner should be seated at the patient's head, forearms resting comfortably on the treatment table. The fingers of both hands should be held without tension and spread out in space forming a hollow in which the patient's cranium can be placed.

The points of contact are specific; incorrect contact may give inaccurate information to the practitioner, and may disrupt the patient's mechanism. The proper points of contact are as follows, using the pads of the fingertips on each side.

1. The little finger is placed on the squamous portion of the occiput.
2. The ring finger is placed in front of the ear with pad on the temporal mastoid region.
3. The middle finger is placed in front of the ear so that the fingertip is in contact with the zygomatic process of the temporal bone.
4. The index finger is placed on the greater wing of the sphenoid.
5. The thumbs rest against each other above the cranium, forming a base for the flexor muscles of the fingers.

Fronto-occipital hold (second vault hold)
The objectives are the same as the vault hold. The different contacts allow the practitioner to use whichever technique is the therapeutically appropriate.

The position of the patient is also the same as the vault hold. The practitioner is seated to either side of the patient's head with the lower hand resting on the table. This hand holds the patient's occipitosquama area. The upper hand is placed over the frontal bone.

The points of contact are as follows.

1. The lower hand is cupped so that the tips of the fingers are on the opposite occipital angle. The angle of the occipital squama closest to the practitioner rests on the thenar and/or hypothenar eminences.
2. The upper hand also forms a cup, enveloping the frontal bone without touching it, making contact with the two external surfaces of the greater wings of the sphenoid. This is accomplished by placing the pad

of the tip of the thumb on the practitioner's side and the pad of the tip of the index finger or middle finger on the side opposite the practitioner.
3. If the practitioner's hand is small relative to the patient's head, it may contact the lateral angles of the frontal bone.

The craniosacral rhythm

The following is a description by Upledger (1991) of his first experience with the craniosacral movement.

> After we had removed the backsides of these cervical vertebrae, there it was in all its glistening glory – the dura mater membrane. And there was our calcium plaque looking at us from right in the centre of the operative field. The nurse now took over my job and held the muscles to the side, while I took a pair of forceps in each hand. Now all I had to do was hold the dura mater membrane perfectly still for Jim as he very carefully removed the calcium plaque. Everything was going well until I tried to stop the movement of the dura mater membrane. It wouldn't hold still no matter what I did. It kept moving toward and away from us rather slowly but rhythmically and irresistibly. I don't recall the exact conversation that Jim and I had, but it was full of comments about my inability to perform a simple task. My responses cast a few aspirations upon anyone who thought this was such a simple task. My pride was hurt. I was embarrassed at my own ineptitude. But, I also became very curious about this strange phenomenon that I was witnessing. Ultimately, Jim removed the plaque without a slip of the knife in spite of the irrepressible moving membrane. I discovered that this rhythmically moving membrane's performance to which I was so intimately connected was new to everyone else in the operating room. It was not synchronous with Delbert's (the patient) breathing. That fact was clearly seen on the breathing machine. It did not synchronise with the heart rate (pulse) that I could see in the cardiac monitor. It was another bodily rhythm at about 10 cycles per minute that seemed very reliable and consistent. I had never seen nor read about this rhythm nor had the neurosurgeon, the anaesthesiologist, the nurses or the intern. Little did I know we were looking at the 'core' of Delbert.

According to Dr W.G. Sutherland (1967) the craniosacral mechanism consists of the brain and spinal cord, the meninges, the cerebrospinal fluid and the articular mobility of the cranium, sacrum and coccyx. These parts, each having its own peculiar and essential function yet operating with others as a unit, form the 'primary respiratory mechanism'. Action of the primary respiratory mechanism is essential to life and is initiated by the inherent contractile motility (characteristic of living tissue) of the brain and spinal cord. Impulses or waves of force are generated by contractions of the brain and cord and transmitted by an essential factor in the healthy function of every cell, tissue and organ, including the nervous system itself. If these waves are normal in rhythm, rate and intensity and are unimpeded during transmission, the tendency is towards health; but if they vary materially from normal for a considerable time, the tendency is towards disturbance of function. Moreover, localized restrictions of the craniosacral mechanism may affect the health of nerve tissue in local areas, altering nerve control to specific parts of the body and in time causing local malfunction and pathological changes in tissue. Cranial malrelations mechanically disturb the functions of the parts and organs of the head, and sacral and coccygeal malrelations and functions of the pelvic area.

Craniosacral treatment is usually directed to regulation and normalization of the motion of the mechanism by freeing from restriction its articulations and membranes. Usually when restrictions are freed, there is an accelerated fluctuation of the cerebrospinal fluid, but occasionally treatment must be directed towards control and slowing of excessive fluctuation. Emphasis is upon securing normal action of the whole primary respiratory mechanism and so delivering normally fluctuating cerebrospinal fluid to all parts of the body (Hoover, 1969).

Lumbosacral decompression technique

1. Place the lower extremities of the patient in approximately 30° of abduction so that the sacroiliac joints are relaxed and the motion is allowed to move to its potential maximum.
2. Hold the sacrum so that the palm of one of your hands rests at the sacral apex and your fingers reach approximately to the fourth or fifth lumbar vertebrae.
3. Place the other hand in a curled-up position so that the spinous processes of L4 and L5 are between the thenar and hypothenar eminences and your fingers.
4. Conform to the sacrum and lumbars to allow movement without influencing it.
5. Note that with flexion the sacral apex will move anteriorly as the lumbar curve straightens slightly. The opposite occurs with extension.
6. Follow the sacrum into flexion while gently applying a cephlad traction on the lumbar vertebrae. This will separate and decompress the lumbosacral junction.
7. Resist extension by becoming immovable but don't try to flex the sacrum further when the craniosacral rhythm is extending.
8. Repeat this procedure until you feel the sacrum release, or the motion becomes disorganized or you sense an unwinding phenomenon or the rhythm disappears. This can take from seconds to minutes.
9. Eventually the sacrum will make a strong effort to extend and you will follow it without resistance and again monitor the motion.
10. Note that the new rhythm is usually stronger and more symmetrical. Do not leave the sacrum before the rhythm returns.
11. This is an excellent 'shotgun' technique for the entire lumbosacral–pelvic area.

Chapman's reflexes

It is appropriate to mention Chapman's reflexes here. The following is an extract from Zucker (1993).

> Chapman's nodes are small individual or groups of nodular, super-ficial masses, found in specific body locations, that quite often are sensitive to palpation. They are related to alterations of visceral function, and they can – in theory – be used in both the diagnosis and treatment of the disturbed organs.
>
> Chapman's nodes are localized changes in the neurolymphatic end structures that produce the palpatory change. The nodes are found where the nerves from organs pass through fascial layers on their way to the surface. They feel like BBs [small pellets] or large globules of tapioca. The specific pathologic nature of these changes is yet to be identified. But, they are excellent diagnostic tools; for some conditions almost unerring. They are also reliable in treatment. One treats the nodes by exerting pressure against them with the fingers, to make them 'melt away.' Chapman does not explicitly say so, but if this is treatment of more than the node, that is, treatment of the condition signified by the node, then making the node 'melt away' must produce changes in the distant organ affected, just as excising the 'genital spots' helped to cure problems of a psychosexual nature according to the nasogenital reflex theory.

One must accept the empiric quality of the nodes; this is the nature of medicine. This last point is put clearly by Owens (1942):

> As a result of many years experience wrestling with the human body, the writer has found that not being overly bright has its advantages . . . Without much sense to start with, such an individual occasionally blunders into a way of doing things in a simple, unscientific way that works, which a man of good sense would hesitate to try . . . The only excuse we have for presenting the simple procedures set forth, herein, is that they work, and frequently have given relief where the more scientific methods evolved by men of intelligence and notional reputation in this field have failed.

The pragmatic concerns of medicine allow for different criteria of acceptance for certain principles of practice. Full understanding can take a backseat to clinical success in some circumstances, but not as a general rule. The notion of clinical success, however, is relative and fragile enough to make one pause. What I and a patient take to be a success may well be due, in large part, to what we already believe about what works. Thus, it behoves medicine (as much as science) to make every effort to substantiate the principles of clinical practice.

Osteopathy is not an alternative medicine, it is an alterative medicine.
Harold Hoover, DO

PSYCHOLOGY

> We find no new tools because we make some venerable but
> questionable proposition as an indubitable starting point. Now, if
> a man will begin with certainties, he shall end in doubts; but if he
> be content to begin in doubts, he shall end in certainties.
>
> Francis Bacon

If we can explain to the athlete why they are feeling what they are feeling
at that particular time, then we have overcome more than half the
problem of athletic health care. We try to standardize treatment, but
when the athlete becomes frustrated when things are not going well we
tend to blame the athlete's attitude. When we fail in our approach to a
problem and the athlete resigns him or herself to continue to get better,
we say 'what a good athlete' and leave them to it.

It was not until a few years ago that people in many professional sports
began to realize the important role played by psychology in winning and
losing 'the edge'. While this has been taken on in a big way in some sports,
in others there does not seem to have been time for such trivial
distractions: I have heard 'if they want to play, they will' many times over
the years. Fortunately, psychology in sport is not just about winning or
losing. The scope covers training, coaching (especially where children are
concerned) and having fun. It is this aspect of having fun that seems to
have been forgotten.

Psychology is usually the last coaching aid to be applied to athletic
activity and health care and is the first to go when things are going wrong.
Psychology in sport should not be wasted by applying it solely to the
aspect of winning; it should be applied all day every day in the life of the
athlete and should be taught in that way. This will lead to well-balanced
athletes with winning as their objective not just on the field, but in their
life as a whole. In addition it is important that athletes develop professional relationships between one another leading to more respect from
outside the sporting world.

Conditioning is the key to behaviour – it is what we are used to and
expect to happen. All athletes after a time become conditioned to respond
and react in a certain way. Any alteration in this routine due to
circumstances beyond their control, depending on the personality of the
athlete, may lead to change in personality. Personality changes present
themselves as lack of concentration, depression etc. If the 'primary
machinery' of life is the musculoskeletal system and the 'vital organs' are
there for support, then the major reason for the change in our neurohormonal system must be as a response to our neuromusculoskeletal needs.
A.T. Still described the osteopathic philosophy of disease as Hippocrates
had centuries before, calling for an approach to psychosomatic disorders

to be the same as any other disturbance in the total body economy (Adams, 1849; Still, 1899). Athletes need feedback, otherwise they suffer from the signs and symptoms of acute and chronic deprivation.

Stress

No work on psychology would be complete without a basic understanding of the work of Hans Selye, the Canadian endocrinologist/physiologist. Selye has influenced thoughts on stress since the mid-1930s, with work that he himself described as an extension of the concepts of Bernard and Cannon, combining adaptation and homeostasis, respectively.

The stress agents can be any stimuli, external or internal, such as heat, light, cold, infections, toxins, haemorrhage, muscular exercise, drugs, injury, surgery etc. In its simplest form, Selye realized that any stimulus can become a stress factor depending on the situation of its input and the exposure time of the individual.

There are both specific and general responses to stressors. Specific responses include vasodilatation to local heat and the immune response to infection. Selye's work is based on plasticity in the organism, especially when the stimulus is non-specific. This non-specific input could be in the form of neurogenic or psychogenic stimulation. As a result there is a modification of the bodily processes, e.g. digestion, metabolism or neuroendocrine response, in an attempt to normalize the stress being imposed on the system. Selye called this the general adaptation syndrome (GAS).

The general adaptation syndrome

Today we are well aware of work in the areas of plasticity in systems of the body from the CNS to the immune system. These system changes are all very well, but it is also important not to lose sight of the fact that we are treating an individual who we need to communicate with. Selye noted some patterns of changes in the total system. These were considered in three main stages:

1. an alarm reaction, including an initial shock phase of lowered resistance and a countershock phase, in which defence mechanisms begin to operate;
2. a stage of resistance, in which adaptation is optimal;
3. a stage of exhaustion, marked by the collapse of adaptive responses.

We are today aware of these changes and their presentation in the forms of arousal performance, burnout, fatigue etc.

The alarm reaction stage presents as excitability of a reflex nature. This can be looked at in the light of Korr's facilitation of the spinal cord. Further, anxiety and neural autonomic excitability begin to present as increased adrenaline release, increased resting heart rate, decreased body temperature and muscle tone, anaemia, acidosis, transitory blood sugar increase followed by a decrease, transitory blood leukocyte decrease followed by an increase, and gastrointestinal ulceration (facilitating bacterial multiplication and plasticity in an acidic environment). Neuroendocrine attempts at homeostasis are what Selye referred to as countershock, i.e. a response to continued stimulation. This is the second phase of the alarm reaction, shown by the enlargement and hyperactivity of the adrenocortical glands and rapid 'shrinkage' of the thymus and lymph nodes (reflecting immune response).

Adaptation of the systems continues until the organism as a whole seems to resign itself to the stimuli, reducing the alarm reaction response or resisting it. This involves the pituitary–adrenocortical axis. This reaction can only be kept up for so long, until the final stage of 'giving-in' and exhaustion. An alarm reaction tends to reappear after this.

Plasticity and conditioning of the neuroendocrine and neurovisceral systems have been recorded as long ago as 1957 (by Bykov), when conditioning, similar to the Pavlovian response, was shown. Conditioned diuresis was established to a particular room, to a distinct stimulus (a horn), following injection of water into the stomach; inhibition of this response was likewise able to be controlled as a result of systematic pairing stimuli. In addition there were demonstrations of cardiac and vascular conditioning, splenic conditioning, respiratory conditioning, and conditioning of hydrochloric acid secretion.

All individuals have their own way of dealing with stresses due to their own past experiences, interpretation of the stimuli, and what they believe is the right form of information from other athletes. The majority of athletes in a distressed state will be in a stage of arousal presenting as distress due to their inability to perform, or due to an injury that 'seems' not to get better within their expectations. The athlete who tends to be distressed or even depressed will invariably have an unqualified, hearsay foundation for the opinion they have arrived at. You have to put them back on track.

Motor skill learning

All physical activities, e.g. football, soccer, golf and OMT, are motor skill activities that generally follow the same phases. While they are going through these phases, we have to recognize the potential not only for overwork and burnout, but in the rehabilitation (physical and psychological) of the athlete back to full performance.

The simplest approach to the stages of motor skill learning was put forward by Fitts (1964), in which he described the phases as cognitive, associative and autonomous.

1. The cognitive phase is where the athlete should be taught the aims and objectives of the act to be performed. The coach or teacher must take into consideration that the athlete has to 'think', and the demonstration you give will be mimicked as the individual tries to emulate

your requests. Feedback analogies are vital for the athlete to relate kinaesthetically to the feel of the movements.

2. The associative phase: once the athlete has the basic skill under control then they should be allowed to practise. This is also a dangerous period in which the individual can develop bad habits that will be programmed into their system making it harder to correct later. This is why it is important to have structured training or teaching environments that are controlled. Naturally, I am not proposing that athletes are never left alone to enjoy their newly acquired skills; they have to develop their individuality. Developing individuality facilitates the subconscious or reflex performance. It begins to show as not so much a higher centre activity but a lower CNS activity, leading to the autonomous phase.

3. The autonomous phase is where the athlete or student performs the skills needed not just without thinking, but in response to changing circumstances, without thinking. Known as the phase of mastery, it still needs the feedback of a coach or teacher. All top athletes have a coach who is the prime source of feedback, tailormade for their needs. Here, the athlete is conditioned.

Conditioning the athlete is the objective, but the danger is of specific conditioning when the athlete is too young. Specific conditioning too early in children leads to specific neural conditioning. It has been shown again and again that children should be trained generally in different activities, and should always have fun if they are to survive mentally and physically.

The most common coaching or teaching error in motor skill learning is making the athlete or student perform the action again and again. The general finding is not that the individual cannot perform the act, but the individual needs to understand the principles of performing the act. The 'why' and 'what for' is not understood by the athlete. Some individuals can go through the motions, but their teaching becomes a form of stress and confusion that gets worse.

Imagery and visualization

Imagery and visualization go hand in hand with the performance of psychomotor skills. Ability to 'see in the mind's eye' is a way of building a mental picture based on information from other senses and/or information when the sense of actually seeing is reduced or non-existent. For example, have you ever tried to find your way around your room at night when the lights are out? You know the room, you remember where the chair and table are, and the light switch is on the other side of the room, etc. It is amazing how all your other senses come to life. Your knowledge of the layout is still there and the other senses back up your memory of what is where. Feedback from your sense of posture in space, tactility and arousal all contribute, and hearing becomes acute. You will probably be able to walk across the room.

As another example, all the senses contribute to the memory of what it was like to have that cola on that hot day last week, and what it would be like to get another at that same shop ahead of you. That shop functions as a stimulus to re-create the memory of an experience. In sport the re-creation of an event or situation and the imagery that results allows us to catalogue the experience before and after that situation. To learn from this situation we tend to analyse what took place before the experience, like scoring a try or touch down. How many times have you seen athletes describing the actions after the try or touch down to each other? This debriefing is important so that athletes can share the experience. Even if something goes wrong they will still talk about it, probably with a little less excitement. The resultant emotional and physical experiences are discussed openly so that members of a team can 'imagine' the situation and later can continue 'imagining' situations that have not even taken place. It is easy to reduce this input of information and execution of output into some clinical psychology formula.

Research on the neural systems underlying imagery brings a new source of evidence to bear on these cognitive science controversies, as well as on the cerebral localization of imagery processes. Emerging from this work is the view that mental imagery involves the efferent activation of visual areas in prestriate occipital cortex, parietal and temporal cortex, and that these areas represent the same kinds of specialized visual information in imagery as they do in perception (Farah, 1989).

Motivation

One of the most important aspects of behaviour is motivation. Some of the best works on the theory of motivation have been written by those in the fields of psychology. Some of the best writings, in my opinion, have been written outside of official texts, for example work by Koestler and Arnold. For years there has been discussion on regarding human responses as simply stimulus–response (S–R). This is without a doubt not only simplistic but dangerous. Computers work in an S–R manner and have no emotion. Is motivation a response to the knowledge of success? The word 'reflex' was also used, by B.F. Skinner, not in an anatomical or neurological sense but as a purely psychological, descriptive term for the unit of behaviour.

The physiological concept of the reflex arc, which even Sherrington (1940) considered as no more than a 'useful fiction', has become an anachronism. The Pavlovian conditioned reflex was another useful fiction which exercised at first a stimulating and then a paralysing effect – a phenomenon frequently met in the history of science. In Hebb's words: (1949) 'Pavlov has deservedly had a great influence on psychology, and his theory has not been rejected because it is too physiological, but because it does not agree with experiment' (Koestler, 1964).

Since the beginning of the century the theory of motivation has been associated with and developed from the study of learning and behaviour theories. To understand motivation states, theories were developed on the basis that the organism worked on the effectiveness of rewards, and the

S–R theory was used to demonstrate this factor in a 'one has to win' situation. In 1929 a series of papers by Clark L. Hull were published concerned with trial and error learning and conditioning. Hull made a major contribution to current theories. A Hullian theory of motivation will be presented mainly for the need to understand the historical perspective. During this period one of his colleagues, K.W. Spence, further developed the theory into an S–R reinforcement theory, sometimes called the drive reduction theory. Again there are overtones of dominance of one system over the other. This is similar to the approach of the concept of the parasympathetic and sympathetic nervous system fighting to out-do each other. Numerous formulae were put forward to illustrate the S–R theory. One example is the response to a stimulus (S_a), for example a light, in a simple locomotor situation, associated with a turn to the right (R_{rt}) rather than to the left. The fractional element of the process was referred to as r_g and s_g, the reaction goal and stimulus goal, respectively. This formula is a simple representation, and therefore it has stuck. We have been conditioned to think by our own attempts to understand conditioning:

$$S_a \rightarrow r_g \rightarrow s_g \Rightarrow R_{rt}$$

The interpretation of Pavlov's work is another example of how prejudiced social ideas have corrupted the sciences. Pavlov is commonly thought to have discovered operant conditioning with reinforcement (i.e. carrot-and-stick training). For the sake of simplicity and because it is merely the other side of the same coin, I do not distinguish here between the carrot (conventional operant conditioning with reinforcement by reward) and the stick (reinforcement by punishment). Both methods have been used since time immemorial to control and manipulate individuals and populations. This is the basis of the stimulus/response, input/output approach in all sciences, which Pavlov showed to work scientifically in a behavioural setting. He made it possible for twentieth-century psychologists like F.W. Taylor, J.B. Watson, B.F. Skinner and H. Eysenck to disguise their authoritarianism with scientific jargon, thus rationalizing long-established methods in education that stupefy perfectly intelligent people. Pavlov's studies led directly to behaviourist psychology, perhaps the most corrupting influence in the social sciences because it institutionalizes conformity and group-think – the enemies of independent thought and reason (Arnold, 1992).

The concept of motivation is reflected in the response of one athlete compared with others. A highly motivated athlete could be the presentation of an overreaction to anxiety, becoming out of control; a kind of pathological motivation.

Arousal–performance

Figure 2.5 shows the factors that affect arousal–performance relationships.

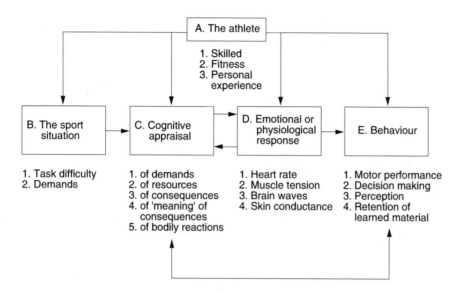

Fig. 2.5 A model illustrating factors that affect the arousal–performance relationship (Landers and Boutcher, 1986).

Inverted-U hypothesis

The inverted-U hypothesis represents a simple relationship between arousal and performance. This theory basically puts forward the principle that with an increase in arousal there will be an increase in ability and vice versa, up to a point. The highest point is the individual's maximum ability to perform; following this, performance decreases in a downward arch (Fig. 2.6).

Drive theory hypothesis

'Since a need, either actual or potential, usually precedes and accompanies the action of an organism, the need is often said to motivate or drive the associated activity. Because of this motivational characteristic of needs they are regarded as producing primary animal drives' (Hull, 1943, p. 57).

The drive theory suggests a linear relationship that relates the athlete's arousal to performance as an ever-increasing relationship known as drive (Fig. 2.7). Hull and Spence made the biggest contributions to the behavioural theories of drive between the 1930s and 1960s. Hull divided drive into primary and secondary. Primary drives are those associated with hunger, thirst, air, temperature regulation, defecation, urination, rest (after exertion), sleep (after wakefulness), activity (after inactivity), sexual intercourse, nest building, care of the young, and avoidance of or relief from pain (tissue injury). Hull wrote:

> [most primary needs] appear to generate and throw into the blood stream more or less characteristic chemical substances, or else to

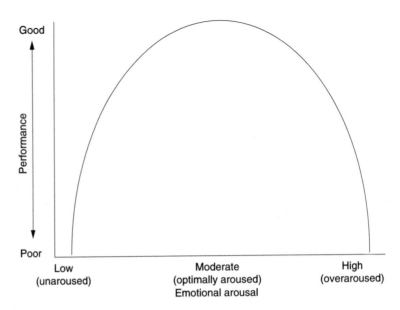

Fig. 2.6 The inverted 'U' relationship between arousal and performance (from Williams, 1986).

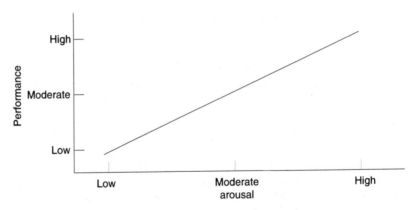

Fig. 2.7 The linear relationship between arousal and performance as suggested by the drive theory (from Williams, 1986).

withdraw a characteristic substance. These substances (or their absence) have a selective physiology effect on more or less restricted and characteristic parts of the body (e.g., the so-called 'hunger' contractions of the body) which serves to activate resident receptors. This receptor activation constitutes the drive stimulus, S_D. In the case of tissue injury this sequence seems to be reversed; here the energy producing the injury is the drive stimulus, and this action causes the release into blood of adrenal secretion which appears to be the physiological motivating substance.

(Hull, 1943, p. 240)

Hull conceived drives as stimuli, and then went on to describe the law of primary reinforcement:

> If, however, any of the evoked movements chances to reduce the receptor (stimuli have to have receptors) discharge characteristic of a need (S_D), the stimuli and the stimulus traces operating . . . at the time acquired an increment of connection of such a nature that on subsequent occasions if any of these stimuli recurs in conjunction with the drive the reaction will tend to be evoked.
>   (Hull, 1951, p. 15; Hull, 1952, pp. 5–6)

Hull spoke of deprivation (C_D), which developed into a drive state. The secondary motivation or drive can be demonstrated in the secondary drive of fear. For example, consider a tissue injury, as might arise from being burned. There will be responses which escape (by withdrawal) the injurious stimulus. These responses will become associated with the stimuli of the situation because of the reinforcement due to the cessation of pain. An example would be hand withdrawal from a hot surface, which avoids further burning. Because of this learning, the stimuli of the situation can arouse the withdrawal responses, ahead of injury, on future occasions. These stimuli, then, are viewed as the conditions of drive arousal in the case of an acquired drive of fear. The responses they arouse also cause proprioceptive stimulation (many of the responses aroused by the situational stimuli would be internal ones – 'fear'), and this proprioceptive stimulation comprises the drive stimulus, or stimuli, of the learned fear drive. These stimuli, being intense, are able to motivate behaviour (Hull, 1951, p. 21). We now know that this secondary or learned drive occurs at spinal cord level, being learned and 'handed down' to the cord, thus allowing it to become a reflex activity. As with primary reinforcement, the secondary reinforcement theory states that neutral stimuli, present during primary reinforcement, acquire the property of being reinforcing stimuli. Thus, they may maintain behaviour when primary reinforcement no longer occurs, or they may serve as 'rewards' for learning acts which are never followed by primary reinforcement.

Psychology and injury

It is important that the physician communicates to the patient that all is not lost; that he is not giving up because of a certain diagnosis, and that it is a battle they are going to fight together – patient, family and doctor – no matter the end result. This is a point taken from the book by Elizabeth Kübler-Ross, *On Death and Dying*. The writings of Dr Kübler-Ross have been used many times in sports medicine to help the athlete who is facing the problem of the consequence of injury or illness. For years, I thought it excessive to relate terminal cancer patients to the athlete who has a groin strain. It was not until some years ago when I had my first amateur soccer player who had aspirations to become a professional, that I realized the similarity was very close. This 18-year-old male university student had been prescribed antidepressants by his general practitioner due to the fact that he had a groin strain lasting for 10 weeks. He would not even look at me in my surgery when he was talking to me; it was as if he had given up all hope but came to me because somebody had told him to.

Dr Kübler-Ross describes five main stages:

1. denial and isolation;
2. anger;
3. bargaining;
4. depression;
5. acceptance and resignation with a degree of hope.

These stages are important as a baseline for making a broad judgement about an athlete. This particular athlete had reached the fifth stage. What was I to do? The important factor was to try and break the ice without making him feel that I was making a joke out of his situation and not taking him seriously. As Dr Kübler-Ross mentioned in her book, it is important to communicate. I had to find out why he was depressed. This may seem a stupid remark, as we know why. But we do not know **why**. As we began to talk about his injury and what he felt with regard to his general health, he said, 'I have rested it for 6 weeks and every time I try to play it hurts again; I know it is not going to get better'. I then asked him why he thought it was not going to get better and reminded him at this point that he had not seen anybody for his condition before. 'Because I know that all injuries only get better if you rest', was his reply. Where did he get this idea from? He just assumed it because everybody at his club had told him. What were their qualifications for these statements, I inquired? This is when he started to look at me.

Many athletes, especially those who 'live for' their sport, are often only exposed to and only respond to this 'sporting' world. This man was 18 years of age and intelligent, but it is possible that his awareness that he was intelligent helped to reinforce his belief. Because others had rested and got better, rest was the only treatment and if it did not work you were in trouble.

After he began to look at me I understood that at this point it was important not to make him feel that he had made an unintelligent decision. I proceeded to break down the rationale of his assumptions and show him that under the circumstances he had made the wrong decision. Then I had to reorder his list of assumptions to show him why the chances and elements for a full recovery were still there. It was a debriefing session. After two visits he said that running for the bus and taking stairs two at a time no longer hurt. Was he ready to play? I told him that he had to test himself, and that if it hurt it did not matter as this would show us that we had a little more work to do. He trained, and felt a little sore. Within another three visits he played a full game with no pain. In retrospect, his overall reason for the depression came out in further conversations. The groin injury was the physical trauma that broke the emotional camel's back.

It is vital to try and use these stages to explain to the athlete that you understand what they are going through, but also remind them that it is their injury and you obviously cannot feel the same way. Telling a depressed and angry athlete that you know how he or she feels, even if you think you do, is a formula for disaster. Never patronize an athlete and never show head tilting, smiling sympathy. They need somebody to take over for a little, while things are rearranged in front of them. They generally work hard at what they do and over the years have been told, usually by a friend or coach, what to do. Make them understand what is going on and get them involved. There is nothing better than hands on treatment when dealing with a depressed athlete. Leaving any athlete alone in a room plugged into the mains is not treatment: it is procedure.

The essential difference between animate and inanimate matter is that in the former, reaction to stress follows as an awareness in a two-part process. First, there is some change in the physical nature of the animal, as when photons initiate retino-chemical changes, or carcinomatous cell division energizes interoceptive neural activity in adjacent tissue. Second, the CNS receives such information and interprets it within the dynamic matrix developed by the life experience of the individual, before bringing it into awareness (Harward, 1985).

Osteopathic manipulative therapy

In his development of the theory of systemic desensitization, Wolpe (1958) drew on the important pioneering work of Jacobson (1938). Over the years, Jacobson had noted that anxious patients typically show elevated levels of muscle tension. On the basis of clinical observations, he developed the parallel idea that cultivating a condition of thorough muscular relaxation could be useful in reducing a patient's anxiety. Specifically, he postulated that a condition of muscular relaxation is physiologically incompatible with an anxiety response. On the strength of this postulate, muscle relaxation came to play a central role in systematic desensitization (Stoyva and Budzynski, 1972). Perhaps memory is in the soft tissue, an organic tape recorder? 'It's common for patients to spontaneously laugh or cry during or after OMT', Dr Edward A. Luke Jr pointed out, 'I once had a woman who started to cry after I gave her OMT. When I asked her why she was crying, she said that she had suddenly remembered a personal loss and that the thought had come to her during manipulation' (Sprovieri, 1992).

Fear, anger, hate, smouldering resentment, anxiety, strong desire for attention, libido, family or job worries – all these alert the protective mechanisms of the whole body. If the nervous tension is not frequently relaxed, unphysiological stress and congestion appear in the reflex areas of the posterior pillar of the spine in the suboccipital area (related to the superior cervical sympathetic ganglia), the upper thoracic (cardiac) area, the mid-thoracic (adrenal) area, and sometimes in the lumbar (gonadal) area. Jacob Wasserman has said, 'the body volunteers to suffer on behalf of the mind'. William James defines emotion as follows: 'It is the state of mind that manifests itself by a perceptible change in the body.'

In osteopathic manipulative practice it is recognized that among the first and universal changes which emotion produces in the body is reflex contraction in the muscles of the upper thoracic spinal area and the suboccipital triangle. In osteopathic manipulative practice, reflexly produced congestion with soreness in spinal joint tissues is commonly observed. Many years ago it was said, 'First the thought; then the emotion; then the congestion; and then the tumor' (McCole, 1972).

We do not control ourselves; we are controlled by our habit patterns. What we deprecate as present irrelevancies are the imprints of past relevances. We think with our habits, and our emotional training determines our thinking. Consciousness is like a moving picture. The emotional patterns of infancy are projected into awareness. We sit in the audience, and insist we're in the projection booth. Children are interesting because they are emotionally outgoing. A childish childhood is a happy childhood. The baby is born free, but his parents soon put him in chains. The tragedy of the drama of psychology is that all of the villains have friendly faces (Salter, 1949). Operant conditioning has been institutionalized in all cultures since time immemorial. When individuals or groups of people condition themselves or let others condition them for long enough and with sufficient reinforcement (either by expectation of a reward, fear of punishment, by imagined unconditional freedom or by mindless imitation) they can be forced (or allow themselves) to become psychologically or physically dependent, self-destructive and a menace to others. Operant conditioning works for training the mentally handicapped, domestic animals, creating human monsters like Stangl, or brainwashing people to be willing victims. Operant conditioning can turn naturally intelligent human beings into imbeciles (Arnold, 1992).

Where does all this lead? Personally, I feel it leads to the area of operant conditioning, where the athlete is trapped. We are all conditioned in one way or another. The responses we make, the words we say, sounds we hear, objects we see, aromas we smell, pain we feel etc. all have to be interpreted; this is an individual factor. Every athlete not only has a story to tell, but in themselves is a story covering all the criteria of fear, comedy, anger, love, depression, hate, joy etc.

NUTRITION AND FLUIDS

For years it has been recognized that the simple process of meeting your calorific output with your calorific intake balances out your energy needs. However, this is not as simple as eating pasta. Athletes often manipulate their diets to the extreme in the hope that it will give them the edge over their competitors. This can develop into a nutritional obsession with a tendency to forget about the quality of the food eaten. Powders, liquids and tablets replace fresh vegetables, fresh fruit, fresh fish and meat and fresh water. That is not to say that these powders etc. which are composed of the essential extracts are not useful. The risk is that they take up too much of the athlete's intake and the athlete is then living on a non-vitalistic diet. One of the main nutritional factors that is overlooked by many athletes is the adequate intake of water. Here I will briefly review nutrition, its basic components and its relevance in sports.

Depending on the activity, an athlete may want to increase or keep up a calorie intake, e.g. a footballer, or undernourish him or herself to keep weight low, e.g. a ballet dancer. Different disciplines do require different calorific and nutritional balances. It should also be realized that it does not matter if you are professional or amateur at your particular sport, it is the amount of training that is undertaken that is relevant. As in the examination of an athlete's physical problems, the general health of the athlete should be considered first. The calorific and nutritional needs of the athlete should not be reduced to simple protein and vitamin intake and usage.

The objectives of the osteopath from a calorific and nutritional aspect should cover the following.

1. To educate the athlete and provide him/her with constant updated information on fluid, calorific, nutritional, and training technique changes that affect health and performance.
2. Not to assume the athlete knows anything about these subjects.
3. When travelling, to check and control the types of foodstuffs and the methods of cooking and storage that will be available to the athlete, from a fluid, calorific, nutritional and psychological aspect.
4. To manipulate the fluid, calorific and nutritional status of the athlete when recovering from injury or resting from training.

The basic concept of good calorific, nutritional and fluid intake should be the starting point, and then adjusted to the individual needs of the athlete. The basic needs for all of us differ mainly through habitual likes and dislikes. As we know, the diet consists basically of the following main groups: carbohydrates, fats, protein, vitamins, minerals and water.

Carbohydrates

These are the sugars in their simple and complex forms. Simple sugars include glucose, fructose, disaccharides, sucrose, maltose and the poly-saccharides, e.g. starch and glycogen. As we know, even the most complex sugars have to be broken down to simple sugars to be of any use. The body has reserves in the form of glycogen in muscles and liver but they are depleted during athletic activity.

Not all carbohydrates have been found to be beneficial to athletes. In contrast to sucrose and glucose, ingestion of a 6% fructose solution during exercise is associated with gastrointestinal distress, compromised physio-logical response, and comparatively poor exercise performance. The reasons why fructose ingestion fails to affect exercise performance in a manner similar to sucrose and glucose intake are not easily identified. The gastrointestinal discomfort with fructose ingestion is thought to be related to the absorptive mechanism of fructose in the small intestine. Unlike glucose, which is actively transported across the intestinal epithelium, fructose is absorbed via facilitated diffusion. Consequently, fructose is absorbed from the proximal small intestine at a lower rate than glucose, resulting in comparatively slower fluid absorption rates. This is considered the cause of the gastrointestinal distress and diarrhoea often reported with fructose feeding.

The rise in plasma fructose levels with fructose and sucrose intake indicates that some fructose escapes hepatic metabolism and is available to peripheral tissues. Although fructose is taken up by skeletal muscle, the extent of its metabolism is thought to be minimal because (a) muscle lacks fructokinase and (b) peripheral fructose levels are too low to compete effectively with glucose for phosphorylation by hexokinase, which has only one-tenth the affinity for fructose as for glucose. Therefore, it appears unlikely that fructose exerts a peripheral effect that could explain the impairment in exercise performance associated with fructose intake (Murray *et al.*, 1989).

The following is a list of good carbohydrate sources:

- cereal grains
- molasses
- beans
- potatoes
- fresh fruit
- peas
- dried fruit
- jams, jellies
- pancakes
- breads
- syrups
- honey
- pasta
- fresh vegetables.

Carbohydrate loading

It is now recognized that regular training causes physiological changes that increase and enhance the lifespan of fuel stores, putting into focus the principle of carbohydrate loading. The body adapts to use less fuel, so even energy consumption shows signs of plasticity.

Fats

Many athletes know what fats are but get confused between the different kinds. Variations depend on chemical make-up of the fat and whether it allows more hydrogen atoms to attach or not. The three types are saturated, unsaturated and polyunsaturated. The fats with chemical formulae that do not allow any more hydrogen atoms to combine are called saturated. This is because they are already saturated with hydrogen atoms and have no more room. The fats with available spaces for hydrogen atoms are unsaturated or polyunsaturated depending on the number of spaces available. We should avoid saturated (animal) fat and should be eating unsaturated and polyunsaturated fats of vegetable origin.

Proteins

Proteins are amino acid-based complexes with elements of carbon, hydrogen, oxygen, sulphur, phosphorus and iron. They are in an available form in the free tissue amino acid pool. The balance between synthesis and degradation determines the size of this pool. Of the 20 or so amino acids, nine are not synthesized in the body – histidine, isoleucine, leucine, lysine, methionine, phenylalanine, threonine, tryptophan and valine – and must be taken from an external source. The recommended daily intake of protein is 0.8 g/kg body weight for adults, with higher levels recommended for growing children (Salvin *et al.*, 1988). There is a history of athletes, especially in contact and collision sports, taking much more protein than they need, especially in the form of red meat. Too much protein leads to weight gain, dehydration and loss of urinary calcium. The rates of protein synthesis are depressed in muscle, liver and throughout the body during acute exercise. Naturally, this depends on the intensity and duration of the exercise (Hood and Terjung, 1990).

Nitrogen balance

Changes in skeletal mass can be caused by changes in the rate of protein synthesis and degradation, although these do not always occur in opposite directions. The parallel increase in rates of protein synthesis and degradation in muscle during growth and during recovery after exercise has been ascribed to the need for extensive remodelling of this highly organized tissue. Nutritional control of muscle protein turnover, in addition to that by certain amino acids, is mediated by hormones, such as insulin, corticosteroids and thyroid hormone. Insulin increases protein synthesis and decreases protein degradation, corticosteroids have the opposite effect, and thyroid hormone stimulates both protein synthesis and degradation, with a relatively greater effect on the former than on the latter. Nutritional control of liver protein turnover, in addition to that by amino acids, mainly occurs through the actions of insulin and glucagon (Meijer *et al.*, 1990).

Vitamins

These act as catalysts, i.e. enzymes and co-enzymes. The word 'vitamin' is derived from 'vital amines' which they were thought to be by the Polish biochemist, Funk. Vitamins have a major tendency to work better individually if combined daily requirements are met.

Vitamin A (retinol)

There are two forms of vitamin A, retinol and dehydroretinol (A_1 and A_2, respectively). The green and yellow parts of plants synthesize precursors for vitamin A, which are classified as carotenoids and are soluble in fat and fat oils, but not in water. A carotene precursor, β-carotene, is converted into vitamin A in the wall of the small intestine. Excessive vitamin A intake leads to hypercalcaemia and bone resorption. The best sources of vitamin A include the liver oils, e.g. cod liver oil, ox liver and halibut liver oil. Other sources include butter, milk, cheese, carrots and spinach. Cooking methods affect availability of vitamin A. Frying in deep fat, for example, will result in the removal of the vitamin into the fat. Steaming vegetables, rather than boiling, is a far better cooking method. Deficiency of vitamin A is noticeable when the athlete has problems seeing in dim light. This is caused by a deficiency in an aldehyde of retinol that is essential for the visual purple (rhodopsin) in the rods of the retina. Deficiency of vitamin A also affects general growth, new bone formation and cell turnover. Where cell turnover is concerned, the epithelial layers develop problems in shedding cells, leading to thickening. A common presentation of this is in the cornea of the eye, where this thickening leads to an opacity known as keratomalacia.

The recommended daily allowance is quite small, around 1.0 μmol for children and 2.5 μmol for adults.

The vitamin B complex

Thiamin (B_1)
This vitamin is water-soluble, and is present in the seeds and outer coats of grains, such as bran, the pulses, nuts and yeast. Therefore, wholemeal products such as bread, rice and spaghetti are good sources. It is also found in animal cells. Obtaining these foodstuffs fresh is important as canning, freezing and dehydration have a tendency to reduce the vitamin content. Cooking fresh foods reduces vitamin content. Deficiency of thiamin leads to an inability to metabolize pyruvic acid, leading to an accumulation in the fluids and tissues of the body. Therefore, analysis of blood levels of pyruvate can be helpful in the detection of this deficiency. Lack of vitamin B intake leads to the condition of beri-beri, which is sometimes seen in alcoholics on a poor diet. This condition presents with polyneuritis, i.e. weakness, poor coordination, altered sensations, and atrophy; cardiac enlargement and eventual cardiac failure; and general oedema.

Recommended daily allowances are around 3.3 μmol.

Riboflavin (B_2)
This was discovered in 1932 when a 'yellow enzyme' was isolated from yeast by Warburg and Christian, i.e. riboflavin phosphate. Riboflavin combines with proteins to form flavoproteins. These flavoproteins are important hydrogen carriers in biological oxidation systems and are

absorbed from the upper intestinal tract. Large amounts of the vitamin are found in the liver, kidneys and heart, even in states of general source deficiency. It is present in urine as a pigment, uroflavin.

As with B_1, good sources of B_2 are grains, peas and beans. Additionally, good animal sources are milk, egg yolk and liver, kidney and heart muscle. Normal cooking does not significantly reduce the amount of this vitamin, but boiling may reduce vitamin content. Deficiency of this vitamin is known as ariboflavinosis; the skin become rough and scaly with the lips becoming red, swollen and developing cracks (cheilosis) and the corner of the mouth becoming fissured and painful (angular stomatitis). The tongue can also become enlarged, tender and a magenta colour. Recommended daily allowance is around 1.7 mg, with an increase during pregnancy.

Pyrodoxine (B_6)

Vitamin B_6 is a generic term for a group of naturally occurring derivatives of pyridine. It is present from both animal and vegetable sources. The major members of this group include pyridoxol, pyridoxal and pyridoxamine. Pyridoxal phosphate is involved in the haem synthetic pathway, and catalyses the synthesis of tryptophan from indole and serine in the conversion of tryptophan to nicotinic acid.

Deficiency is rare in humans, but in animals can lead to anaemia, dermatitis and convulsions. The recommended daily allowance is about 1 mg.

Cobalamin (B_{12})

Vitamin B_{12} is one of a group of compounds known as corrinoids. The bonding of dimethylbenzimidazole to cobamide forms cobalamin which like other B group vitamins is converted in the body into a co-enzyme. Cobalamins bond to β-globulin, with some still free in the plasma. If not metabolized they are stored in the liver bound to β-globulin. B_{12} is important in haemopoiesis. Good sources are the bovine kidney and liver, fresh meat and dairy produce. There is no B_{12} in plants.

Recommended daily allowance is in the region of 0.5 mg.

Laetril (B_{17})

Vitamin B_{17} is found mostly in apricots, but in very minute amounts.

Niacin

This is a generic name that covers nicotinic acid and nicotinamide. The amide form of this vitamin is converted into nicotinamide adenine dinucleotide (NAD) and nicotinamide adenine dinucleotide phosphate (NADP). It can be synthesized in the body from tryptophan by the action of intestinal flora. Nicotinamide is a very stable vitamin that is not destroyed by oxidation, alkali, heat or light. Sources of nicotinic acid include the wholefoods, e.g. barley, maize, rice, oatmeal, bran etc. In addition animal sources include fresh meat, fresh liver, kidney, fish and milk.

Deficiency leads to the condition known as pellagra. This usually develops after a lengthy period of general illness where the athlete may have lethargy, irritability and weight loss due to diarrhoea. With this kind of general problem there will be other vitamin deficiences that complicate the picture. Pellagra presents with soreness, roughness and scaly skin of body areas that are exposed to heat and light. The tongue and mouth become swollen and red.

Recommended daily allowances are around 20 mg.

Panthothenic acid

This is so widely available that it is rarely described in a deficiency context. It combines with mercaptoethylamine forming pantotheine, which then forms co-enzyme A which is essential in the metabolic processes of fat and carbohydrates. Daily requirements are around 20 mg.

Biotin

This acts as co-enzyme in fixing carbon dioxide in carboxylation reactions. Raw egg white tends to bond with biotin forming a stable compound which is not absorbed. This vitamin is found in yeast, liver, kidney and in human intestinal bacteria.

Choline

Important in the synthesis of acetylcholine (ACh) and phospholipids, deficiency is very rare because lecithin contains choline and is present in all animal and vegetable foodstuffs.

Vitamin C (ascorbic acid)

In its pure form, vitamin C is white, crystalline and soluble in water. It is not synthesized in the body so it needs to be obtained from food. This vitamin belongs to a group of reversible oxidation–reduction systems and acts as a hydrogen carrier or respiratory catalyst. It is present in all body fluids and is present in large amounts in the pituitary, corpus luteum and thymus. The liver, lungs and heart muscles have small amounts and the skeletal muscles have traces. When there is a lack of ascorbic acid in the body the content of leukocytes and platelets is reduced over a period of months.

Ascorbic acid deficiency affects the laying down of collagen fibres of connective tissue which is important in the successful healing of wounds. Deficiency also affects bone formation, and causes scurvy which is quickly cured with the administration of vitamin C.

Good sources of vitamin C include rose hips, blackcurrants, green vegetables and citrus fruits.

Recommended daily allowances are in the 100 mg region.

Vitamin D (calciferol)

These are a group of heat-stable compounds, the most important being D_2 (ergocalciferol) and D_3 (cholecalciferol). Vitamin D_2 does not occur naturally, but is produced artificially by the action of ultraviolet light on the plant sterol ergosterol. Cholecalciferol is produced in mammals by ultraviolet irradiation of provitamin 7-dehydrocholesterol. Good sources of vitamin D are the fish livers, halibut liver oil and cod liver oil. Ox liver, egg yolk and white fish are other sources. Loss of vitamin D from foodstuffs during storage, preparation, canning or dehydration is minimal. Deficiency occurs when both dietary sources and sunlight are lacking. This results in rickets and osteomalacia, i.e. poor deposition of calcium salts in newly formed bone. The best source is sunlight so that no real supplementation of vitamin D is necessary.

Vitamin E

A generic term for a number of compounds of which α-tocopherol is the most active. This is a yellow oil that is insoluble in water. It is a stable compound that is not destroyed by cooking and its richest sources are vegetable oils and wheat germ.

The consumption of vitamins increases significantly when people have to perform under conditions of elevated psychoemotional and physical stress. Consumption of large amounts of high calorie food products significantly impairs uptake of vitamins, particularly those that are fat soluble, and may lead to the development of vitamin insufficiency. It should also be noted that consumption of such food products is also associated with a subnormal ingestion of potassium, magnesium, phosphorus, iron, cobalt, manganese, copper and zinc. Only the intake of calcium is reduced less significantly (Udalov, 1992).

Minerals

Iron

Iron is present in organ meats, dark green vegetables, wholegrains, fruits, fish and molasses. It is an important mineral for pregnant women, menstruating women, sufferers of chronic haemorrhoids and performers of long-distance events. Iron deficiency in pregnancy will show as a deficiency in the newborn. Signs and symptoms of deficiency include generally looking unwell, tiredness and fatigue. Athletes need about 18 mg/day.

Calcium

The best sources of calcium are a combination of sesame seeds and dolomite, with magnesium. A pint of milk contains around 600 mg calcium. This is the most common mineral in the body, due to its presence in bones and teeth, and it is vital for nerve function, blood clotting and heart muscle enzyme reactions. It is taken up in the small intestine (duodenum) by a process of active transportation. It is an important mineral for athletes, especially post partum. Deficiency presents as osteoporosis and rickets. Daily intake should be around 700–1000 mg.

Magnesium

Magnesium is an important mineral for muscle function, protein synthesis and the nervous system. It is also an activator for the enzymes involved in the oxidative phosphorylation of ADP to ATP. Therefore, it is important in cellular processes. It is important that this mineral is balanced with the intake of calcium because both are absorbed by active transport at the same sites. An increase in the intake of one will lead to an interference in absorption of the other. The best source is dolomite tablets. Deficiencies can result from alcoholism, cirrhosis of the liver and diabetes. Signs and symptoms of deficiency include muscle cramps, constipation, pre-menstrual symptoms and insomnia. Daily requirements are around 300–500 mg, but there should be a higher intake, around 800 mg, where there is an increased intake of protein, calcium, phosphate and vitamin D.

Zinc

Good sources of zinc include red meat, green peas, shellfish, carrots, pork, beans, eggs and potatoes. Zinc is an important mineral in general enzyme function, e.g. mobilizing of vitamin A from the liver. Deficiency has been shown to lead to hair loss, a low sperm count, night blindness and an inability to taste foods. Signs and symptoms of deficiency include poor wound healing, white spots or lines under brittle nails, and a lack of appetite. Other situations that lead to deficiency include alcoholism, anorexia and a strict vegan diet. Poor absorption of zinc occurs with high fibre diet, excess iron intake and coeliac disease. Daily allowance should be around 10–50 mg.

Potassium

This is present in the body in large amounts along with sodium and is important in fluid balance, nerves and muscles. Deficiency results in cramps and oedema. There is a balance between the amount of potassium and sodium in the body: an increase of sodium will lead to a loss of potassium as sodium is stored and potassium is excreted from the body. Potassium is important for converting glucose to glycogen when bound with phosphate, but it is then released during glycogenolysis. Best sources include green leafy vegetables and fruit, especially bananas. A good daily intake is around 10–100 mg.

Sodium

The commonest source of this mineral is in table salt. As with potassium, it is important in fluid balance, muscles and nerve cells. Many athletes make the mistake of thinking that they have to take extra salt in their food to prevent cramp; if anything they are making the situation worse. Generally, athletes are in a dehydrated condition, suffering from water depletion not salt depletion. As they lose more water the relative salt concentration increases, leading to an increased risk of cramps. Salt is present in practically everything we eat.

Supplementation

In the last few years creatine monophosphate has been the latest form of supplementation to enter the arena. There is at the time of writing no conclusive evidence, from literature reviews, that this form of supplementation is beneficial (McEwan, 1994). Creatine is formed in the liver and kidney from the amino acids arginine, glycine and methionine. It combines with phosphates by a chemical bond that provides the energy supply for the contraction – relaxation process of muscular action. Athletes have told me how they can work harder, for longer and recover more quickly when taking creatine monophate. Where does the excess go? Would the excess be found in fascia and connective tissue? Does it weaken these tissues? These questions have yet to be answered.

Water

The majority of athletes are in a constant state of chronic voluntary dehydration. Water (fluid) loss from the body does not only occur due to sweating in hot environments, it also occurs in swimmers, high altitude climbing, and in athletes suffering from chronic pain. The chronic pain factor is vitally important to the success of treatment in myofascioskeletal presentations that have become a burden to the athlete. Pain increases the ventilatory rate. An athlete may be bordering on hyperventilation syndrome, which leads to increased fluid loss and hypersensitivity to the chronic condition, leading to a vicious circle of pain and dehydration. It is important to ask injured athletes how much water they drink.

Since tissue cells are constantly 'turning over', hydration of tissues is vital in the synthesis and degradation of protein, protein being the building blocks of tissues. An increase in cellular hydration (swelling) acts as an anabolic proliferative signal, whereas cell shrinkage is catabolic and antiproliferative. The cellular hydration state is mainly determined by the activity of ion and substrate transport systems in the plasma membrane. Hormones, substrates and oxidative stress can change the cellular hydration state within minutes, thereby affecting protein turnover. It is postulated that a decrease in cellular hydration in liver and skeletal muscle triggers the protein catabolic states that accompany various diseases (Häussinger *et al.*, 1993).

Pre-game meals

It is important to realize that the pre-game meal is not as important as a good nutritious diet during the week. The pre-game diet of an athlete is important, but too much emphasis is placed on this psychodietary boost before an event. Players often say 'I have to have my favourite meal before a game'; the problem is that they sometimes have not eaten properly since the last game. Some coaches believe that it does not make a great deal of difference what an athlete eats prior to competition or heavy training as long as the food tastes good and the stomach is not too full when exercise begins. However, current research indicates that nutrition during the 4 hours before competition can affect performance significantly, and athletes should pay close attention to what they eat (Wheeler, 1989). Types of carbohydrate consumed before an event are important. Fructose is less readily available for oxidation than glucose or corn starch, and pure corn starch does not offer any advantage over glucose as a pre-exercise meal (Guezennec *et al.*, 1989).

Cooking

The majority of athletes do not understand the effects of cooking. Many athletes will be pleased to inform you that they have a very good diet, but do not realize that storage and cooking methods destroy the nutrients in the food. There is also the aspect of hygiene and reducing the risk of food poisoning especially when dealing with a large number of athletes eating together. Cooking usually involves direct heat, as in grilling and baking, heated water (boiling and steaming) and frying. All processes of cooking degrade the structure of food so that it is more palatable and digestible. The only problem is that in the majority of cases nutrient values can be drastically reduced.

The cooking of meat removes water, soluble protein is coagulated and collagen is changed to gelatin, and the fibres shorten and become softer making it easier to chew. Overcooking has the opposite effect, making it harder to chew. Starch, cereals and potatoes swell and burst during cooking, again allowing for easier digestion and chewing. Vegetables that are boiled will lose soluble nutrients into the water. This nutrient-rich water can then be drunk or used in a soup or stew. Steaming vegetables and fish is the preferred method, with its higher temperatures and shorter cooking times. Reduced loss of nutrients in grilling and frying is due to the short time of exposure to the heat which also seals the outside of the meat. The origin of foods needs to be considered; there is much discussion on the choice of free range foodstuffs.

Eating disorders

Eating disorders in athletes are often seen. It is becoming apparent that the causes of the majority of eating disorders are far deeper than a desire to lose weight. Pressure from coaches, dance teachers and the media can overwhelm the individual. They may believe they will perform better, and look better, if thinner. The most important factor is for the osteopath to recognize the 'at risk' athlete. It is also important to remember that male athletes are at risk as well as females.

The athlete may attend the surgery for an injury that he or she does not associate with an eating disorder. Always consider the athlete's general health first. A poor or improper diet could be the underlying factor in both the injury and the reason that the athlete is not recovering. As far as ballet dancers are concerned, one of the main precipitating factors of eating disorders is the environment in which they work and socialize. It is not uncommon to see ballet dancers in the canteen, after a 2 hour class, drinking strong coffee, smoking cigarettes and eating a miniscule fruit salad for lunch. They eat together, and will watch what each other is eating. Dancers do not consider themselves athletes, but artists. However, they are in fact the highest form of athletes. Fitness and health magazines do not direct their products at dancers. It is important that coaches and teachers are aware of the problems and that they change or adapt the environment in which their athletes perform and eat. An overall view to this is given in Figure 2.8.

Basic diagnostic criteria for anorexia nervosa and bulimia

Anorexia nervosa:

- Refusal to maintain body weight over a minimal normal weight for age and height (for example, the athlete works to keep his or her weight 15% below the target weight, so growth does not occur as expected during childhood or teen years, which results in a body weight 15% below average).
- Intense fear of becoming obese, even when underweight.
- Inability to accurately see one's body weight, size or shape (i.e. the person claims to feel fat even when emaciated). Belief that one area of the body is too fat even when the person is obviously underweight.
- Absence of at least three menstrual cycles in a row.

Bulimia:

- Binge eating (i.e. the hurried eating of large amounts of food usually in less than 2 hours).
- Fear of not being able to stop eating during binges.
- Regularly engaging in either self-induced vomiting, use of laxatives, or rigorous dieting or fasting in order to get rid of the food or the calories from the food eaten during binges.
- At least two binge eating sessions per week for at least 3 months.
- Abrasions on the back of the hand caused by teeth due to putting fingers down the back of the throat.
- Foul smelling breath.
- Mouth ulcers, angular stomatitis, discoloration of teeth.

(Adapted from Grandjean, 1991.)

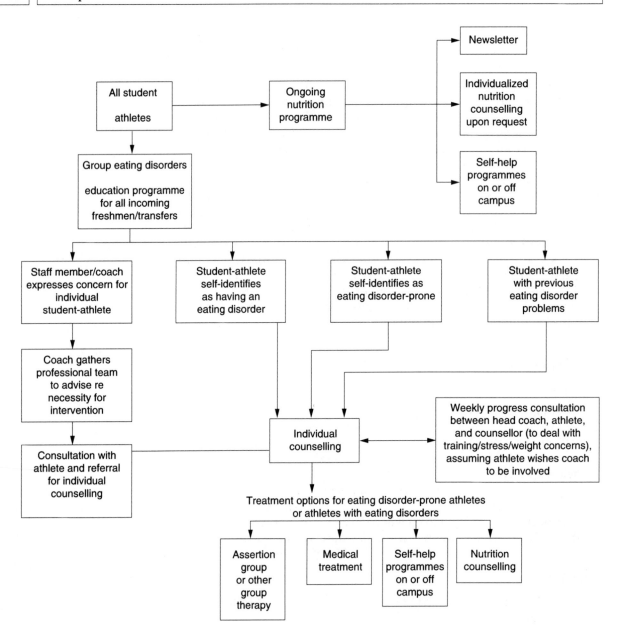

Fig. 2.8 University of Texas Performance Team Algorithm: illustrates a working algorithm for the prevention and treatment of eating disorders among student athletes.

Osteopathic manipulative therapy

Tissue texture is an important guide to the general health of the patient. In cases of poor quality and/or inadequate nutrition, tissues generally present with signs ranging from fluid retention to a fibrotic dryness. This is controlled by the autonomic nervous system. As with psychosomatic conditions, the effects of even the gentlest OMT procedure can be unpredictable under these circumstances. It is always good practice to advise the patient of possible soreness and possible emotional reactions.

Conclusion

At the end of the day the basic approach to healthy eating is that the athlete should choose food first before supplements. The old-fashioned wholefoods, bread, fruit and vegetable diets, supplemented with chicken, fish, minerals and vitamins is a good combination. It is important that athletes drink plenty of water. Excessive supplementation, chronic dehydration and carbohydrate overloading are a common presenting combination in too many athletes. Developing a diet on a calorie intake basis is all very well, but most athletes become unwell and suffer from poor nutritional support. Every athlete should be looked at from the view of health before any other factor. Therefore, good nutrition and adequate fluids are vital, especially in the pregnant athlete.

BASIC PHARMACOLOGY

Pharmacology is as important to the osteopath as it is to the allopathic physician. Drugs in sports are being used more and more, and restrictions on generic types of drugs may cause problems for athletes. An athlete in need of any medication should consult somebody who has a list of restricted medications. Also, side effects of prescribed medications should be considered, and a history of the athlete's condition and past and present medication is relevant. Abuse of drugs is a growing problem in sports, as it is in general practice. The incidence of abuse may be declining, but the preparations used are becoming more dangerous.

Definitions

Pharmacology is the study of both the physiological and biochemical aspects of drugs and their effects. These effects include absorption, distribution, metabolism, elimination, toxicity, and specific mechanisms of drug action. **Pharmacokinetics** is the study of the quantitative mechanisms of drug absorption, distribution and excretion. **Sites of action** depend on the specific binding sites of the cell, known as receptors. Receptor sites can be either in a cell or on the cell surface and they will mediate the action of the drug.

Pharmacokinetics

Absorption

The action of drugs can take place either outside or inside membranes. Route of administration is an important factor in absorption. For example, drugs may have to cross too many membranes or be subjected to chemicals that may break them down. Another factor is dosage. Generally, the higher the dose the greater the effect. Dosage can be increased to achieve its maximum effect, i.e. the **dose–response effect**. Of greater importance to the clinician than absorption is a factor known as **bioavailability**. This term informs the clinician about the extent to which a drug reaches its site of action or a biological fluid from which the drug has access to its site of action. When a drug is absorbed it may have to pass through an organ, like the liver, before it reaches the systemic circulation. This will decrease its bioavailability, and is called the **first-pass effect**. Other factors that affect bioavailability include physical, pathological and anatomical factors. For example, anatomically there may be some distance between the site of absorption and the receptor site, or if there is structural alteration due to autonomic disruption, there could be an alteration in fluid movement, membrane function or local metabolism. In the case of injury or infection there will be aberrant reflex activity. It is important to reduce this reflex pattern to increase the drug bioavailability.

The solubility of the drug affects its transport across membranes. Obviously, the smaller the particles the greater the absorption, especially if the drug is given in aqueous solution rather than in an oil-based solution or solid form. The higher the concentration of a drug and the more soluble it is the greater the absorption. As mentioned above, local factors play a major role in drug absorption. This is important osteopathically in both acute and chronic presentations. To influence the local absorption of a drug does not mean using OMT only on a local level. Local circulation of blood and lymph, and soft tissues are under the control of the autonomic nervous system. Stomach circulation can be improved by OMT at the neck. In addition, the application of heat to a nerve root or over the site of pain will improve the local absorption. The opposite response will occur if cold is applied at the site of injury or at the nerve root. Similar responses occur in shock and vasoconstriction leading to a decrease in absorption. Surface areas affect the absorption rate, e.g. a large surface area like the lungs and intestines provides a good area for absorption.

Common routes of administration include gastrointestinal and parenteral routes. Gastrointestinal methods are:

- oral
- sublingual
- rectal.

Like any route of administration, there are advantages and disadvantages to gastrointestinal methods. The advantages include a slow release of the drug into the circulatory system, thus avoiding a rapid build up which might cause undesirable effects. Sterility is less important with this route. The disadvantages include variable rate of absorption, irritation of mucosal surfaces, patient compliance, and the first-pass effect due, for example, to hepatic metabolism. Sublingual administration avoids this.

Parenteral routes are the following:

- intravenous
- intramuscular

- subcutaneous
- intraperitoneal
- intra-arterial
- intrathecal
- transdermal.

Advantages with these routes are a generally rapid response, more accurate dose delivery, and it provides an alternative when the GI route cannot be used, e.g. the patient may be unconscious. Disadvantages are that the rapid absorption may lead to undesirable effects, sterility is important, and local irritation may result at the injection site.

Other routes of administration include topical preparations for local administration, but having little system absorption, and inhalation, which is a common and rapid route used in bronchodilators and for anaesthetics.

Transportation

The method by which a drug passes through the cell membrane is of great importance. As we have discussed there are many factors involved in the drug reaching its target, e.g. first-pass effect, bioavailability etc. When the drug reaches the cell it can cross the membrane by passive diffusion, carrier-mediated diffusion, active transport or endocytosis.

Passive diffusion
There are two types of passive diffusion, simple diffusion and filtration.

Simple diffusion This is based on Fick's law:

$$\mathrm{d}Q/\mathrm{d}t = (-D)\,(A)\,(\mathrm{d}c/\mathrm{d}x)$$

Where $\mathrm{d}Q/\mathrm{d}t$ is the rate of drug flux (the change in concentration of a drug within a given time), D is a temperature-dependent diffusion constant of the molecule, A is the area of the absorbing surface and $\mathrm{d}c/\mathrm{d}x$ is the concentration gradient. As we can see, the greater the concentration gradient, the greater the rate of absorption, and the larger the absorbing surface, the greater the drug flux. The diffusion constant, D, is directly proportional to the temperature and is inversely related to the molecular size. The greater the lipid–water partition coefficient, the greater the drug flux.

Simple diffusion molecules cross the lipid cell membrane in an uncharged form, and distribution of this uncharged form is a function of the pK_a of the compound and the pH of the medium, and is expressed by the Henderson–Hasselbalch equation:

if the drug is a weak acid:

$$pK_a = pH + \log \frac{\text{concentration of unionized acid}}{\text{concentration of ionized acid}} \qquad (1)$$

if the drug is a weak base:

$$pK_a = pH + \log \frac{\text{concentration of ionized base}}{\text{concentration of unionized base}} \qquad (2)$$

The pH of the medium affects the absorption and excretion of a passively diffused drug. For example, aspirin, which is a weak acid, is best absorbed in the acidic environment of the stomach. Basic drugs are best absorbed in the small intestine. Since urine is acidic, any drug that is acidic can be reabsorbed into the body, as long as the pH does not rise. If this occurs then excretion of the drug increases.

Filtration In this form of passive diffusion, water, ions and some polar and non-polar molecules of low molecular weight diffuse through membranes. This has fuelled suggestions that pores or channels may exist. For example, filtration occurs in capillaries of the kidneys, allowing the movement of large protein molecules.

Carrier-mediated facilitated diffusion

Here, movement through a membrane is aided by a macromolecule. This type of diffusion is specific for chemical structure, requires no energy and cannot move against a concentration gradient, keeping it a diffusion process. It is saturable, i.e. external concentrations are achieved when increasing the internal–external concentration gradient will not increase the rate of influx.

Active transport

Like carrier-mediated facilitated diffusion, active transport across membranes is mediated by macromolecules, it is a saturable process, and it is specific for particular chemical structures. The differences in active transport compared with passive transport are that it requires energy (metabolic), which is generated by the enzyme Na^+K^+-ATPase, and the molecules move against a concentration gradient.

Endocytosis

This is a method of minor importance by which some drugs are transported into cells. Fluid phase endocytosis takes place for substances such as sucrose, and absorptive phase endocytosis occurs for substances such as insulin.

Distribution

Once in the circulatory system drugs can bind non-specifically and reversibly to various plasma proteins, e.g. albumin or globulins. As well as the bound drug there is the free drug element, and an equilibrium is set up between the bound and free drug. It is the free drug that has a biological effect; the bound drug is neither metabolized nor eliminated.

As we know from studying bioavailability, the distribution of a drug to a particular area or organ depends on circulation and the physical and chemical properties of the preparation. Because of this circulation dependence there are some areas of the body that are not readily accessible to drugs, e.g. the brain because of the blood–brain barrier, and the placenta; these are generally known as anatomic barriers. Lipid-soluble drugs will deposit in fatty tissues; this is known as being **sequestered**. Again, an equilibrium is set up between the deposited drug and the free circulating drug. This tissue-bound drug will eventually be in a free state and will be excreted before or after it has been metabolized. We can use compartment models that give us a basic understanding of what might be happening when a drug enters a compartment. These models can be single, double or multiple.

The single compartment model is the easiest to understand and relies on the assumption that the drug is uniformly distributed and absorption and elimination of the drug occur rapidly:

$$V_d = \frac{\text{total amount of drug in the body}}{\text{concentration of drug in the plasma}} \qquad (3)$$

The above equation is used to find the apparent volume of distribution (V_d). When the V_d is high it is an indication that many receptor sites are allowing the drug to become attached or there is a high lipophilicity.

Equation (4) below is used to find the total body clearance, which is the volume of blood or plasma that is cleared in a specific unit of time:

$$\text{clearance} = V_d(k) = \frac{V_d\,(0.693)}{t_{1/2}} \qquad (4)$$

This formula assumes a fixed value for V_d, which in reality changes over time. Therefore, the total body clearance in this simple model is V_d times the constant (k), 0.693, divided by half the time ($t_{1/2}$) actually taken. As the number of compartments increases the results of equations tend to approach reality and obviously become more complicated. In the two compartment model there is better representation of the distribution and elimination of the drug, especially in intravenous administration. This model has a distribution rate constant known as the alpha half-time ($t_{1/2\alpha}$) and an elimination rate constant known as the beta half-time ($t_{1/2\beta}$). The elimination rate is the most important of the two. As you can imagine, the multicompartment model is even more complex. This model is important where a number of drugs are stored in body depots and where drugs have an extensive metabolism or elimination mechanics.

Repeated doses

Drugs accumulate in the body, especially when the time interval between doses is less than four half-times. This accumulation of drugs in the body stores increases exponentially until it forms a graphic plateau, known as the **steady-state concentration**. This steady-state concentration should be maintained, as it is the minimum concentration needed to be of therapeutic value and below the concentration that would produce toxicity. This plateau is maintained when the infusion of the drug equals the rate of elimination. The time between doses, the dosing interval, relies on two basic considerations: first, smaller intervals result in minimal fluctuations in plasma concentration, and second, if the interval is a relatively standard number of hours it will assist patient compliance and medical staff.

Metabolism

The main site of metabolism for the majority of drugs is the liver, but the lungs, kidney and adrenal glands also have a role. As mentioned above, lipid-soluble drugs are not easily eliminated from the body; these include weak organic acids and bases. They have to be conjugated or metabolized. The process generally results in inactivation of the preparation, but can also result in being activated. Drugs which need activating to have effect are called prodrugs.

The following factors affect drug metabolism:

- chemical properties
- route of administration
- genetics
- diet
- age
- gender
- disease
- species differences
- circadian rhythm.

The biochemical processes in drug metabolism are generally quite straight-forward, involving oxidation, hydrolysis, reduction and conjugation.

Oxidation

By definition, an oxidation reaction requires the transfer of one or more electrons. This is the most common type of reaction and the majority of these reactions are thought to take place under the cytochrome P_{450} mixed function oxidase system. Oxidation can be subdivided into microsomal and non-microsomal oxidation. Microsomal oxidation takes place within the subcellular components of the endoplasmic reticulum (ER), the microsomes, where the primary components of the enzyme system, cytochrome P_{450} and cytochrome P_{450} reductase are present. Non-microsomal oxidation takes place in the cytosol or mitochondria of cells and involves alcohol dehydrogenase, aldehyde dehydrogenase, xanthine oxidase and monoamine oxidase.

Hydrolysis

Non-microsomal hydrolysis takes place in a number of tissues including the liver, plasma and the gastrointestinal tract. Hydrolases include esterases, which are non-specific for drugs such as ACh and procaine, as well as peptidases, phosphatases and amidases such as lidocaine.

Reduction

This again occurs in both microsomal and non-microsomal systems. Enzymes in both the ER and cytosol in the liver reduce nitro and azide groups.

Conjugation

This involves the coupling of another group to the drug, in the presence of a drug-metabolizing enzyme, resulting in a product with greater water solubility or easier biliary and renal elimination. Energy is needed for this process to take place and this is provided by high energy phosphate compounds that 'activate' the reaction. The most common conjugation reaction involves glucuronide. Glucuronic acid can be conjugated, in the presence of the enzyme uridine diphosphate-glucuronosyl transferase, after the acid has been activated. The acid is the product of the activation process between glucose-1-phosphate and uridine triphosphate. The conjugation process results in the formation of ROH-glucuronide where ROH is the drug. Other conjugation reactions occur with activated glycine, sulphate and acetate.

Elimination

Renal excretion of drugs and metabolites is the most important route out of the body. This involves glomerular filtration, active tubular secretion and passive tubular reabsorption. Biliary and faecal excretion metabolites and drugs usually come from the liver, when bile is excreted into the intestinal tract. Other routes of elimination of drugs are excretion in sweat, saliva and tears.

Concentration–response relationship

The concentration–response relationship allows us to work out how much drug is needed to obtain the right magnitude and duration of the response we desire.

Quantal dose–response

This is an all-or-none response. This means that we are looking for a factor that gives us a response to an amount of drug given, not in an individual patient, but in a population of people. It is an overall look at the amount of drug that has to be administered to become effective in a cross-section of individuals. So, the quantal response is the minimum concentration necessary to produce the desired drug effect. Naturally, this does not suit everybody.

Graded dose–response

When a drug is administed the amount of drug in the individual or tissue increases; this is the graded dose–response. As administration continues there is a point when the amount of drug reaches a maximum level; this is the ceiling effect. This maximum effect of a drug is known as its efficacy, which should be distinguished from potency. If we take two or three drugs which have the same potency, the amount of drug needed to have the same effect may be different, i.e. they have different efficacy, referring to the maximum effect of that drug. So, the maximum effect of one drug may not be the same as another but the potencies may be the same. An example of this is aspirin and morphine: they produce the same basic effect, analgesia, but they have different levels of efficacy.

Drug–receptor interactions

When a drug (D) binds to a receptor (R) on the surface or within the cell, a drug–receptor complex state is set up. This moves backwards and forwards between the free floating state and the receptor bound state:

$$D + R \longleftrightarrow DR$$

The maximum amount of drug bound to receptor sites (DR) that will produce an effect (E) is the maximum effect that we are looking for. Therefore, for E to be at its maximum, DR has to be at its highest possible. This can be expressed as:

$$E = \alpha[DR]$$

Alpha (α) in this expression is a given constant for the drug. The ability for a drug to produce an effect is known as its intrinsic activity, which is determined experimentally. It is also known as the alpha (α) factor. When the α factor is zero then the drug has no intrinsic pharmacological effect.

Agonists and antagonists

An agonist is a drug that activates a receptor when it binds to it. An antagonist is a drug that reduces or cancels the effect of another drug. Also, an antagonist may prevent another drug (the agonist) from actually binding with the receptor site; this occurs pharmacologically either competitively or non-competitively. Competitive antagonism is where the antagonist drug can be overcome if the dose of agonist is high enough. They compete for the same sites and the effect of the antagonist is reversible. When the antagonist is overcome the dose–response curve changes; this is known as **parallel shift**. Non-competitive antagonism is where the effect of the antagonist is irreversible at the receptor site, i.e. no amount of agonist will displace the antagonist. This results in a **non-parallel shift**. Physiological antagonism occurs when drugs act at different receptor sites with their actions causing a physiological-dose shift. An example of this is where one drug acts on the parasympathetic nervous system and another drug exerts a pharmacological effect on the sympathetic nervous system. Antagonism, in the pharmacological sense, cannot really be occurring in this case as the two parts of the autonomic nervous system do not work against each other. So, the shift will depend on which drug is the most effective. Lastly, there is chemical antagonism (or antagonism by neutralization) where the combination of two drugs results in an inactive compound.

Enhancement

Generally, there are three types of enhancement. First, where the combination of two drugs results in an effect (E) that is the sum of their two capabilities:

$$E_{ab} = E_a + E_b \; (1 + 1 = 2)$$

So, the result E_{ab} (of magnitude 2) is due to the combination of E_a and E_b (both of magnitude 1). This effect is known as **equal magnitude**.

Second is **synergism**, where two drugs when combined result in a greater than equal magnitude.

Lastly, **potentiation** occurs when one drug which has a weak effect on its own activates another drug to a value greater than their individual values.

The therapeutic index

Practically all drugs have toxic capabilities, so it is important that the amount that is administered is of therapeutic value and is safe. The calculation of this amount of drug is termed the therapeutic index (TI) and is expressed in the following formula:

$$TI = \frac{LD_{50}}{ED_{50}}$$

where LD_{50} is the amount of the drug that is lethal for 50% of the population and ED_{50} is the amount that is effective for 50% of the population. Obviously, the LD is higher than the ED, making the TI large.

Common drugs used in sport

Antacids

These are designed to counteract/neutralize the effects of gastric acids in the gastric lumen. The common components of antacids include carbonate, bicarbonate, citrate, phosphate and trisilicate. Hydroxide compounds like aluminium and magnesium hydroxide are the basic preparations. The effectiveness of antacids in acid neutralization depends on the pH of the preparation and whether the stomach has food in it or not. Food in the stomach can elevate the pH to around 5 for about 1 hour. Table 2.3 lists

Table 2.3 Antacids, antispasmodics and ulcer preparations

Brand name	Active ingredient(s)
Actal	Alexitol sodium
Actonorm Gel	Dried aluminium hydroxide gel, magnesium hydroxide and activated dimethicone
Alexitol sodium	Magnesium alginate, aluminium hydroxide/magnesium carbonate co-dried gel, magnesium carbonate and potassium bicarbonate
Algicon	Magnesium alginate, aluminium hydroxide/magnesium carbonate co-dried gel, magnesium carbonate and potassium bicarbonate
Almasilate suspension	Almasilate
Altacaps	Hydrotalcite and activated dimethicone
Altacite Plus	Hydrotalcite and activated dimethicone
Alu-cap	Dried aluminium hydroxide gel
Aludrox	Aluminium hydroxide gel
Aluhyde	Aluminium hydroxide gel, magnesium trisilicate and belladonna liquid extract
Andursil	Aluminium oxide, magnesium hydroxide, aluminium hydroxide/magnesium carbonate, co-dried gel and activated dimethicone
Antepsin	Sucralfate
APP	Papaverine hydrochloride, somatropin methylbromide, calcium carbonate, magnesium, carbonate, magnesium trisilicate, bismuth carbonate and aluminium hydroxide gel
Asilone	Activated dimethicone and dried aluminium hydroxide gel
Bellocarb	Belladonna dry extract, magnesium trisilicate and magnesium carbonate
Biocastrone	Carbenoxolone sodium
Buscopan	Hyoscine butylbromide
Cantil	Mepenzolate bromide
Carbellon	Belladonna dry extract, magnesium hydroxide, charcoal and peppermint oil
Caved-S	Deglycyrrhizinized liquorice, aluminium hydroxide gel, magnesium carbonate and sodium bicarbonate
Colofac	Mebeverine hydrochloride
Colpermin	Peppermint oil
Colven	Mebeverine hydrochloride and ispaghula husk
DeNol	Tripotassium di-citrato bismuthate
DeNoltab	Tripotassium di-citrato bismuthate
Diovol	Aluminium hydroxide, magnesium hydroxide and dimethicone
Droxalin	Alexitol sodium and magnesium trisilicate
Duogastrone	Carbenoxolone sodium
Dynese	Magaldrate
Gastrocote	Alginic acid, dried aluminium hydroxide gel, magnesium trisilicate and sodium bicarbonate
Gastron	Alginic acid, dried aluminium hydroxide, sodium bicarbonate and magnesium trisilicate
Gastrozepin	Pirenzepine
Gaviscon	Alginic acid, magnesium trisilicate, dried aluminium hydroxide gel and sodium bicarbonate
Gelusil	Magnesium trisilicate and dried aluminium hydroxide gel

Table 2.3 Continued

Brand name	Active ingredient(s)
Kolanticon	Dried aluminium hydroxide gel, magnesium oxide, dicyclomine hydrochloride and dimethicone
Kolantyl	Dried aluminium hydroxide gel, magnesium oxide and dicyclomine hydrochloride
Libraxin	Chlordiazepoxide and clidinium bromide
Loasid	Dried aluminium hydroxide, magnesium hydroxide and activated dimethicone
Maalox suspension	Dried aluminium hydroxide gel and magnesium hydroxide
Malinal	Almasilate
Maxolon	Metoclopramide hydrochloride
Merbentyl	Dicyclomine hydrochloride
Metramid	Metoclopramide hydrochloride
Metox	Metoclopramide
Mintec	Peppermint oil
Mucaine	Oxethazaine, aluminium hydroxide gel and magnesium hydroxide
Mucogel	Dried aluminium hydroxide gel and magnesium hydroxide
Nacton Forte	Poldine methylsulphate
Neutradonna	Hyoscyamine and aluminium sodium silicate
Nulacin	Whole milk solids combined with dextrins and maltose, magnesium trisilicate, heavy magnesium oxide, calcium carbonate and heavy magnesium carbonate
Parmid	Metoclopramide hydrochloride
Peptard	Hyoscyamine sulphate
Phazyme	Activated dimethiocone and pancreatin
Piptal	Pipenzolate bromide
Piptalin	Pipenzolate bromide and activated dimethicone
Polycrol	Revised formula: dried aluminium hydroxide gel and light magnesium oxide
Primperan	Metoclopramide hydrochloride
Pro-Bathine	Propantheline bromide
Prodexin	Aluminium glycinate and magnesium carbonate
Pyrogastrone	Carbenoxolone sodium, magnesium trisilicate and aluminium hydroxide gel
Rabro	Deglycyrrhizinized liquorice, magnesium oxide, calcium carbonate and frangula
Robinul	Glycopyrronium bromide
Roter	Magnesium carbonate, bismuth subnitrate, sodium bicarbonate and frangula
Siloxyl	Dried aluminium hydroxide gel and activated dimethicone
Simeco	Aluminium hydroxide/magnesium carbonate co-dried gel, magnesium hydroxide and dimethicone
Spasmonal	Alverine citrate
Stelabid	Trifluoperazine hydrochloride and isoproamide iodide
Tagamet	Cimetidine
Topal	Dried aluminium hydroxide gel, light magnesium carbonate and alginic acid
Unigest	Dried aluminium hydroxide gel and dimethicone
Zantac	Ranitidine hydrochloride

Table 2.4 Antidiarrhoeal preparations

Brand name	Active ingredient(s)
Arobon	Ceratonia and starch
Celevac	Methylcellulose
Deseril	Methylsergide
Dioralyte	Sodium chloride, potassium chloride, sodium bicarbonate and dextrose
Imodium	Loperamide hydrochloride
Kaopectate	Kaolin
Lomotil	Diphenoxylate hydrochloride and atropine sulphate
Norit	Activated charcoal
Questran	Cholestryramine
Rehidrat	Sodium chloride, potassium chloride, sodium bicarbonate, citric acid, glucose, sucrose and laevulose

available antacid, antispasmotic and ulcer preparations, under both brand and generic names.

Antidiarrhoeals

Diarrhoea is characterized by the excessive faecal loss of water and electrolytes. This has been attributed to many infectious and non-infectious disorders. The manipulative approach to diarrhoea is very effective, especially when abdominal bloating is present. Drugs themselves can induce diarrhoea as a side effect of therapeutic administration. The usual course of action is dosage alteration.

Non-specific treatment of diarrhoea tends to be with opioid antagonists like diphenoxylate and loperamide, which are piperidine opioids. The most common of these that is on the permitted list is Imodium, which contains loperamide hydrochloride. Imodium is available in 2 mg capsules and as a liquid (1 mg/5 ml). Over-the-counter preparations play a major part in antidiarrhoeal preparations. Bismuth subsalicylate-based preparations are some of the most commonly used. Cellulose-, laevulose-, and starch-based preparations are easily available. The most common oral rehydration powder currently used is Dioralyte. Table 2.4 lists antidiarrhoeal preparations available.

Migraine treatments

These are based on the ergot alkaloids and are weak α-adrenergic blockers, constricting both arteries and veins in their actions. Their other area of use is in obstetrics. They provide symptomatic relief for migraine where drugs such as naproxen and aspirin are not satisfactory. A major contraindication to the use of ergotamine is sepsis (vascular disease and diseases of liver and kidney) as many patients have incurred gangrene with its administration. Due to the cardiovascular nature of the drug action, undesirable effects may include nausea, vomiting, muscle pains, and numbness and tingling in the hands and feet. Table 2.5 lists migraine preparations.

Table 2.5   Migraine

Brand name	Active ingredient(s)
Cafegot	Ergotamine tartrate and caffeine
Deseril	Methysergide
Dihydergot	Dihydroergotamine mesylate
Dixarit	Clonidine hydrochloride
Lingraine	Ergotamine tartrate
Medihaler-Ergotamine	Ergotamine tartrate
Midrid	Isomethepthene mucate, dichloraphenazone and paracetamol
Midgravess Forte	Metoclopramide hydrochloride and aspirin
Migril	Ergotamine tartrate, cyclizine hydrochloride and caffeine hydrate
Paramax	Paracetamol and metoclopramide hydrochloride
Sanomigran	Pizotifen

Bronchodilators and other anti-asthma drugs

There is a surprising number of young athletes who suffer from asthma or cold-induced bronchospasm. The use of inhalers in an emergency or comfort situation is vital. Enough stress and anxiety can build up in a few minutes or even seconds from the inability to breathe to be fatal. Long-term usage of these drugs can lead to toxicity, presenting as susceptibility to infections and pituitary–adrenal suppression.

Becotide (beclomethasone dipropionate) is an adrenocortical steroid, and long-term usage is not desirable. Ventolin (salbutamol or albuterol) is a selective β_2-adrenergic agonist usually administered by inhalation and it produces bronchodilatation in about 15 minutes, lasting for around 3 hours. Undesirable effects result from the over-activation of β-adrenergic receptors, but the selectivity of this preparation results in a lower incidence of cardiovascular and CNS toxicity. See Table 2.6.

Hypnotics, sedatives and anxiolytics

Sleep is a natural phenomenon. Children need more sleep than adults. An upset in the athlete's sleeping pattern can alter their judgement and therefore performance. In this age of country hopping, the athlete's circadian rhythm is easily altered. Sleep during air travel, especially when injured, can be difficult and drugs such as Halcion were popular in inducing a short sleep, relief from anxiety, muscle relaxation and anticonvulsant effects. Other uses include administration in cases of chronic pain that causes a fragmented sleeping pattern.

The use of these drugs is based on the patient's needs, and classification is dependent on the type of insomnia: transient, short-term or chronic. These hypnotics are mainly benzodiazepines, chloral hydrates and their derivatives.

The main effect of the benzodiazepines is on the central nervous system, in varying degrees. Unlike barbiturates the benzodiazepines are

Table 2.6 Anti-asthma drugs

Brand name	Active ingredient(s)
Atrovent	Ipratropium bromide (inhaler)
Becloforte	Beclomethasone* dipropionate (inhaler)
Becotide	Beclomethasone* dipropionate (inhaler)
Berotec	Fenoterol hydrobromide (inhaler)
Bextasol	Betamethasone* valerate
Biophylline	Theophylline hydrate
Bricanyl	Terbutaline sulphate
Bronchodil	Reproterol hydrochloride
Choledyl	Choline theophyllinate
Cobutolin	Salbutamol
Duovent	Fenoterol hydrobromide and ipratropium bromide (inhaler)
Exirel	Pirbuterol hydrochloride
Intal	Sodium cromoglycate. NB Intal compound also contains isoprenaline and hence is not allowed
Lasma	Theophylline
Nuelin	Theophylline
Nuelin SA	Theophylline
Phyllocontin continus	Aminophylline
Pro-vent	Theophylline
Pulmadil	Rimiterol hydrobromide (inhaler)
Pulmicort	Budesonide* (inhaler)
Sabidal SR	Choline theophyllinate
Slo-Phyllin	Theophylline
Theodrox	Aminophylline and dried aluminium hydroxide gel
Theo-Dur	Theophylline
Theograd	Theophylline
Tilade	Nedocromil sodium
Uniphyllin Continus	Theophylline
Ventide	Salbutamol and beclomethasone* dipropionate (inhaler)
Ventolin	Salbutamol
Zaditen	Ketotifen

* Steroid warning.

not general neural depressants; their action is selective. A few benzodiazepines cause muscle hypotonia without affecting normal movement. Benzodiazepines are fairly safe as they have a self-limiting action when they cause neural depression, unlike barbiturates, which in higher doses severely depress the CNS. They have a slight effect on respiration, decreasing alveolar ventilation and PO_2 and increasing PCO_2, and they may cause CO_2 narcosis in patients with chronic obstructive pulmonary disease. Benzodiazepines exert little effect on the cardiovascular system, except in severe intoxication. It has been found that benzodiazepines may have an indirect effect on gastrointestinal anxiety-related disorders. Diazepam is the most common of the anxiolytic preparations, being widely used as a muscle relaxant.

Side effects of benzodiazepines include menstrual irregularities, ataxia, drowsiness and sedation, especially when combined with other CNS depressing agents. Overdoses are seldom fatal.

Table 2.7   Hypnotic drugs (see MPA warning)

Brand name	Active ingredient(s)
Dalmane	Flurazepam
Dormonoct	Loprazolam
Halcion	Triazolam
Heminevrin	Chlormethiazole edisylate
Lorazolam	Loprazolam mesylate
Mogadon	Nitrazepam
Nitrados	Nitrazepam
Noctamid	Lormetazepam
Noctec	Chloral hydrate
Noctesed	Nitazepam
Normison	Temazepam
Remnos	Nitrazepam
Rohypnol	Flunitrazepam
Sominex	Promethazine hydrochloride
Somnite	Nitrazepam
Surem	Nitrazepam
Trancopal	Chlormezanone
Unisomnia	Nitrazepam
Welldrom	Dichloralphenazone

Chloral hydrate and its derivatives are basically similar to benzo-diazepines. They have little analgesic action, are relatively safe hypnotic preparations, and are used mainly in children. Sleep can be induced in about half an hour and lasts for around 6 hours. The CNS depression is potentiated by alcohol (a combination known as 'Mickey Finn'). Chloral hydrate and its derivatives can irritate skin and mucous membranes including the gastrointestinal tract. This is more likely to occur if the drug is not sufficiently diluted or is taken on a empty stomach. Addiction can occur, which may present with skin eruptions and gastritis.

Hypnotic and anxiolytic preparations are listed in Tables 2.7 and 2.8, respectively.

Antidepressants

These comprise two major types of preparation: the tricyclics and monoamine oxidase inhibitors. The tricyclic antidepressants are effective in treating moderate to severe depression, and oral and facial pain may respond particularly if associated with depression. These preparations produce an immediate reduction in the firing rate of neurones containing noradrenaline and exert their principle effect on the function of the autonomic nervous system. This is believed to be the result of inhibition of noradrenaline transport. In the non-depressed patient sleepiness is the usual experience. Therapeutically, tricyclics have a significant effect on the cardiovascular system, with orthostatic (postural) hypotension and arrhythmias being common. In addition to this mild sinus tachycardia is a frequent occurrence. Antidepressant drugs are listed in Table 2.9.

Table 2.8 Anxiolytics (see MPA warning)

Brand name	Active ingredient(s)
Abboxapam	Oxazepam
Almazine	Lorazepam
Alupram	Diazepam
Anxon	Ketazolam
Atarax	Hydroxyzine hydrochloride
Atensine	Diazepam
Ativan	Lorazepam
Centrax	Prazepam
Diazemuls	Diazepam
Evacalm	Diazepam
Frisium	Colbazam
Integrin	Oxypertine
Lexotan	Bromazepam
Librium	Chlordiazepoxide
Motipress	Fluphenazine hydrochloride and nortriptyline
Motival	Fluphenazine hydrochloride and nortriptyline
Nobrium	Medazepam
Oxanid	Oxazepam
Solis	Diazepam
Stesolid	Diazepam
Tensium	Diazepam
Tranxene	Chlorazepate dipotassium
Tropium	Chlordiazepoxide
Valium	Diazepam
Valrelease	Diazepam
Xanax	Alprazolam

Side effects of tricyclics include blurred vision, sweating, constipation, and urinary retention. Rare side effects include skin rashes, cholestatic jaundice and orgasmic impotence. Figure 2.9 lists precautions advised for patients taking monoamine oxidase inhibitors (MAOIs).

Anti-emetics and prokinetic agents

The control of nausea and vomiting falls to the use of anti-emetic and prokinetic agent preparations (Table 2.10). Vomiting requires the coordination of the vomit centre in the lateral reticular formation of the medulla which receives input from the chemoreceptor trigger zone (CTZ) in the floor of the fourth ventricle.

Analgesics and antipyretics

The action of the non-steroidal anti-inflammatory drugs (NSAIDs) is based on the fact that when cells are damaged they release, amongst other chemicals, prostaglandins. Inhibition of cyclo-oxygenase, the enzyme responsible for the biosynthesis of prostaglandins, is thought to be the mechanism of action of aspirin and aspirin-like drugs. NSAIDs are not thought to affect any of the other inflammatory exudates as a result

TREATMENT CARD

Carry this with you at all times. Show it to any doctor who may treat you other than the

doctor who prescribes this medicine, and to your dentist if you require dental treatment.

....

INSTRUCTIONS TO PATIENTS

Please read this carefully

While taking this medicine and for 14 days after treatment finishes you must observe the
following simple instructions:-

1. Do not eat CHEESE, PICKLED HERRING OR BROAD BEAN PODS.

2. Do not eat or drink BOVRIL, OXO, MARMITE or ANY SIMILAR MEAT OR YEAST

EXTRACT

3. Eat only FRESH foods and avoid food that you suspect could be stale or "going off".

This is especially important with meat, fish, poultry or offal. Avoid game.

4. Do not take any other MEDICINES (Including tablets, capsules, nose drops, inhalations

or suppositories) whether purchased by you or previously prescribed by your doctor,

without first consulting your doctor or your pharmacist.

N.B. *Treatment for coughs and colds, pain relievers, tonics and laxatives are medicines.*

5. Avoid alcoholic drinks and de-alcoholized (low-alcohol) drinks.

Keep a careful note of any food or drink that disagrees with you, avoid it and tell your

doctor. Report any unusual or severe symptoms to your doctor and follow any other advice

given by him.

M.A.O.I.   Prepared by the Pharmaceutical Society and the British Medical Association

on behalf of the Health Department of the United Kingdom.

Fig. 2.9 Treatment card: listing the necessary precautions for MAOI's patients (source: *British National Formulary*, March 1991).

Table 2.9 Antidepressants (see MPA warning)

Brand name	Active ingredient(s)
Allegron	Nortriptyline
Anafranil	Clomipramine hydrochloride
Aventyl	Nortriptyline
Bolvidon	Mianserin hydrochloride
Camcolt	Lithium carbonate
Concordin	Protriptyline hydrochloride
Domical	Amitryptyline hydrochloride
Elavil	Amitriptyline hydrochloride
Evadyne	Butriptyline
Fluanxol	Flupenthixol
Gamanil	Lofepramine
Lentizol	Amitriptyline hydrochloride
Limbitrol 5	Amitriptyline and chlordiazepoxide
Liskonum	Lithium carbonate
Litarex	Lithium citrate
Ludiomil	Maprotiline hydrochloride
Marplan	Isocarboxazid
Marsilid	Iproniazid
Molipaxin	Trazodone hydrochloride
Motipress	Fluphenazine hydrochloride and nortriptyline
Motival	Fluphenazine hydrochloride and nortriptyline
Nardil	Phenelzine
Norval	Mianserin hydrochloride
Optimax	L-Tryptophan, pyridoxine hydrochloride and ascorbic acid
Optimax WV	As Optimax but vitamin free
Pacitron	L-Tryptophan
Parnate	Tranylcypromine
Parstelin	Tranylcypromine and trifluoperazine
Pertfran	Desipramine hydrochloride
Phasal	Lithium carbonate
Priadel	Lithium carbonate
Prondol	Iprindole
Prothiaden	Dothiepin hydrochloride
Sinequan	Doxepin
Surmontil	Trimipramine
Tofranil	Imipramine hydrochloride
Triptafen	Amitriptyline hydrochloride and perphenazine
Tryptizol	Amitriptyline hydrochloride
Vivalan	Viloxazine

of tissue damage. Infection and tissue damage cause the synthesis of prostaglandin E_2 (PGE_2) in vascular organs in the preoptic hypothalamic area, which produces an elevation of body temperature, i.e. fever. Aspirin-like drugs inhibit this PGE_2 synthesis.

Some of the most common NSAID medications include naproxen (Naprosyn, Synflex (UK), Anaprox (USA)) and ibuprofen. Table 2.11 lists those and other analgesics available.

Naproxen
Absorption of naproxen is influenced by food in the stomach. Its plasma concentration usually peaks at around 2–4 hours and will be greater if

Table 2.10 Anti-emetic and prokinetic agents

Brand name	Active ingredient(s)
Ancoloxin	Meclozine hydrochloride and pyridoxine hydrochloride
Dramamine	Dimenhydrinate
Emetrol	Laevulose, dextrose and phosphoric acid
Maxolon	Metoclopramide hydrochloride
Metox	Metoclopramide
Metramid	Metoclopramide hydrochloride
Motilium	Domperidone
Parmid	Metoclopramide hydrochloride
Primperan	Metoclopramide hydrochloride
Serc	Betahistine dihydrochloride
Stelazine	Trifluoperazine hydrochloride
Stemetel	Prochlorperazine maleate
Sturgeron	Cinnarizine
Torecan	Thiethylperazine maleate
Valoid	Cyclizine hydrochloride
Vertigon spansule	Prochlorperazine maleate

combined with sodium, i.e. Synflex or Anaprox. It is approximately 99% bound to plasma proteins. Naproxen is able to cross the placental barrier and appears in the milk of lactating women. It is almost totally excreted in the urine as metabolites.

Side effects of naproxen are mostly gastrointestinal or on the central nervous system. They include nausea, vomiting, heartburn, headache, dizziness, fatigue and sweating.

Ibuprofen

The oral administration of this preparation causes a peak plasma concentration in about 1–2 hours. Like naproxen, ibuprofen is 99% bound to plasma proteins. It passes slowly into the synovial spaces and even when the plasma concentration decreases the concentration in the synovial spaces is maintained. The excretion of ibuprofen is rapid and complete; about 90% of the ingested drug is excreted in urine as metabolites (no ibuprofen is present in the urine).

Ibuprofen has a better record with patients with gastric ulceration, so it is preferred to other aspirin-like medications. Undesirable effects include nausea, epigastric pain, a feeling of 'fullness', and consipation.

Local anaesthetics

The action of local anaesthetics is to reduce the generation and conduction of nerve impulses. This is known as **conduction block** and affects the cell membrane by decreasing or suspending the permeability of excitable membranes to Na^+ as a result of slight depolarization of the membrane. This group includes cocaine and lidocaine. Lidocaine is the most commonly used local anaesthetic.

Table 2.11 Analgesic preparations

Brand name	Active ingredient(s)
Acupan	Nefopam hydrochloride
Apsifen	Ibuprofen
Aspav	Aspirin and papaveretum
Benoral	Benorylate
Brufen	Ibuprofen
Cafadol	Paracetamol and caffeine
Calpol Infant	Paracetamol
Claradin	Aspirin
Dispol Paediatric	Paracetamol
Dolobid	Diflunisal
Ebufac	Ibuprofen
Fenbid spansule	Ibuprofen
Fenopron	Fenoprofen
Ibumetin	Ibuprofen
Laboprin	Aspirin and lysine
Medised	Paracetamol and promethazine hydrochloride
Meptid	Meptazinol hydrochloride
Motrin	Ibuprofen
Nu-seals Aspirin	Aspirin
Paldesic	Paracetamol
Pameton	Pamacetamol and methionine
Panadol	Paracetamol
Panasorb	Paracetamol
Paxofen	Ibuprofen
Paynocil	Aspirin and glycine
Ponstan	Mefanamic acid
Progesic	Fenoprofen
Sarapryn	Aspirin and paracetamol
Salzone	Paracetamol
Solprin	Aspirin
Synflex	Naproxen sodium
Tegretol	Carbamazepine
Unigesic	Paracetamol and caffeine

Non-steroidal anti-inflammatory drugs

Alrheumat	Ketprofen
Ananase	Bromelains (proteolytic enzymes)
Apsifen	Ibuprofen
Artracin	Indomethacin
Benoral	Benorylate
Brufen	Ibuprofen
Caprin	Aspirin
Chymar	Chymotrypsin
Chymoral Forte	Trypsin
Claradin	Aspirin
Clinoril	Sulindac
Deanese D.C.	Delta-chymotrypsin
Disalcid	Salsalate
Distamine	Penicillamine base
Dolobid	Diflunisal
Ebufac	Ibuprofen
Feldene	Piroxicam

Table 2.11 Continued

Brand name	Active ingredient(s)
Fenopron	Fenoprofen
Fenbid spansule	Ibuprofen
Fenopron	Fenoprofen
Froben	Flurbiprofen
Ibumetin	Ibuprofen
Imbrilon	Indomethacin
Indocid	Indomethacin
Indoflex	Indomethacin
Indolar	Indomethacin
Indomod	Indomethacin
Laraflex	Naproxen
Larapam	Piroxicam
Lederfen	Fenbufen
Levius	Aspirin
Lodine	Etodolac
Motrin	Ibuprofen
Mycrisin	Sodium aurothimalate
Naprosyn	Naproxen
Nu-seals aspirin	Aspirin
Orudis	Ketoprofen
Oruvail	Ketoprofen
Paraprin Forte	Aloxiprin
Paxofen	Ibuprofen
Paynocil	Aspirin and glycine
Pendramine	Penicillamine
Plaquenil	Hydroxychloroquine sulphate
Ponstan Forte	Mefanamic acid
Ramodar	Etodolac
Rheumox	Azapropazone dihydrate
Safapryn	Aspirin and paracetamol
Salazopyrin EN-tabs	Sulphasalazine
Solprin	Tiaprofenic acid
Surgam	Tiaprofenic acid
Synflex	Naproxen
Tolectin	Tolmetin
Trilisate	Chlorine magnesium trisalicylate
Voltarol	Diclofenac sodium

Local hydrocortisone

Hydrocortisone (cortisol) has a reputation in sports medicine as a drug that 'gets you back out on the field'. Its main action is the suppression of the inflammatory response, however it must be remembered that the underlying problem is still there. Intra-articular injections can be used in extreme cases, ensuring the minimum number possible. The more that is administered the greater the risk of painless joint destruction, similar to Charcot's arthropathy. Suppression of the inflammatory response is by action against oedema, capillary dilatation, fibrin deposition, leukocyte migration into the inflamed area and phagocytic activity. The anti-inflammatory action also prevents the joint/tissue injury from healing naturally. Eventually, the proliferation of capillaries and fibroblasts and collagen deposition are compromised. Improvement will be short lived and reduce the athlete's life in sport.

Abused drugs in sport

The controversy continues in sport about the use of certain drugs that may or definitely do give one athlete the advantage over another. Common drugs and groups that have to be restricted or banned outright include the following:

- anabolic steroids
- amphetamines
- barbiturates and benzodiazepines
- phenylpropanolamine and ephedrine
- amyl nitrite
- human growth hormone
- narcotics
- cocaine
- marijuana
- caffeine
- alcohol
- tobacco
- beta blockers
- phosphate loading
- NSAIDS
- analgesic injections
- diuretics
- caritine
- bicarbonate doping

Anabolic steroids

> I honestly believe that if I'd told people back then that rat manure would make them stronger, they'd have eaten rat manure
>
> Dr John Ziegler, one of the early developers
> of anabolic steroids in the USA

These drugs are most widely known in connection with body builders, but there is increasing evidence that anabolic steroid abuse is prevalent in the business world. Sports such as American football were renowned for anabolic steroid abuse, especially in linemen. These drugs, derivatives of testosterone, can more accurately be called 'androgenic–anabolic steroids' as they are capable of producing both androgenic (masculinizing) and anabolic (tissue building) effects. Commonly used anabolic steroids are listed in Table 2.12.

Testosterone is secreted by the testes and is the main androgen in humans. In women, small amounts are synthesized by the ovary and adrenal glands. In prepubesent males and women the plasma testosterone concentrations are much lower than in adult males – 15 to 65 ng/dl

Table 2.12 Commonly used androgens (anabolic–androgenic steroids)

Brand (and generic) name	Dosage
Parenteral	
Testoject-50 (testosterone)	10–50 mg 3 × weekly (aqueous suspension for i.m. use)
Testex (testosterone propionate)	10–25 mg 2–3 × weekly (oil for i.m. use)
Delatestryl (testosterone enanthate)	50–400 mg every 2–4 weeks (oil for i.m. use)
Depo-Testosterone (testosterone cypionate)	50–400 mg every 2–4 weeks (oil for i.m. use)
Deca-durabolin (nandrolone decanoate)	50–100 mg every 2–4 weeks (oil for i.m. use)
Durabolin (nandrolone phenpropionate)	50–100 mg weekly for breast carcinoma (oil for i.m. use)
Oral	
Danocrine (danazol)	200–800 mg daily (capsules)
Halotestin (fluoxymesterone)	2.5–20 mg daily (tablets)
Dianabol (methandrostenolone)	2.5–5 mg daily for osteoporosis
Methadren, Oreton Methyl (methyltestosterone)	10–50 mg daily (capsules and tablets) 5–25 mg daily (buccal tablets)
Anavar (oxandrolone)	2.5–20 mg daily (tablets)
Anadrol-50 (oxymetholone)	1.5 mg/kg daily for anaemia (tablets)
Winstrol (stanozolol)	6 mg daily (tablets)
Teslac (testolactone)	250 mg 4 × daily for breast carcinoma (tablets)

compared with 300–1000 ng/dl. Testosterone can be converted into many different forms, both inactive and active. The active component represents around 2% that is not plasma bound.

The process of testosterone release begins in the hypothalamus, which produces hormones that control the release of the pituitary gonadotrophins, follicle stimulating hormone (FSH) and luteinizing hormone (LH). These hormones initiate a complex series of reactions in the testes and seminiferous tubules resulting in spermatogenesis and the release of testosterone.

At target tissues, testosterone is reduced to its active forms of dihydrotestosterone and oestradiol, and the inactive forms androsterone and etiocholanolone. Dihydrotestosterone is the principle intracellular mediator, and binds to protein receptors ten times more tightly than testosterone.

Anabolic steroids become bound to cytoplasmic receptors after entering the cell by diffusion as free testosterone. It is here in the cytoplasm that testosterone is converted to dihydrotestosterone. There are a limited number of binding sites, e.g. in skeletal muscle. Therefore, supraphysiological doses of anabolic steroids will have no further effect once these sites are occupied.

Testosterone, taken by mouth, is rapidly absorbed and metabolized by the liver before it reaches the systemic circulation. Testosterone injected in a oil-based solution is also absorbed, metabolized and excreted. Two basic modifications of the androgen have to take place to cause a reduction in metabolization, i.e. esterification and alkylation. Excretion of the compounds, metabolites and conjugates occurs in the urine and faeces.

Side effects of anabolic steroids
These are categorized into three main groups: virilization, feminization and toxicity.

Virilization Anabolic steroids that are taken by women put them at risk of masculinizing effects. In addition to this there are further undesirable changes such as acne, facial hair, deepening of the voice and menstrual irregularities. In children advanced epiphyseal closure occurs which may continue for some months after the drug has been stopped. These drugs can also cross the placental barrier and can cause masculinization of a female foetus.

Feminization The most common feminizing effect is gynaecomastia in males. Feminization can be severe in children and adults who have liver disease.

Toxicity The taking of anabolic steroids results in retention of water and sodium chloride. This oedema results in weight gain and the appearance of looking bigger. Jaundice is a clinical feature due to the disturbance of the biliary capillaries in the central portion of the hepatic lobules. The severity of the jaundice seems to be dose related; the larger the amounts taken the greater the severity. Carcinogenic liver tumours result from long-term administration; it is common for athletes to develop these tumours years after they have stopped taking the drugs.

The question of the effect of androgens on athletic performance is not easy to resolve scientifically for several reasons (Goodman and Gilman, 1991):

1. The side effects of the doses taken by athletes are so pronounced as to preclude truly blinded studies of efficiency.
2. Only a small subset of users may have a beneficial response, making it difficult to identify the rare responder.
3. Effects on athletic performance become more difficult to assess as the calibre of the athlete increases.

Amphetamine (racemic β-phenylisopropylamine)

This sympathomimetic amine, which shares a common chemical structure with catecholamines, has most of its effects on the CNS. This drug is described as an 'upper'. Its cardiovascular effects are raised systolic and diastolic blood pressure, heart rate is often reflexly slowed, and cardiac arrhythmias, occurring with large doses. Cerebral blood flow changes minimally. In the central nervous system, it stimulates the medullary respiratory centre, probably by cortical stimulation and possibly stimulation of the reticular activating system. Doses between 10 and 30 mg lead to wakefulness, alertness and a decreased sense of fatigue; elevation of mood, with increased initiative, self-confidence, ability to concentrate, and often elation and euphoria; and increase in motor and speech activity. There is an increase in the number of tasks performed but also in the number of mistakes made. The drug is also commonly used as an appetite supressor, the action site probably being in the lateral hypothalamic feeding centre. Effects on the gastrointestinal tract are negligible.

Side effects of amphetamine are an extension of the therapeutic effects of the drug, notably restlessness, dizziness, tremor, hyperactive reflexes, talkativeness, irritability, weakness, insomnia, fever and sometimes euphoria. Cardiovascular responses include headache, shivering, pallor or flushing, palpitation, cardiac arrhythmias, anginal pain, hypertension or hypotension, and circulatory collapse. Excessive sweating may occur, which is a response of the autonomic nervous system. Gastrointestinal side effects include dry mouth, metallic taste, anorexia, nausea, vomiting, diarrhoea and abdominal cramps. Fatalities usually result from cerebral haemorrhage after convulsions and coma.

Benzodiazepines and barbiturates

The barbiturates are lipid soluble. The main compound is barbituric acid, which does not have a central depressant activity. The actual barbiturate does depress excitable central nervous system activity and in the peripheral nervous system depress autonomic ganglia transmission. Barbiturates seem to inhibit the central nervous system in two ways:

1. by facilitating the effects of gamma-aminobutyric acid (GABA), which is an inhibitory neurotransmitter, opening the chloride ion channels and hyperpolarizing neuronal membranes.
2. it also influences cortical depression which is unrelated to GABA inhibition.

The overall clinical effects of benzodiazepines and barbiturates are muscular relaxation, reducing tremors and thus having a beneficial effect on nervousness. This has been shown to enhance the athlete's performance.

Side effects: as amphetamines, including respiratory depression.

Phenylpropanolamine and ephedrine

These sympathomimetic amines are structurally similar to amphetamines. Their action is indirectly on the sympathetic nervous system by displacing noradrenaline and other monoamine transmitters from storage sites. This results in the stimulation of heart rate and cardiac output; as a result ephedrine, for example, usually increases blood pressure. Because they are similar to amphetamines they are also known as 'look-alikes', and also by many other names, e.g. black beauties, white crosses, Christmas trees, greens and clears.

These agents commonly come in the form of oral preparations, as expectorants, nasal and sinus decongestants, and compound cough preparations. They are thought to have very little therapeutic value. Some of the commonest preparations are Sudafed and Actifed (pseudoephedrine hydrochloride), and Triogesic and Triominic (phenylpropanolamine hydrochloride).

The use of phenylpropanolamine and ephedrine has been shown to have no effect on athletic performance. The main reason why they are banned is that they are easily open to abuse as ergogenic aids. The banned sympathomimetic compounds include:

- chlorprenaline
- ephedrine
- etafedrine
- isoetharine
- isoprenaline
- methoxyphenamine
- methylephedrine
- phenylpropanolamine
- and related compounds.

Acute but mild adverse effects of these drugs include nervousness, irritability, insomnia, anorexia, dizziness, headaches, tachycardia, palpitations and mild hypertension. More severe acute effects include agitation, confusion, paranoia, mania, hallucinations, stroke/TIA, cerebral vasculitis, cerebral haemorrhage, severe hypertension, myocardial ischaemia, ventricular arrhythmia and rhabdomyolysis.

Amyl nitrite (isoamyl nitrite)

This organic nitrate is used therapeutically as an antianginal preparation. It is a volatile liquid at room temperature that is inhaled. It does not affect the course of the pathology. Like all nitrates it relaxes smooth muscle and reduces venous tone, thus increasing venous capacitance and reducing venous return to the heart. Other effects include vasodilatation of cerebral vessels, causing occasional headache, and dilating blood vessels in the skin, causing a flush.

The drug usually comes in a small bottle, and is inhaled and thus absorbed through the lungs, but it can also be absorbed through the mucous membranes, the skin and the gastrointestinal tract. Side effects include, as mentioned above, headache, dizziness and weakness. Acute nitrate poisoning leads to circulatory collapse or respiratory failure.

Human growth hormone

Growth hormone is present in the anterior pituitary, accounting for around 10–15% of the gland's dry weight. The main form of human growth hormone is a single chain, 191-amino acid protein. It is produced biosynthetically by recombinant DNA technology and is marketed as synthetic growth hormone (somatrophin). An identical protein containing an additional amino-terminal methionine residue is marketed as synthetic methionyl-growth hormone (somatrem).

Actions of growth hormone

Growth Growth hormone affects every organ and tissue in the body except the brain and eyes. It acts to increase the number of cells rather than increase the size of the cells. The use of growth hormone has mainly been studied in dwarfs. On administration of the hormone, bone growth increases; skin also grows along with arms and legs; and the skeletal muscles enlarge. Continued use can lead to classical eunuchoid proportions (long limbs and short trunk). These proportions occur because sex steroids are responsible for promoting growth of the vertebral bodies.

Nitrogen metabolism For growth to occur an assimilation of protein and nitrogen is necessary. Growth hormone causes nitrogen to be retained, therefore allowing the anabolic effect to take place by increasing the conversion of amino acids into protein. Other changes that take place are an accretion of Ca^{2+}, Mg^{2+}, K^+, Na^+, phosphate, and in connective tissue, an increase in collagen synthesis.

Carbohydrate and lipid metabolism Although an oversimplification, growth hormone seems to switch over the source of fuel for the body from carbohydrate to fat.

Excess growth hormone
In children this may lead to giantism. In adults and children the effects include myopathy, cardiovascular disease, peripheral neuropathy, thickening of skin, soft tissue swellings and hirsutism as well as others.

Narcotics

These are the opiates from the poppy plant *Papaver somniferum*. The most common form, consisting of around 20 alkaloid derivatives, is morphine, named after Morpheus, the Greek god of dreams. Morphine was readily available in the USA in the 19th century. It was even more commonplace during the civil war, especially after the invention of the hypodermic needle in 1856. The year 1898 saw the discovery of a semisynthetic opiate more powerful than morphine, heroin (diacetyl-morphine). Because of the rising number of addicts the USA enacted the Harrison Act of 1914 prohibiting opium, heroin and morphine from non-prescription preparations.

The main effects of morphine are on the CNS and the gastrointestinal tract. CNS opioid receptors are located exclusively in the grey matter, in the periaqueductal grey, limbic cortex, hypothalamus and the basal ganglia. The main effects of morphine and other narcotics are analgesia, euphoria or dysphoria, drowsiness, mental clouding and decreased bowel motility.

The signs of narcotic withdrawal include sweating, rhinorrhea, yawning, tremor, vomiting, nausea, muscle cramps, restlessness etc.

Narcotics have no known ergogenic properties but may be open to abuse due to the pressures imposed by athletic competition. An athlete who is injured may want to participate so desperately that he or she uses these drugs again and again.

Cocaine

Cocaine is an alkaloid derivative of the coca plant, *Erythroxylon coca*. The acid and solvent extraction of the leaves leads to the production of many alkaloids, which after hydrolysis yields ecgonine, an amino alcohol base. Esterification of ecgonine by methanol/benzoic acid leads to cocaine hydrochloride. If ammonia is added, with or without sodium bicarbonate, to an aqueous solution of cocaine hydrochloride (alkalinization) the result is 'crack'. This is pure cocaine. If on the other hand a buffered ammonia and a solvent, like ether, is added, the result is 'freebase cocaine' (benzoyl methylecgonine).

This drug has its primary effects on the brain 'pleasure centres' – the mesocortical and mesolimbic dopamine tracts. This leads to friendliness, elation, vigor and generally a positive mood state. Further usage leads to dysphoria and craving attributed to the depletion of presynaptic dopamine. Continued use leads to tremors and convulsive movements as it begins to affect the subcortical and brain stem areas. Extremely high doses of cocaine lead to an excessive stimulation of the nervous system resulting in elevated body temperature, with shivering.

Common side effects and complications of cocaine use include the following:

- cardiac: ventricular arrhythmia, angina pectoris, myocarditis, myocardial infarction, sudden death;
- neuropsychiatric: cerebrovascular events, addiction, seizures, Tourette's exacerbation, headache, optic neuropathy, behavioural alterations;
- obstetric/gynaecological: spontaneous abortion, abruptio placentae, congenital foetal malformations, placental transfer to infant, breast milk transfer;
- general: sexual dysfunction, liver toxicity, nasal septal perforation/necrosis, osteolytic sinusitis, gastrointestinal ischaemia, pneumomediastinum, anosmia (loss of smell), hyperthermia and tachycardia.

Cocaine is generally mixed with other substances when it is abused. These include caffeine, phenylpropanoline, strychnine, procaine, lidocaine, LSD, PCP, diazepam, talc, sugars, quinine and sodium bicarbonate. Street terminology for the drug in its mixed forms included dama blanca, flake, snow, gold dust, C girl, Charlie, candy girl, nose candy, lady, green gold, coke and toot. Use of cocaine in sports is generally recreational. Due to its short action and feeling of euphoria, it has little if any effect as an ergogenic aid.

Marijuana

Otherwise known as hashish and cannabis, marijuana comes from the hemp *Cannabis sativa,* which originated in China. It is a green plant that is tall and strong smelling. The main active ingredient of marijuana is delta-9-tetrahydrocannabinol (Δ-9-THC). This constituent mainly affects the CNS, affecting a number of neurochemical pathways. Although no receptor site has been localized, the chemical changes after this drug has penetrated the blood–brain barrier include the following.

1. An increase in catecholamine synthesis.
2. Alterations in the uptake of chemicals at synaptic levels. These include noradrenaline and serotonin in the hypothalamus, and dopamine and GABA in the striatum and cerebral cortex, respectively.
3. There is a dose-related decrease in acetylcholine synthesis and release, especially in the hippocampus.

The most common mode of use is smoking. Here the dried brown leaves or resin are rolled in tobacco paper and can either be smoked 'straight' or mixed with tobacco. Other methods include eating the leaves or resin mixed in food such as cake. Blood levels increase in minutes after when smoking, while it may take hours with eating. Physiological changes peak around 20–30 minutes after smoking a marijuana cigarette and can last from 2–4 hours. Eating the drug can delay physiological effects from anything between 30 minutes and 2 hours, persisting for 2–3 hours. Δ-9-THC is highly lipid soluble and blood levels can drop fairly quickly. This means that there is a slow release of the chemical back into the circulation from the fat deposits. To eliminate the drug totally may take up to 1 month.

Side effects may present as some of the following:

- neuropsychiatric: panic attacks, delirium, psychosis, depression;
- respiratory: rhinitis, pharyngitis, bronchitis, bronchospasm, bronchial squamous metaplasia, pulmonary fibrosis, pneumomediastinum;
- immunological: impaired cell-mediated immunity, impaired monocyte maturation;
- endocrine: decreased sperm production, inhibition of ovulation, gynaecomastia;
- cardiovascular: tachycardia, orthostatic hypotension, increased carboxyhaemoglobin.

Withdrawal signs and symptoms include anorexia, anxiety, agitation, depression, sweating, restlessness, irritability, tremor, insomnia and cannabinoid craving.

Marijuana is subject to compulsive abuse, but tolerance and physical dependence do not occur (Wolstenholme and Knight, 1965).

Caffeine

We are all well aware of the effect that a strong cup of coffee has on us by stimulating the CNS. This is due to the fact that caffeine blocks adenosine receptors, therefore blocking the sedative effects of adenosine. It also affects the translocation of intracellular calcium, and increases the available cyclic AMP. In addition to the effects of increasing alertness, shortening the reaction time, clearer thinking and increasing concentration, it also has a diuretic effect and causes relaxation in smooth muscles. Too much caffeine leads to restlessness, insomnia and nervousness.

Chronic and acute ingestion of caffeine is known to precipitate peptic ulcers, sinus tachycardia, hypertension, gastrointestinal irritation and increased serum cholesterol.

Caffeine's effects on athletic performance seem to be positive in endurance events rather than short, high intensity activity.

The National Collegiate Athletic Association (NCAA) urine limit for caffeine is 15 μg/ml, but it has been suggested that levels above 10 μg/ml indicate ingestion to improve performance.

Alcohol

Ethanol (CH_3CH_2OH) works on the CNS exerting its effect as a depressant. It is a general anaesthetic that inhibits synaptic function rather than neural impulses. Alcohol also reduces the sodium current underlying the action potential, alters the resting permeability and active transport, stimulates neurotransmitter release, and alters the postsynaptic excitatory current. Chronic alcohol usage leads to increased tolerance and dependence.

Alcohol is not regarded as an ergogenic aid. The chronic use of alcohol interferes with psychomotor skills, as occurs while under the influence of alcohol. Psychomotor skill impairment usually occurs around the 35 mg/100 ml blood level. The skills that are impaired include reaction time, visual tracking, balance, fine and complex motor coordination and judgement. Anaerobic activity may be affected, but this is not consistent. Endurance is generally not affected by alcohol consumption.

Tobacco

There are two main ways in which tobacco is taken, by smoking and by chewing (smokeless). The alkaloid nicotine is the compound responsible for the effects of tobacco. This weak base has both stimulant and depressant actions on the central and peripheral nervous systems. In the peripheral nervous system low doses of nicotine lead to autonomic ganglia stimulation, while high doses lead to depression. Norepinephrine and dopamine are released in the CNS after the administration of nicotine. Acetylcholine may be increased or decreased, and reflects dosage. Relaxation and improved concentration, memory and alertness have been recorded after the administration of nicotine. Dependency on nicotine has been demonstrated in both humans and animals. Withdrawal symptoms include craving, anxiety, irritability, restlessness, trouble in concentration, upset in appetite and gastrointestinal complaints.

The effects of nicotine on athletic ability have not yet been established. Many argue that the use of smokeless tobacco enhances psychomotor skills, as has been demonstrated in animal models. The appetite reduction effects of nicotine could be useful in weight control. Nicotine has been shown to impair oxygen transport secondary to increases in carboxyhaemoglobin, which would have a detrimental effect on performance.

Some of the adverse effects of chronic smokeless tobacco are peridontol destruction, teeth abrasion, oral mucosal hyperkeratosis, gingival inflammation, leukoplakia, decreased taste perception, oral cavity squamous cell carcinoma, addiction/withdrawal, halitosis, dysgeusia and dysosmia. (See also mouth ulcers, p.252.)

Beta blockers

These are otherwise known as 'beta-androgenic blockers' as they block beta-androgenic receptors. Androgenic receptors are divided into two types: alpha receptors and beta receptors. Beta receptors are further divided into beta-1 and beta-2. Generally, beta-1 receptors control cardiac effects (tachycardia) and beta-2 receptors are responsible for bronchodilatation and peripheral vasodilatation. Therapeutically these preparations are commonly used for treating hypertension, angina and some cardiac arrhythmias. They are also used as a preventive measure in calming patients, for stage fright, when they will reduce tremor, and they are used in the prophylaxis of migraine.

Beta blockers are selective or non-selective. Low dose selective beta-1 blockers inhibit beta-1 activity causing bradycardia, without associated bronchospasm. Higher doses may lead to bronchospasm in certain individuals. Non-selective beta blockers tend to lead to bradycardia and inhibit bronchodilatation and peripheral vasoconstriction.

The anti-tremor and calming effects are the main reason for the use of these drugs by athletes. A steady hand and arm may make a major difference for the participant of sports such as snooker and archery. This is the main reason for their being banned.

Adverse effects include bradycardia, heart failure, bronchospasm, peripheral vasoconstriction, gastrointestinal disturbances, fatigue and sleep disturbance. Beta blockers can cause slightly reduced glucose tolerance in diabetics; they also interfere with metabolic and autonomic responses to hypoglycaemia. Their use is therefore contraindicated in diabetics, and they should be avoided altogether in those with frequent episodes of hypoglycaemia. Cardioselective beta blockers may be preferable.

Phosphate loading

When an athlete trains at altitude and then returns to sea level there is an increase in the levels of plasma phosphate and 2,3-diphosphoglyceride

(2,3-DPG). Basically, this change allows the off-loading of oxygen for tissue availability. Studies have shown that there is an increase in the levels of 2,3-DPG after phosphate loading.

NSAIDS

NSAIDs are used for their analgesic, anti-inflammatory, and antipyretic properties. Although NSAIDS are ergogenic by definition, i.e they limit pain in performance, they are not banned by the International Olympic Committee.

REFERENCES

Adams, F. (1849) *The Genuine Works of Hippocrates*, The Sydenham Society, London.

Ader, R. and Cohen, N. (1981) *Psychoneuroimmonology*, Academic Press, Orlando, FL p. 281.

Arnold, A. (1992) *The Corrupted Sciences. Challenging the Myths of Modern Science*, Paladin, London.

Beal, M. (1980) Osteopathic basics. *Journal of the American Osteopathic Association*, **79** (7), 456/81–459/84.

Beal, M. (1989) Louisa Burns Memorial Lecture: perception through palpation. *Journal of the American Osteopathic Association*, **89** (10), 1334–52.

Blalock, J.E. (1989) A molecular basis for bidirectional communication between the immune and neuroendocrine systems. *Physiological Reviews*, **69** (1), 1–32.

Brooks, G.A. (1987) *Exercise. Benefits, Limits and Adaptations* (eds Macleod, Maughan *et al.*), E. &. F.N. Spon, London.

Bulloch, K. and Moore R.Y. (1981) Innervation of the thymus gland by the brain and spinal cord in mouse and rat. *American Journal of Anatomy*, **162**, 157–66.

Bulloch, K. (1985) Neuroanatomy of lymphoid tissue: a review, in *Neural Modulation of Immunity* (eds R. Guillemin, M. Cohn and T. Melnechuk), Raven Press, New York, p. 111–41.

Burns, L. (1933) Principles of therapy dependent on the osteopathic pathology of sprains and strains. *Journal of the American Osteopathic Association*, **July**, 100–2.

Buskirk, E. (1974) Nutrition for the athlete, in *Sports Medicine* (eds A. Ryan and F. Allman), Academic Press, New York, p. 146.

Bykov, K.M. (1957) *The Cerebral Cortex and the Internal Organs* (ed. transl. W.H. Gantt), Chemical Publ. Co., New York.

Cassone, V.M. (1990) Effects of melatonin on vertebrate circadian systems. *Trends in Neuroscience*, **13** (11), 457–64.

Cathie, A.G. (1974) The fascia of the body in relation to function and manipulative therapy, in *1974 Year Book*. American Academy of Osteopathy, pp. 81–4.

Cyriax, J.M. (1980) *Textbook of Orthopaedic Medicine. Treatment by Manipulation, Massage and Injection*, 10th edn, Vol. 2, Bailliere Tindall, London.

Denslow, J.S. and Hassett, C.C. (1944) *The Central Excitatory State Associated With Postural Abnormalities*. Still Memorial Research Trust, Kirksville, Missouri, pp. 393–402.

Eichner, E.R. (1988) Circadian timekeepers in sports. *The Physician and Sports Medicine*, **16** (2), 79–84.

Farah, M.J. (1989) The neural basis of mental imagery. *Trends in Neuroscience*, **12** (10), 395–9.

Fitts, R.M. (1964) Perceptual–motor skills learning, in *Categories of Human Learning* (ed. A.W. Melton), Academic Press, New York.

Frymann, V.M. (1963) Palpation: its study in the workshop, Part I–IV. *Academy of Applied Osteopathy Year Book*, pp. 16–31.

General Council and Register of Osteopaths (1993) *Competencies Required for Osteopathic Practice*.

Goodwin, A.W. (1993) The code for roughness. *Touch. Current Biology*, **3** (6), 378–9.

Goodman and Gilman (1991) *The Pharmacological Basis of Therapeutics*, 8th edn, Macmillan, London, p. 1425.

Gordon, J.E. (1987) *Structures or Why Things Don't Fall Down*, Penguin, London.

Grandjean, A.C. (1991) Eating disorders – the role of the athletic trainer. Athletic training. *Journal of the National Athletic Training Association*, **26**, 105–10.

Guezennec, C.Y., Satabin, P., Duforez, F. *et al.* (1989) Oxidation of corn starch, glucose, and fructose ingested before exercise. *Medicine and Science in Sports and Exercise*, **21** (1), 45–50.

Guyton, A.C. (1961) *Textbook of Medical Physiology* 2nd edn, Saunders, Philadelphia.

Harward, L.R. (1985) The stress and strain of pain. *Stress Medicine*, **1**, 41–6.

Hässinger, D., Roth, E., Lang, F. and Gerok, W. (1993) Cellular hydration state: an important determinant of protein catabolism in health and disease. *Lancet*, **341**, 1330–2.

Hazzard, C. (1938) The basis of immunity, natural, and acquired. *Journal of the American Osteopathic Association*, **37** (8), 389.

Hebb, D.O. (1949) *The Organization of Behaviour*, Wiley, New York.

Heilig, D. (1981) The thrust technique. *Journal of the American Osteopathic Association*, **81** (4), 61–5.

Heilig, M., Irwin, M., Grewal, I. and Sercarz, E. (1993) Sympathetic regulation of T-helper cell function. *Brain, Behavior and Immunity*, **7**, 154–63.

Hoag, J.M., Cole, W.V. and Bradford, S.G. (1969) *Osteopathic Medicine*, McGraw-Hill, New York.

Hood, D.A. and Terjung, R.I. (1990) Amino acid metabolism during exercise and following endurance training. *Sports Medicine*, **9** (1), 23–35.

Hoover, H.V. (1969) Craniosacral therapy and the general practitioner. *Academy of Applied Osteopathy 1969 Year Book of Selected Osteopathic Papers*.

Howell, J.N., Binder, M.D., Nichols, T.R. and Loeb, G.E (1986) Muscle spindles, Golgi tendon organs, and the neural control of skeletal muscle. *Journal of the American Osteopathic Association*, **86**(9), 599/119–602/118.

Hull, C.L. (1943) *Principles of Behavior*, Appleton-Century-Crofts, New York.

Hull, C.L. (1951) *Essentials of Behavior*, Yale University Press, New Haven.

Hull, C.L. (1952) *A Behavior System: An Introduction to Behavior Theory Concerning the Individual Organism*, Yale University Press, New Haven.

Hunt, C.C. (1990) Mammalian muscle spindle: peripheral mechanisms. *Physiological Reviews*, **70**(3), 643–63.

Hunter S.L. *et al* (1987) Malignant hyperthermia in a college football player, *The Physician and Sports Medicine*, **15**(12), 77–81.

Isaacson, P.R. (1980) Living anatomy: an anatomy basis for the osteopathic concept. *Journal of the American Osteopathic Association*, **79**(12), 745/51–759/65.

Jacobson, E. (1938) *Progressive Relaxation*, University of Chicago Press, Chicago.

Jami, L. (1992) Golgi tendon organs in mammalian skeletal muscle: functional properties and central actions. *Physiological Reviews*, **72**(3), 623–67.

Jehue, R. Street, D. and Huizenga, R. (1993) Effect of time zone and game time changes on team performance: National Football League. *Medicine and Science in Sports and Exercise*, **25**(1), 127–31.

Johnston, W.L. (1982) Passive gross motion testing: Part I. Its role in physical examination. *Journal of the American Osteopathic Association*, **81**(5), 298/59–303/64.

Kapler, R.E. (1982) Postural balance and motion patterns. Postural Balance and Imbalance: Clinical and theoretical significance of posture and imbalance. American Academy of Osteopathy.

Kappler, R.E. (1981) Direct action techniques. *Journal of the American Osteopathic Association*, **81**(4), 53–7.

Katch, F.I. and Katch, V.L. (1984) Symposium on profiling: the body composition profile – techniques measurement and applications. *Clinics in Sports Medicine*, **3**(1), 31–63.

Keeler, J.A. (1948) Introduction to soft tissue technic. *Journal of Osteopathy*, May, 19–25.

Kennedy, W.R. and Wendelshafer-Crabb, G. (1993) The innervation of human epidermis. *Journal of Neurological Sciences*, **115**, 184–90.

Kimberly, P.E. (1980) Formulating a prescription for osteopathic manipulative treatment. *Journal of the American Osteopathic Association*, **79**(8), 506–13.

Koestler, A. (1964) *The Act of Creation*, Arkana, London.

Koestler, A. (1967) *The Ghost in the Machine*, Arkana, London.

Kraus, H. (1947) Therapeutic exercises in pediatrics. *Medical Clinics of North America*, **31**, 629.

Krause, D.N. and Dubocovich, M.I. (1990) Regulatory site in the melatonin system of mammals. *Trends in Neurological Science*, **13**(11), 464–70.

Kübler-Ross, E. (1963) *On Death and Dying*, Tavistock/Routledge, London.

Landers, D.M. and Boutcher, S.H. (1986) Arousal–performance relationship. Personal growth to peak performance, in *Applied Sports Psychology*, (ed. J.M. Williams), Mayfield Publishing Company, California.

McCann, S.M. (1994) *Neuroimmunomodulation*. Editorial. **1**(1), 1.

McCole, G.M. (1972) The osteopathic contribution to somaticopsychics, in *American Academy of Osteopathy Year Book*, Ch. 18.

McEwan, G. (1994) Creatine supplementation – review of the literature. Presentation at the 2nd Annual Scientific Meeting of the Department of Sports Medicine, 15 October, The Royal London Hospital.

Meijer, A.J., Lamers, W.H. and Chamuleau, A.F.M. (1990) Nitrogen metabolism and ornithine cycle function. *Physiological Reviews*, **70**(3), 701–48.

Melion, M.B., Walsh, W.M. and Shelton, G.L. (1990) Youth sports leagues, in *The Team Physician's Handbook*, Ch. 18, Hanley and Belfus (Mosby Year Book).

Metal'nikov, S. and Chorine, V. (1926), Rôle des Réflexes Conditionnels dans L'immunité. *Annuals Institut Pasteur*, Paris, 40, pp. 893–900.

Miles, K., Quintans, J., Chelmicka-Schorr, E. *et al.* (1981) The sympathetic nervous system modulates antibody response to thymus-independent antigens. *Journal of Neuroimmunology*, **1**, 101–5.

Minors, D.S., Scott, A.R. and Waterhouse, J.W. (1986) Circadian arrhythmia: shift work, travel, and health. *Journal of Social and Occupational Medicine*, **36**, 39–44.

Murray, R., Paul, P.L., Seifert, J.G., Eddy, D.E. and Halaby, G.A. (1989) The effects of glucose, fructose, and sucrose ingestion during exercise. *Medicine and Science in Sports and Exercise*, **21**(3), 275–82.

National Institutes of Health (1985) Consensus Development Conference Statement. Health implications of obesity. *Annals of Internal Medicine*, **103**, 981–1077.

Nelson, C.R. (1948) Postural analysis and its relation to systemic disease. American Osteopathic Association.

Nowak, J.K., Zurawska, E. and Zawilska, J. (1989) *Neurochemistry International*, **14**, 397–406.

Olcese, J. and Moller, M. (1989) *Neuroscience Letters*, **102**, 235–40.

Owens, C. (1942) *Chapman's reflexes at your finger tips*. Chatanooga, TN, Chapmans Reflexes Foundation Clinics, p.3.

Page, L.E. (1927) *Osteopathic Fundamentals*. Journal Printing Co., Kirksville, MO, p. 181.

Puhl, S.M. and Clark, K. (1992) Exercise intensity and body fat. *National Strength and Conditioning Association Journal*, **14**(6).

Roscoe, R.S. (1948) Dynamics of therapy. *Journal of the American Osteopathic Association*, **47**(7), 341–50.

Salter, A. (1949) *Conditioned Reflex Therapy. The Direct Approach to the Reconstruction of Personality*, Creative Age Press, New York.

Salvin, J.L., Lanners, G. and Engstrom, M.A. (1988) Amino acid supplements: beneficial or risky? *The Physician and Sports Medicine*, **16**(3).

Sathian, K. (1989) Tactile sensing of surface features. *Trends in Neurological Sciences*, **12**(12), 513–19.

Schiowitz, S. (1990) Facilitated positional release. *Journal of the American Osteopathic Association*, **90**(2), 145–55.

Schmidt, I.C. (1982) Osteopathic manipulative therapy as a primary factor in the management of upper, middle, and paraspinal infections. *Journal of the American Osteopathic Association*, **81**(6), 83–9.

Selye, H (1936) Thymus and adrenals in the response of the organism to injuries and intoxications. *British Journal of Experimental Pathology*, **17**, 234–8

Sharp, C.N.C. (1986) Some aspects of exercise physiology of children, in *The Growing Child in Competitive Sport* (ed. G. Gleeson), Ch. 9, Hodder & Stoughton, London.

Sherrington, C.S. (1894). On the anatomical constitution of nerves of skeletal muscles; with remarks on recurrent fibers in the ventral spinal nerve-root. *Journal of Physiology, London*, **17**, 211–58.

Siehl, D. (1984) Andrew Taylor Still Memorial Lecture: the osteopathic difference – is it only manipulation? *Journal of the American Osteopathic Association*, **83**(5), 47–51.

Snyder, G.E. (1956) Fasciae – applied anatomy and physiology, in *Academy of Applied Osteopathy Year Book*, Kirksville College of Osteopathy and Surgery, Kirksville, MI.

Sprovieri, J. (1992) Osteopathic philosophy applies to specialities, AAO Members Told. *The DO*, June, 83–5.

Sprovieri, J. (1992) OMT has a role in psychiatry, AAO told. *The DO*, 86–7.

Still, A.T. (1899) *Philosophy of Osteopathy*. Kirksville, MO.

Sutherland, W.G (1967) *Contributions of Thought*, The Sutherland Cranial Teaching Foundation.

Stoyva, J. and Budzynski, T. (1972) From abridged presidential address by the first author at the Fourth Annual Meeting of the Biofeedback Research Society, November, Boston, MA.

Stryer, L. (1981) *Biochemistry*, 2nd edn, W.H. Freeman & Co. p. 827.

Szentivanyi, A. (1989) The discovery of immune–neuroendocrine circuits in the fall of 1951, in *Interactions Among CNS, Neuroendocrine and*

Immune Systems (eds J.W. Hadden, K. Mašek and G. Nistico), Pythagora Press, Rome.

Tyrell, G.N.M. (1963) *Apparitions*, revised edn, Collier books, New York.

Udalov, Y.F. (1992) Vitamins in the nutrition of athletes. *Sports Medicine, Training, and Rehabilitation*, **3**, 79–86.

Upledger, J.E. (1991) *Your Inner Physician and You, Craniosacral Therapy Somatoemotional Release*, North Atlantic Books, Berkeley, CA.

Van Buskirk, R.L. (1990) Nociceptive reflexes and the somatic dysfunction. *Journal of the American Osteopathic Association*, **90**(9), 792–809.

Wells, J.P., Fisk, R.M. and Finn, W. (1980) Proceedings of the Twenty-Fourth Annual Osteopathic Research Conference: Part 2. Functional anatomy of human locomotion and posture – A symposium. *Journal of the American Osteopathic Association*, **80**(4), 276–89.

Wheeler, K.B. (1989) Sports nutrition for the primary care physician: the importance of carbohydrate. *The Physician and Sports Medicine*, **17**(5), 106–17.

Wiechmann, A.F. (1986) *Experimental Eye Research*, **42**, 507–27.

Williams, J.M., Peterson, R.G., Shea, P.A. *et al.* (1981) Sympathetic innervation of murine thymus and spleen: evidence for a functional link between the nervous and immune systems. *Brain Research Bulletin*, **6**, 83–94.

Winget, C.M. (1984) A review of human physiology and performance changes associated with desynchronosis of biological rhythms. *Aviation, Space and Environmental Medicine*, **54**, 132–7.

Winget, C.M., DeRoshia, C.L. and Holley, D.C. (1985) Circadian rhythms and athletic performance. *Medicine and Science in Sports and Exercise*, **17**, 498–516.

Wolpe, J. (1958) *Psychotherapy by Reciprocal Inhibition*, Stanford University Press, Stanford.

Wolstenholme, G.E.W. and Kinght, J. (eds) (1965) *Hashish: Its Chemistry and Pharmacology*, Ciba Foundation.

Woolbright, J.L. (1991) An alternative method of teaching strain/counterstrain manipulation. *Journal of the American Osteopathic Association*, **91**(4), 370–6.

Woolf, C.J. and Walters, E.T. (1991) Common patterns of plasticity contributing to nociceptive sensitization in mammals and aplysia. *Trends in Neuroscience*, **14**(2), 74–8.

Zucker, A. (1993) Chapman's reflexes: medicine or metaphysics? *Journal of the American Osteopathic Association*, **93**(3), 346–52.

FURTHER READING

Finke, R.A. (1986) Mental imagery and the visual system. *Scientific American*, **254**, 76–84.

Johansson, R.S. and Vallbo, Å.B. (1979) Tactile sensibility in the human hand: relative and absolute densities of four types of mechanoreceptive units in glabrous skin. *Journal of Physiology*, **286**, 283–300.

Koestler, A. (1964) *The Act of Creation*. Arkana, London.

Koestler, A. (1967) *The Ghost in the Machine*. Arkana, London.

Korr, I.M. (1987) Osteopathic principles for basic scientists. *Journal of the American Osteopathic Association*, **87**(7), 513/105–515/107.

Nordstrom, M.A. and Miles, T.S. (1990) Fatigue of single motor units in human masseter. *Journal of Applied Physiology*, **68**(1), 26–34.

Olausson, H. and Norrsell, U. (1993) Observations on human tactile directional sensibility. *Journal of Physiology*, **494**, 545–59.

Seals, D.R. (1989) Influence of muscle mass on sympathetic neural activation during isometric exercise. *Journal of Applied Physiology*, **67**(5), 1801–6.

Thomas, C.K., Woods, J.J. and Bigland-Richie, B. (1989) Impulse propagation and muscle activation in long maximal voluntary contractions. *Journal of Applied Physiology*, **67**(5), 1835–42.

3 | The athlete and trauma

INTRODUCTION

The response to an injury varies between athletes. Similar degrees of trauma can make one athlete faint while another would be extremely calm and coherent. Even the neuroendocrine responses will be different, both in release rates and volume. A knowledge of the neuroendocrine response, and the responses of all the other systems, is vital to the osteopath. These responses are an indirect reflection of the athlete's ability to deal with injury, and an indication of his or her psychological ability to deal with recovery from this injury.

There are differences between attending to the athlete on the sideline and in the confines of your practice. General and local reactions to trauma are integrated, and the athlete must, as emphasized earlier, be treated as a whole. The inflammatory response is generally considered as a local reaction indicating the point of injury. This is not however always the case. There are many physiological factors controlling the local inflammatory response. Pain, the major sensory indicator of trauma, is closely linked through the central nervous system to the neuroendocrine system and the neuroendocrine system is paramount in recovery from an inflammatory reaction.

NEUROENDOCRINE RESPONSE

Catecholamines

Catecholamines is the collective term for the hormones **adrenaline** (US epinephrine) and **noradrenaline** (norepinephrine). The normal ratio of adrenaline to noradrenaline is 4:1. These hormones are released by the process of exocytosis from the medulla. This action is controlled by nervous impulses from the hypothalamus, which are conducted via the preganglionic sympathetic nerve fibres from the greater splanchnic nerves, which are cholinergic. Cholinergic means that they act by releasing acetylcholine (ACh) from their endings in the medulla. ACh depolarizes chromaffin cells, increasing their uptake of calcium and releasing adrenaline and noradrenaline from granules into the extracelluar space. Adrenaline produces vasoconstriction in the skin and vasodilatation in the muscles, therefore shifting the blood from the skin to the muscles. It also stimulates the metabolism and mobilizes glycogen as glucose. Cannon (1927) called this the 'fight or flight' response. Noradrenaline produces general vasoconstriction (except of the coronary arteries) and can be regarded as a pressor hormone required for maintenance of blood pressure.

One of the basic principles of osteopathy is that the musculoskeletal system is the primary machinery of life. Many classical evolutionists have suggested that locomotor activity is the dominant theme in animal evolution. Hence, changes in body structures through evolution have occurred as adaptations to facilitate locomotor activity. This is believed to be the case for vertebrates as well as invertebrates. First, sufficient food as raw material should be taken into the body, and second, an active metabolic energy supply for locomotion should be assured. If we examine metabolic pathways, we notice that the biochemical pathways, such as glycolysis and the Krebs' cycle, through which ATP is generated from carbohydrates or fats, do not differ appreciably from invertebrates to vertebrates. This means that new metabolic pathways producing energy did not evolve in parallel with evolution of the body structures which assured higher locomotor activity. In other words, to gain more metabolic energy, animals did not develop more efficient chemical pathways that are completely different from those which prevailed in the ancestral forms. Rather, in my opinion, animals developed systems which stimulate the metabolic pathways to produce energy more actively. This process gave rise to the development of metabolic endocrine organs and their target tissues (Kobayashi, 1980).

Inflammation and pain

Trauma, and pain, can result in an inflammatory response. The inflammatory response can be initiated by:

- physical trauma
- thermal trauma
- foreign bodies
- microorganisms
- immune reactions
- radiation.

Types of inflammation can be broadly grouped into:

- acute
- chronic
- granulomatous.

Acute inflammation

In acute inflammation there is a transient vasoconstriction, followed by arteriolar, capillary and venule dilatation, and increased vascular permeability. The brief arteriolar vasoconstriction near to the injury site is an antidromic neural reflex activity, reducing blood flow to the area. Histamine seems to be the chemical mediator for the dilatation of the vessels, also causing the spaces between the vascular endothelial cells to increase in size. The increased permeability allows for the movement of large protein molecules such as fibrinogen. Due to the dilatation of blood vessels and slowing circulation, a stasis develops in the area. This leads to the classical signs and symptoms of inflammation, i.e. heat, redness, oedema, pain and limitation of joint movement. Exudates, which are proteins from the plasma, contain substances including complement proteins, antibodies (oponins) and fibrinogen, delivered as fibrin, that act as carriers for drugs.

Infection is dealt with through the action of leukocytes in the cellular phase of the inflammatory response. These leukocytes migrate to the outside endothelial surface of the blood vessels, and stick to the endothelial surface, along with platelets and erythrocytes (called 'pavementing'). Once they have adhered to the endothelium they emigrate into the surrounding tissue. The most active of these emigrating cells are the neutrophils, followed by the monocytes and lymphocytes. Red blood cells move out through the vessel walls by a passive process known as **diapedesis**. Cells involved in the acute inflammatory process are neutrophil polymorphs, macrophages, eosinophils, basophils and lymphocytes. Neutrophil polymorphs are the major cell type involved in the acute inflammatory response, their main function being phagocytosis and destruction of microorganisms. Macrophages also have a phagocytic function; they tend to occur later in the inflammatory process and in greater numbers than neutrophils. Eosinophils tend to be present in larger numbers where the reaction is due to a hypersensitivity or allergic reaction. Basophils release histamine on degranulation to mediate early inflammation. Lymphocytes deal with both humoral and cellular immunity. The process by which leukocytes move to the injury site is called **chemotaxis**. Grouping of these leukocytes is more apparent in acute bacterial infection than acute inflammation. The presence of lymphocytes is rare in some kinds of acute inflammation.

Chemical mediation of the inflammatory process results in vasodilatation, increased vascular permeability, smooth muscle contraction, leukocyte attraction and pain. The chemicals involved include histamine, serotonin (5-hydroxytryptamine), peptides and proteolytic enzymes. The reactions occur through the kallikrein–kinin system. Highly vasoactive kinins like bradykinins and N^2-L-lysylbradykinin are produced by this system. These kinins can produce changes in inflammation and pain. The kallikrein–kinin pathway begins by the activation of factor XII to XIIa. These factors are involved early in the process of coagulation.

The complement system is involved in inflammation, usually due to an immune reaction, but can also be involved in inflammation that is not immune reaction based. The complement system causes increased vascular permeability and contraction of smooth muscle. The system can be divided into C3a, C3b, C3c and C5. Other mediators of the

Table 3.1 Sequence of the main events in acute inflammation and their mediators

Event	Mediated by
Injury	
Transient arteriolar construction	Antidromal nerve reflex
Vasodilatation, endothelial separation, and increased permeability of venules	Amines, kinins, prostaglandins
Slowing of circulation	Monoamine oxidase, ?lysolecithin
Migration and pavementing leukocytes	Alteration in leukocyte cell membrane
Leukocyte emigration (± cell diapedesis) and aggregation	Chemotactic factors including complement complexes, fibrin split products, and kallikrein
Phagocytosis	Attachment between leukocytes, bacteria, and foreign materials
Pus formation	Leukocyte proteolytic enzymes

Source: Cawson *et al.* (1982).

inflammatory process include the prostaglandins, specifically PGE (prostaglandin E) and PGI_2 (prostacyclin).

In the cellular phase of inflammation the movement of leukocytes and phagocytosis are influenced by a number of products, including complement complexes (C5, C6 and C7), fibrin split products, kallikrein and chemotactic substances from microorganisms. Table 3.1 shows the sequence of events and mediators involved in acute inflammation.

The types of acute inflammation include:

1. Suppurative (purulent) inflammation, where the inflammatory exudate contains white cells (pus). This form of inflammation results mainly from bacterial infection, often by *Staphylococcus aureus*, *Streptococcus pyogenes* or *Neisseria gonorrhoea*. An example of this is an abscess or boil.
2. Fibrinous inflammation results from the movement of fibrinogen molecules as they escape from damaged vessels and develop as scar tissue from the development of fibrin. Common examples are the formation in visceral and parietal layers of the pleura and pericardium obliterating the cavities after diseases like acute rheumatic fever.
3. Catarrhal inflammation describes the thickening of mucous membranes due to the activity of mucoid glands. For example, this occurs due to the common cold.
4. Cellulitis is an acute inflammation of the subcutaneous tissue due to β-haemolytic streptococcus.
5. Pseudomembranous inflammation occurs on the surface of mucous membranes from an inflammatory exudate of fibrin and white cells with death of the superficial layers of the mucous membrane. An example of this is in diphtheria, and as a reaction to some antibiotics.

Chronic inflammation

Unlike in acute inflammation, where there is an exudative and a cellular phase, in chronic inflammation the reaction is mainly cellular. The length of time for an acute state to reach a chronic state varies. Chronic inflammation can slowly appear without ever having been in an acute phase; on the other hand it is common for a chronic inflammation to have an acute presentation due to irritation. The majority of chronic inflammatory processes have a causal factor, which may be nutritional, infective, repetitive traumatic or structural. Often, chronically inflamed tissue becomes thickened and distorted, destroying the structure of tissue.

Granulomatous inflammation

In this kind of inflammation there is a reaction of a focal distribution in presentation that is characterized by the presence of an epitheloid cell. It is this focus of inflammation that is called granulomous or granulomatous.

It should be noted that inflammation is not always present when pain occurs. Classic signs of inflammation after injury are not always present or identifiable as a reliable guide. Pain is usually identified by anatomical area rather than a particular structure; a painful shoulder, not a painful biceps tendon; and a painful knee, not a painful patella tendon. And although the onus is on the examiner to be competent and accurate in making a physical diagnosis, the elicitation of pain does not necessarily shed light on the exact pathology or mechanism of injury. Traditionally, pain has assumed a disproportionate importance in the clinical definition of inflammation, so that any painful structure is immediately presumed inflamed (Leadbetter, 1993). This immediately puts into question the use of hydrotherapy and ultrasound, in my opinion, in a large number of cases. If there is no inflammatory response then treatment by the usual sports medicine modalities should be brought into question. What we should be asking is 'if these usual modalities are not working then why do the athletes get better?' If the speed at which they get better with non-inflamed (but assumed to be inflamed) presentations is similar to the healing time of inflamed presentations, then are modalities like ultrasound actually as successful in the sports medicine field as we think? All I know is that good osteopathic manipulative therapy (OMT) is much faster at reducing inflammation from tissue than any machine. As an American osteopathic physician once said 'what makes us think that if you boil, bake, and fry the human body it will get better any faster?'

Plasticity

This brings us to the concept of neural plasticity. The work by Korr is paramount to the understanding of the osteopathic interpretation of the body in health and disease. Woolf and Walters (1991) have described the neural changes that take place due to injury, and afterwards. They describe two basic processes, **central sensitization** and **peripheral sensitization**.

> Central sensitization is the term used to describe alterations in the responsiveness of the spinal cord neurones to normal inputs after a

conditioning noxious stimulus or peripheral tissue damage; this is Korr's 'facilitated spinal segment'. More importantly, once other changes were established, a local anaesthetic block of the injury site did not return the facilitation to its reflex baseline, suggesting that the afferent signal associated with the injury could induce a prolonged facilitation in the spinal cord. Peripheral sensitization involves a reduction in the threshold and an increase in the gain of the transduction processes of the primary afferent nociceptors. The most common manifestation of nociceptive sensitization is a hypersensitivity of the site of an injury and of surrounding areas. Recent investigations in a number of different mammals, including humans, show that nociceptive sensitization involves peripheral alterations within the site of the injury and central alterations within the neural circuits representing the injured region. This nociceptive sensitization spreads to areas beyond the site of damage, increasing the sensitivity of uninjured tissue; this phenomenon is known as secondary hyperalgesia.

(Woolf and Walters, 1991)

When treating an injured athlete by OMT, it is paramount to reduce the input of this secondary hyperalgesia, which is making the injury worse. A further effect of OMT is a change in the autonomic response of the tissues in the area, increasing drainage and reducing pain and inflammation. This approach is especially important in chronic pain and inflammation presentations. The athlete's CNS has to be 'set up' so that the injured area has a chance of getting better.

A feature of nociceptive sensitization is its persistence long after the initiating stimulus has terminated. A nociceptive memory has been established, which, by contributing to an animal's exaggerating response to a potentially harmful stimulus, is adaptive. However it should be considered whether this sensitization is always advantageous. Indeed the problem of chronic pain could be the maintenance of a state of nociceptive sensitization where such sensitization no longer has an obvious protective role. Repeated strong shock also leads to morphological changes in these cells, doubling the number of presynaptic varicosities and active zones within the central nervous system. Common features include: enhanced sensitivity of peripheral sensory elements, enlargement of receptive fields, long-term modifications of central neurons, and activity-dependent plasticity.

(Woolf and Walters, 1991)

It is this morphological change that leads to the description of 'plasticity'. As we know, structure governs function.
How far does this plasticity go?

Increases in neural activity, in response to tissue injury, lead to changes in gene expression and prolonged changes in the nervous system. The system becomes re-wired. These functional changes appear to contribute to the hyperalgesia and spontaneous pain associated with tissue injury. This activity-dependent plasticity involves neuropeptides, such as dynorphin, substance P and calcitonin gene-related peptide, and excitatory amino acids, such as NMDA (*N*-methyl-D-aspartic acid), which are chemical mediators involved in nociceptive processing. How does the expansion of the receptive fields of nociceptive neurons lead to hyperalgesia? One hypothesis is that expanded receptive fields will result in greater overlap of receptive fields and, therefore, will lead to a greater number of neurons being activated by a stimulus than the number activated by the same stimulus applied in the absence of receptive field expansion. The increase in neuronal activity may ultimately be perceived as more intense pain. Evidence is accumulating to support the view that NMDA receptor is involved in nociceptive transmission in spinal dorsal horn. The phenomenon of 'windup' (increased responsiveness of dorsal horn nociceptive neurons to frequency-dependent stimulation) is prevented by the administration of NMDA antagonists . . . a large increase in dynorphin gene expression and dynorphin peptide levels in the spinal cord is associated with peripheral inflammation and hyperalgesia. It has been postulated that the large increases in dynorphin gene expression and dynorphin peptide levels following inflammation, as well as following nerve injury, are related to enhanced excitability and development of expanded receptive fields. Small neurons in the superficial dorsal horn exhibit morphological changes suggestive of dysfunction following partial injury. Abnormal function of such neurons could lead to a loss of inhibitory mechanisms and the release of dynorphin-containing neurons from inhibition. The combined effects of excessive depolarisation and loss of inhibition would further contribute to the expansion of receptive fields, hyperexcitability and behavioural hyperalgesia.

(Dubner and Ruda, 1992)

Can an injury that causes plasticity in the CNS affect the function of other systems?

The spinal cord in general, and spinal reflexes in particular, are widely viewed as fixed and inflexible, responding in a stereotyped manner to inputs from the periphery or from supraspinal areas. This common perception is incorrect. Every learning process has a specific goal, an intended change in behaviour. In the present context, the goal is defined by the experimenter, i.e. a larger or smaller spinal stretch reflex (SSR). The memory trace responsible for this behaviour change can be called 'intended plasticity'. Depending on its nature and location, this trace may have additional effects: it may interfere with other behaviours that involve some of the same neurones and synapses. Thus, it may provoke 'compensatory plasticity', modifications that allow the

CNS to continue to perform these other behaviours properly. For example, suppose that up-conditioning causes greater transmitter release at the triceps surae la synapse. In addition to affecting the SSR, greater transmitter release would also affect other behaviours in which this synapse participates, such as walking or jumping. Compensatory plasticity would be needed to maintain proper performance (perhaps by increasing a specific inhibitory input to the triceps surae motoneuron).

(Wolpaw and Carp, 1990)

Symbolic pain

It is sometimes difficult to treat athletes who are involved in contact and collision sports with OMT, even for the simplest injury, due to pain. On application of the slightest pressure to, for example, the posterior thorax with the athlete lying prone, the athlete will tense up. Even when this is not the damaged area, the athlete will tell you that it hurts even though not enough pressure is being applied to cause any degree of damage. This is what I have termed **symbolic pain** – it is there to protect the individual. Symbolic pain occurs through facilitation of the spinal cord (central sensitization). Athletes most likely to present with this condition are those who are exposed to repeated trauma (physical and/or emotional) that is hardly ever, or never, treated. They rest until the pain goes away, reinforcing a change in the receptiveness of the CNS to external stimuli in the future, i.e. compensatory plasticity. Athletes commonly showing this plasticity include club rugby union and league players. Their general lack of stretching, flexibility and social habits often leads to the formation and perpetuation of aberrant CNS input.

Referring back to Leadbetter (1993), we can see that not all pain has to have an inflammatory response. But all pain is subjective, and the athlete's interpretation of his or her pain is not only due to the degree of damage at the site. Slow aberrant silent afferent input is a long-term contributor to the constant adjustment and responsiveness of the central and peripheral nervous systems. Old injuries and/or compensations can make any injury feel far worse than it is. The athlete cannot feel this input, only the pain. It is vital from an osteopathic point of view to search for these sources of aberrant input. They may include a poorly functioning shoulder girdle, flat feet, or even poor neck rotation.

Shock

Shock can occur due to excessive bleeding, tissue loss, infection and any acute stress. A sequence of metabolic and hormonal changes takes place as a consequence of these events or in anticipation of them. The circulating catecholamines from the adrenal glands, and the increased response of the sympathetic nervous system, may subside in a few minutes following minor incidents, but if they continue following major loss of blood or body fluids the athlete will progress to a state of shock. Shock is a haemodynamic shift primarily leading to poor circulation/volume. It is important that the circulating volume of blood is maintained.

Broad clinical features of shock are:

1. a low blood pressure, rapid pulse and reduced pulse pressure;
2. cold, clammy skin, turning ashen (especially in the face), with signs of cyanosis;
3. increased breathing rate (bordering on hyperventilation);
4. dizziness, thirst, nausea and vomiting;
4. irritability, confusion;
5. oliguria;
6. slipping into unconsciousness, coma.

Shock is usually classified according to the type of haemodynamic disturbance that is presented, i.e.

1. oligaemic;
2. vascular;
3. central or cardiac.

Oligaemic shock

This type of shock is the result of a decrease in the circulating blood volume. Both internal bleeding, into cavities or around fractures with large surrounding muscle mass, and external haemorrhage may lead to oligaemic shock. In addition, plasma loss and loss of fluids with electrolytes causes severe dehydration, vomiting and diarrhoea. On average around 70% of circulating blood lies in the venous system. Severe haemorrhage reduces the central venous capacitance, return to the right atrial cardiac chamber, and causes a fall in central venous pressure. This leads to a reduction in diastolic volume of the right ventricle, poor cardiac output and low systemic arterial pressure.

The response depends on the percentage of blood loss. Minor blood loss is compensated for on a local level. When blood loss is more than around 15% in the healthy adult then major haemodynamic changes take place. These include the following.

1. The skin becomes cold and clammy, with oliguria due to regional vasoconstriction in the skin, kidneys and muscles. There may be a rise in blood pressure due to an increase in peripheral resistance, but this is short lived.
2. Compensation of venous return will also be short lived as the central venous and right atrial pressures fall.
3. There is a drop in cardiac output.
4. Both systolic and diastolic arterial pressures fall with an increase in heart rate.
5. There is an increase in the circulation time throughout the capillaries.

Because there is eventually a situation where the peripheral flow does not meet the needs of cellular metabolism of the splanchnic and muscular beds, the type of metabolism becomes anaerobic. The result is production of lactic and pyruvic acids. Pulmonary function becomes compromised with a drop in arterial PO_2, which can fall as low as 50 mmHg, with congestion, and blood being shunted from arterial to venous sides without being oxygenated. The resultant combination of metabolic acidosis and hypoxia affects the respiratory centres, presenting as hyperventilation. A decrease in renal circulation, leading to a drop in glomerular filtration, results in oliguria. Even with regional changes in circulation natural adjustments are made, including the following.

1. A movement of water and salt from interstitial fluid into the circulation, adding fluid to the circulation.
2. The liver secretes albumin leading to osmotic activity, drawing more fluid into the circulation.
3. Vasopressin (ADH) is secreted following the fall in central venous and arterial pressures.
4. Aldosterone is secreted in increasing amounts, reducing sodium excretion.

Infections, for example by *Escherichia coli*, can lead to a form of oligaemic shock as a result of hypoxia of the intestinal mucosa. The endotoxins from the bacteria lead to a reduction in tone in the peripheral circulation.

Vascular shock

Vascular shock can be divided into neurogenic, anaphylactic and toxic shock.

Neurogenic shock
This is the most common reason for fainting, where there is vasodilatation in the splanchnic region with a sudden decrease in peripheral resistance, increasing the capacity of the circulation, resulting in a relative blood loss in the blood vessels leading to a short reduction in venous return. These changes also occur in cases of spinal or brain injury as a reflex sympathetic paralysis.

This is treated as follows. Have the patient lie supine. Do not let the patient sit or stand up; leave them where they are if they are not at any risk due to their location. Oxygen should be administered. In extreme cases they may need fluid replacement, and this is administered quickly by an i.v. crystalloid solution (1 l) for 20–40 minutes depending on the acuteness of symptoms. If the patient becomes unconscious or is unconscious at presentation, initiate cardio-pulmonary resuscitation until help arrives; the patient should then be hospitalized as soon as possible.

Anaphylactic shock
This is an allergic reaction to the administration of drugs or non-human proteins, sera, food or venoms. In the outdoor sporting environment the most common risk factor is insect stings. Response is fairly rapid, with anxiety, apprehension, urticaria, oedema, general aches, cough and bronchospasm. As severity increases there is dilatation of pupils, hypotension, incontinence, convulsion and death.

If an athlete thinks they have been stung or bitten and seems unusually distressed antihistamine medication should be administered as a precaution. Do not assume an athlete is 'over-reacting' to a small sting. If the patient shows signs of slipping into unconsciousness keep airways clear and administer oxygen. If the athlete becomes or is unconscious at presentation initiate CPR until paramedics arrive.

Toxic shock

This is also known as septic shock and endotoxic shock. Severe bacterial infections, usually with Gram-negative bacteria, can be the cause of peripheral circulatory failure and collapse. Other organisms, including fungi, are capable of producing very powerful toxins. For example, a psoas abscess can cause extensive local bacteraemia. Toxins are absorbed leading to what is called toxic shock syndrome. This may be precipitated by trauma, immunosuppressive medication, genitourinary disease, diabetes or leukaemia. As with the other types of shock, there is a reduction in the circulating blood volume (hypovolaemia), pooling in the microcirculation, and loss of fluid from the intravascular space owing to increased capillary permeability. General signs include hyperventilation with hypercapnia, fever (or hypothermia), rigors, petechiae, leukocytosis or leukopenia. Localized signs include abdominal tenderness, perirectal abscess and an extensive pneumonia. Common regional areas of infection include the pelvis, retroperitoneum, perirectal area and biliary system.

Toxic shock syndrome tends to occur due to localized staphylococcal infection or colonization. This can lead to hypotension, a red rash (that does not last very long), vomiting, nausea, diarrhoea and thrombocytopenia. The commonest cause of this in women is use of tampons within a week of their period onset.

Treatment is by restoration of blood volume and the administration of oxygen. Colloid solution should not be used, but a balanced salt solution in the case of short-term fluid replacement. Antibiotic therapy is specific to the organism found. Stabilizing procedures should be the same as for other types of shock.

Cardiogenic or central shock

This is a shock syndrome that results from any cardiac malfunction, that is a failure of the heart as a pump. Cardiogenic shock is usually associated with conditions such as acute myocardial infarction, obstruction to a major pulmonary artery, valvular disease, arrhythmias, etc. This is a form of severe myocardial dysfunction.

FIRST AID AND THE ACUTELY INJURED ATHLETE

A major factor determining success in emergency situations (besides the immediate care) is the preparation at the event in case such a situation arises. I have been to numerous clubs where the sudden 'unexpected' potentially fatal sporting accident has sent players and organizers into a frenzy of disorganized activity. Alternatively, it is not uncommon for precautions to be taken, but procedures not considered. An example of this is arranging for an ambulance to be outside the ground; when an incident takes place the caretaker cannot be found to unlock the gates allowing the ambulance into the ground to transport an injured rugby player to hospital. It is important that lines of communication are set up and a systematic approach to emergency care is understood by all involved, including coaching and management staff.

Many clubs cannot afford an osteopath, or any other medical cover, let alone an ambulance. It is important that you make your own decision whether you work for the love of the sport in the case of amateur and children's activities, or if you consider you need some remuneration in the case of heavily sponsored or professional events. It is important if you take responsibility for osteopathic cover at an event, especially where children are concerned, that you are allowed free access to all areas, and that if there are first aiders or paramedics present you meet with them and make sure you all know who is responsible for what. Here are a few ideas on the preparation of your working environment and the subsequent understanding and care of the injured athlete.

Club, game day and event organization

As an osteopath your duties at any event or club should include the following.

1. Establish written policies of your appointment as soon as possible. Do not get into the habit of casually turning up to help. A written invitation to work as osteopath for a club or event is not a legal contract, but it will make sure that all involved know where you and they stand – for example, that you are there to coordinate and take responsibility for the health care and injury management for the club or athletic programme.
2. Establish any remuneration policy or promises to pay for supplies, no matter how small, in writing, by someone in authority.
3. Make sure that all the players, coaches, management and club staff are aware of your appointment and services to the programme. This is best achieved through the club newsletter, mail outs and/or the notice board.
4. It may be your job to select and hire staff, such as osteopaths, physiotherapists, and/or doctors. If so:
   (a) Make sure everyone is aware of their responsibilities.
   (b) Make sure that the staff you choose are genuinely interested in sports and athletic health care.
   (c) Make sure that they can make the practice and event days (or at least in rotation).
   (d) The first person who comes along is not always the best. It can be difficult to release someone from a programme when you find out they are not what you want.

(e) Choose personnel who have a sense of humour, are understanding, helpful, sympathetic, have enthusiasm, are competent, and most of all show calmness and maturity.

5. It is important at club level to have readily available medical histories for all players. Have some simple forms made up and sent out. You may have to make a decision on a player's ability to continue based on a past history. Keep short notes on the injuries or illnesses incurred. A dictaphone is the most practical way of doing this, filling in the details later.

6. You may have to perform pre-season check-ups and physical fitness level tests. Make sure you know disqualifying parameters for both fitness and general health.

7. It is important that you keep a close observation of all athletic team members at all times.

Telephone numbers/addresses

Some of the sporting events that you may be asked to attend will not be able to afford an ambulance or any other medical cover. One of your main priorities is to get the numbers and addresses of the local hospitals (those that have accident and emergency departments). You may have to get somebody to take a player by car to a local hospital. In an emergency situation call 999 (UK) or 911 (USA) (or other national emergency number depending on the country). Know where you are and the contact number.

To summarize:

1. Know where you are, i.e. telephone number, address and location landmarks.

2. Know telephone numbers, addresses and locations of local hospitals (with accident and emergency departments, that are open). If away from home, a local doctor could be useful.

3. Make sure you have change for a public telephone; you may need to contact a relative or friend to come and collect the injured athlete from hospital.

Transportation

If you have ordered or arranged for an ambulance, it is important that you make sure that it has arrived at the specified time, i.e. at least 30 minutes before your event takes place. When the ambulance crew arrives make sure:

1. that the crew knows who you are, i.e. introduce yourself, especially at a big event;

2. that you know which hospital an injured player will be taken to;

3. that you give them any relevant information about the players.

Medical team members

When there are several medical team members at an event it is important that you organize yourselves into a system so that you know the overall management protocols. It does not matter whose system you use as long as it works and you all know how it works.

1. Make sure you know each other if you have not met before.
2. Make sure you know who is the osteopath, physiotherapist, athletic trainer or physician.
3. Make sure you have your instructions for the day or event. If you do not understand *ask*.
4. If you leave the area, make sure that you leave your expected location with somebody responsible, so that if you are needed people know where to find you.

Communication is of vital importance, particularly at major events, which continue over a number of days, and/or over many locations. Make sure that:

1. you have meetings in the morning;
2. somebody has a radio or mobile phone;
3. if this is not available, then make sure that somebody at base knows all your locations and telephone numbers around the site;
4. all athletes know where your medical facilities are and what times you are going to be available for treatments;
5. leave messages on the door of your medical room if you are at lunch etc. and when you are expected back.

Immediate care of contusions, sprains, strains and bruises

These injuries are progressive for the first 12–24 hours and should receive the following 'RICE' (**R**est, **I**ce, **C**ompression and **E**levation) treatment. This treatment will slow the swelling, reduce the pain and speed up recovery time. Resting an injury is only necessary if the injury is structurally unstable. Even with this RICE approach, all injuries should be diagnosed and treated as soon as possible. The quicker the athlete can use the area the quicker the rate of recovery. Freezing cold should not be applied to the injured area; the object is to control the swelling not freeze the area, which can cause skin and neural damage. If in doubt, make sure the skin is protected with by a thick bandage or towel.

1. Rest: the implication of rest is non-use of the affected area or system. This does not mean that other body areas or system cannot be used, if they do not interfere with the injured part.
2. Ice: apply immediately on appearance of swelling and surround the entire injured area for a maximum of 20 minutes. Reapply when the area shows signs of warming. This should be continued for between 12 and 24 hours.

3. Compression: apply a thick wide bandage. This bandage should be rewrapped several times a day, and more frequently if the swelling is severe, so as not to impair circulation.
4. Elevation: if the injury is to a limb, it should be elevated above the level of the heart.

For minor contusions and bruises, ice applied by massage is all that is needed. Movement of the ice over the skin prevents skin damage. An ice whirlpool is an ideal way of cooling the injured area.

The majority of first aid situations in sports happen at events. All approaches to an athlete who is in any form of distress must be kept simple. Below are some situations that can occur in sport. Luckily, the commonest acute presentations in sport involve minor bumps and scrapes. In these circumstances the athlete is conscious and may be in various degrees of distress based on age, previous trauma experience and the extent of the presenting trauma. All athletes must be assessed and evaluated properly in a quiet environment. You as the practitioner have to reassure the athlete to stay calm and talk to you. And you must listen!

Extremity trauma

Most extremity trauma is of a soft tissue nature, but it may involve fractures. When approaching or presented with an athlete with extremity pain, the following is the basic procedure.

1. Remove clothing.
2. Where is the pain? Get athlete to indicate.
3. Observation (deformity, swelling, discoloration etc.).
4. Any other pain?
5. Active movement (only move until pain or discomfort).
6. Pulses, sensory and motor examination.
7. Palpation (deformity, heat, tenderness, puffiness etc.).
8. Passive examination (joint and soft tissue examination).
9. Weight bearing (upper and lower extremity).

Thoracic trauma

The following is the basic procedure when presented with thoracic trauma.

1. Remove clothing.
2. Where is the pain? Get athlete to indicate.
3. Observation (trachea, abrasions, deformity, swelling, discoloration etc.).
4. Any other pain?
5. Gentle controlled breathing.
6. Pulses, sensory and motor examination.
7. Palpation (deformity, heat, tenderness, puffiness etc.).
8. Auscultation.

The following signs and symptoms should be noted:

- pain on breathing;
- coughing and swallowing;
- displacements.

Abdominal trauma

The following is the standard procedure for abdominal trauma.

1. Remove clothing.
2. Where is the pain? Get athlete to indicate.
3. Observation (distension, abrasions, swelling, discoloration etc.).
4. Any other pain?
5. Gentle controlled breathing, if distressed.
6. Pulses and sensory examination.
7. Abdominal examination and blood pressure.

Back trauma

The following procedure should be followed when back trauma presents.

1. Stop the athlete from moving.
2. Remove clothing.
3. Where is the pain? Get the athlete to indicate.
4. Observation (abrasions, deformity, swelling, discoloration etc.).
5. Any other pain?
6. Motor and sensory examination.
7. Get the athlete to make a gentle attempt to move the limbs.

On the field

When in attendance in an on-the-field or sideline situation for the first time, it is important to put yourself in a situation to be able to do the best you can. You should be prepared for the worst that can happen, i.e. an athlete who has stopped breathing or shows no sign of consciousness. If you are in charge, then is up to you to perform or coordinate any action. Any first aid manual will give you the basics.

It is important in all on-the-field emergencies for one person to take control.

The 'ABC' (**A**irway, **B**reathing, **C**irculation) protocol should employed in an emergency. When an athlete is badly injured, he or she may be face down. The following procedure should be carried out.

1. Attempt communication. Ask the injured athlete (do not shout, unless the stadium is noisy), clearly and directly, 'can you hear me?'; even a grunt is a good sign. Assess level of consciousness.
2. If there is no response, check carotid pulse and breathing at the same time. (Make sure that any pulse you can feel is not your own.) At the same time listen and look for chest and/or mouth movements that indicate breathing.

3. The athlete must be turned on to his or her back. It is important to consider the neck and spine, which may be injured. The neck should be under traction before the athlete is turned over. When 'log rolling' the athlete on to his or her back neck traction should be maintained; this is easier with more than one person in attendance.

Cervical spine injury

It is essential that any medical team working together for the first time practises their emergency protocols. The cervical spine injury protocol is easy to practise. It needs to be rehearsed regularly, and the procedures written down. New people joining the team may have different ways of doing things. Here, I will review cervical spine injury management and a transportation protocol, using American football as an example. Sports such as rugby, soccer etc. will follow the same protocol but do not involve the removal of helmet and shoulder pads which, if the athlete is not breathing, can take time and increase the risk of injury, if there is no practised procedure.

Usually the helmet should not be removed, for several reasons. First, even with the helmet removed, modern shoulder pads with neck restraints may make the application of rigid collars difficult. Second, the field setting does not offer the ideal environment for helmet removal. In hospital the helmet removal procedure can be reviewed and removal performed in a warm, dry, well-lit setting. Third, decisions regarding patient management often can be transferred to the team physician, thus reducing the exposure of those in the field to medico-legal risk. Finally, with the face mask removed, optimal victim packaging and airway management can proceed with the helmet in place. Access to the airway is gained by cutting the lower rubber clips holding the face mask and swinging it out of the way (Denegar and Saliba, 1989).

There are only three circumstances when the helmet should be removed:

1. when the face mask cannot be removed and it interferes with establishing an open airway;
2. when the face mask is removed and the helmet and neck area of the shoulder pads contact so early as to prevent adequate extension of the head to establish an airway;
3. when the helmet is so loose that it cannot be used to stabilize the neck during transportation.

Removal of the helmet
If you have to remove the helmet, follow these basic guidelines (assuming mouth guard is removed).

1. While person A holds the helmet, person B removes the face mask (if not already removed), cuts the chin strap, and removes the cheek pads which have press studs.

2. Person B then places a hand on the player's chin and the other under the player's neck as far up as can be managed to the occiput. Person B applies gentle cervical traction with person A.
3. When person B is comfortable that the amount of traction is adequate, person A pulls the helmet away from the already held ear holes. This releases the traction applied by person A but allows person B to pull the helmet away, rotating the top of the helmet towards the player's nose and dragging the back of the helmet clear of the player.
4. Person B is still applying chin–occiput traction to the athlete; person A takes over by holding the side of the head while person B applies a neck roll or a cervical collar.

Non-removal of the helmet

The helmet (or head) can be used to traction the neck of the athlete while he is being assessed. With fingers in the ear holes, the person tractioning the athlete's neck should kneel down with his or her knees on either side of the athlete's head. They can then sit on their heels and use the inside of their knees to provide additional pressure on the backs of their hands, helping stabilize the neck. The gum shield should be on a tag attached to the face mask. Remove this carefully; it may be stabilizing a broken jaw or broken teeth. The face mask can now be removed by cutting the rubber clips at the side of the helmet. Cut the chin strap. Sweep your finger or non-sterile swab around the inside of the athlete's mouth. At the same time make sure you can see the the upper surface of the tongue. If you see the underside it has dropped back into their throat. Always play safe and clear the airway with your finger either way. You should now be able to use an oro-pharyngeal airway.

Removal of the shoulder pads

In the case of the athlete who has no pulse and needs cardiac compression the chest has to be exposed. Cut the playing jersey in the midline from the collar between the numbers. Then cut the laces at the front of the shoulder pads.

Moving the athlete

Athletes may be stunned or dazed, for example by a knock to the head, blow to the abdomen or knee in the back. They may be moving and complaining of pain. Unless they are in danger due to their location, do not pick them up. Communicate with them: tell them to stay where they are, not to try to get up and ask where the problem is. Get them to touch the area, and keep them talking. If they are dazed due to a knock to the head and/or face, initiate a level of consciousness protocol (see p. 242).

Multiple injured players

When in a situation of multiple injured athletes, and on your own, it is important to assess the situation and pick out your priorities. The general principle is that if they are moving, complaining and shouting they are conscious. Those who are not moving may be in extreme pain, unconscious or not breathing. The presence of blood is always alarming, especially with head injuries. If you have an athlete who is on all fours and bleeding from the head, and another lying motionless on the ground, you should immediately attend to the motionless athlete. When you have help, the most experienced should attend to the motionless athlete. In reality, the sequence will change with experience of the practitioner and the presenting case.

WOUND CARE

In the overall care of athletes, one of the most basic skills for the osteopath is wound care. The vast majority of wound situations will happen at events, but there are a small number who will come to the practice complaining of poor healing or pain elsewhere, not making a connection between a wound and the complaint. The majority of wounds are very simple; often the athlete does not even mention them.

Antisepsis and prevention of infection

The first general area to consider, where open wounds are concerned, is the environment in which the wound occurs and where it should be treated. It would not be proper to discuss this area of medicine without a reference to Joseph Lister (1827–1912). Contrary to popular belief, Lister did not discover antiseptics of any kind. He did however lay down the principles of wound care, infection prevention and treatment. Lister believed (further developing the ideas of Pasteur) that there were microbes in the air and these entered the open wound causing it to degenerate, and compared this to the putrefaction of wine. He developed an 'antiseptic system'. (These ideas were opposed by Robert Lawson Tait (1845–99), a gynaecologist practising in Birmingham.) To prevent microbes from entering the wound he developed a carbolic acid spray, which was initially driven by hand and then later by steam to spray fine particles into the air, reducing air-borne contaminants. His system was first used in March 1865 when treating a compound leg fracture.

Today the principles are basically the same. Any treatment room is a possible environment for sepsis. The main routes are exogenous, i.e. infection from outside sources such as air, hands and instruments, and endogenous, where the source is from the athlete themselves, e.g. their own hands, nose, urinary or gastrointestinal tract.

The treatment room should be well-ventilated and warm, and all surfaces should be cleaned with mild antiseptic (tables, sinks, window-ledges etc.), the most commonly used areas at least once a day, e.g. treatment couches and sinks. The easiest and most convenient method is a small plastic garden spray bottle filled with antiseptic and a little water, with which you can spray and wipe areas quickly. Do not leave the contents in the bottle over night: empty after use and refill before use (i.e. do not make up solution hours before use). All used material should be placed in containers that are either disposable themselves or contain plastic bags. All containers must have covers and must be emptied once a day even if they have hardly anything in them. Surgical instruments that are not disposable should be boiled and dried, not left to air dry. Many training and medical rooms use a large number of towels, for cleaning, doubling as pillows, and to insulate hot packs. Every towel should be used once and then put in the towel bin for laundry that evening.

Personal hygiene is very important for every member of the medical team. The obvious points are short, clean nails and clean hands. On the field wound care always requires the use of surgical gloves, for protection of both the athlete and the osteopath. In the treatment room always wash and dry hands before putting on gloves and after removing them. Masks can be worn where close work is concerned, e.g. draining and packing an abscess. They are particularly useful if the osteopath has an upper respiratory tract infection.

Wounds and mechanisms of injury

Wounds in the day-to-day athletic environment are generally minor. Athletes should be encouraged to treat even minor injuries, thus reducing the possibility of any situation progressing to a more serious state. An osteopath working on the field should have the following available for treating minor wounds: plasters, antibiotic cream, dilute hydrogen peroxide, non-sterile swabs and ice bags.

Wounds are classified by their appearance and how they were caused.

Contusion

The most common wound is the contusion. This is a closed wound caused by blunt impact. Varying degrees of damage may be seen, from simple subdermal capillary damage to major vascular damage where blood leaks into the intercellular soft tissue spaces, causing a **haematoma**. Skin appearances are of the classic bruise, especially at the surfaces inferior to the point of pain/damage, where there is tracking of blood with gravity. The larger and deeper the haematoma the longer it will take to heal and the greater the risk of infection. Surgical intervention where there has been poor ligation of blood vessels or the secondary injury health factors can also lead to haematoma formation.

Abrasions

These wounds are the result of the skin being rubbed against an abrasive surface. They are especially common on knees, elbows, the outside upper thigh and over the femoral trochanter due to sliding on grass (grass burn) or synthetic turf (turf burn). In addition for these wounds to occur there has to be varying degrees of force and rubbing; this is important to understand as deeper structures could be involved, with subdermal damage wider than is immediately visible. For example, abdominal or back abrasions may in addition incur organ damage.

Lacerations

A wound that has well-defined edges and is long and gaping is generally defined as a laceration. These are usually the result of contact with a sharp object, e.g. sharp studs/cleats. Blunt impact can also result in laceration, e.g. head-to-head contact resulting in a facial or scalp laceration or tear. These can be very deep. Again the subdermal damage may be wider than the visible appearance of the cut and deeper structures may be involved.

Penetrating wounds

These are stab and bullet types wounds and are rare injuries in sports. Deep structures are especially vulnerable. Large vessels and organs will bleed excessively, and bowel damage can lead to peritonitis.

Sunburn

Light-skinned athletes should always be protected from ultraviolet (UV) rays. Prevention is always the best situation. Most burn situations will occur during light practice sessions when the athlete does not think about the effect of sunshine, especially when there is light cloud cover where UV rays can still cause problems. Baseball or similar caps should be worn. In addition small light towels can be placed under the caps to drape over the back of the neck. White long-sleeved shirts and light shorts should be worn. Sun block should always be used, anti-glare face cream and perhaps sunglasses.

Sunburned skin is inflamed, warm and red. Cooling the skin is important. Even an apparently mild case of sunburn can precipitate into a very painful condition. Always get the athlete to visit the medical room for treatment. Make sure they do not have headache, nausea, loss of appetite or seem to be agitated, which indicate a more severe problem.

Healing

Wound healing is a response to acute tissue damage, and has the same vascular and cellular reactions as the inflammatory response. Wound healing can be classified as primary and secondary (Fig. 3.1)

Primary wound healing

This can be illustrated by the healing process after a surgical incision. Tissue within the incision is less than a millimetre thick. As the wound begins to heal a blood clot fills it. In this ideal situation, cells move under

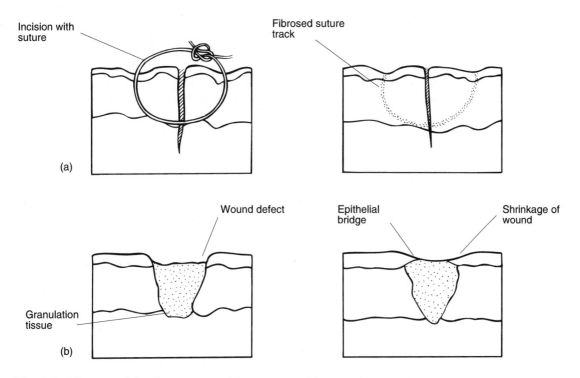

Fig. 3.1 The wound healing process. (a) Primary wound healing; (b) secondary would healing.

the clotted blood pushing it to the surface. The wound should be well on the way to healing in about 48 hours, especially in an area of good vascularity. The mild inflammatory reaction calms and a fibroblastic infiltration with new capillaries takes place. Collagen accumulation shrinks the incision and strengthens the healing wound. Hair does not grow back over the wound but sweat glands do. In this kind of incision sutures can be used to bring the two edges together. If the tissue incised is not prone to excessive movement or can be kept still adhesive strips are preferable to suturing. Tissue congregates around the suture forming a fibrosed suture track, which does not happen with adhesive strips. The wound should be strong enough within a few days to allow a return to activity.

Secondary wound healing

Secondary wound healing takes place where the skin tissue is damaged to the extent that the surfaces cannot be brought together. Again an inflammatory reaction takes place, but this time granulation tissue is formed to 'fill' the area. It may be possible to suture deep tissue to encourage primary healing. Epithelial tissue tends to form over the granulation tissue and the whole process causes a shrinking and reduction of the surface area. This kind of healing can take around 2 weeks, and may leave a scar. Deep rough stud/cleat injury and deep abrasions generally result in this kind of wound. Movement of tissue should be kept to a minimum and antisepsis is a primary consideration. Since this is a wide and deep wound, strengthening of the healing tissue will take weeks. Light training can be resumed within days if the wound is strong enough.

Wound strength

Osteopathically contributing to the nutrition of a wound locally and generally is of primary importance. Like any injury, a wound is an inflammatory process. Factors affecting any tissue injury are similar in response to a wound and are influenced by OMT. Reduction in local joint and soft tissue tension will improve local circulation. In the case of large wounds that lead to immobilization or reduction in joint movement OMT can again help with circulation and enhance drug action. Strength of the wound is provided by collagen, a fibrous protein, and healing is influenced by hydration and vitamin C content of the athlete. Whitby (1995) suggests an overall cascade towards a healing wound (Fig. 3.2).

Treatment of wounds

The majority of wound presentation situations in sports will be during an event or at practice. The following protocol should be followed.

1. Reduce the flow of blood by using sterile gauze (if possible, otherwise non-sterile is generally safe enough). If this measure is not enough to reduce the flow of bleeding, use a sphygmomanometer or, for a finger, a rubber catheter. Never use a non-elastic tourniquet around the limb. There is a risk when non-elasticated material is used, and even elastic material should not be applied for more than about 1 hour.
2. Find and expose the full extent of the wound. This is particularly important in scalp wounds where blood and hair will be matted together.
3. Examine the wound and surrounding area for secondary injury features, e.g. underlying fractures in scalp injuries, joint damage etc.
4. Clean the wound (debridement). This does not just involve removing dirt but also removing tissue in jagged tears that will interfere with healing. When cleaning a wound the general approach is to use cold running water and a very mild antiseptic. Where cold running water is unavailable, a plastic garden spray bottle labelled 'clean water' is useful. This can be sprayed on the wound while being swabbed with gauze or cotton bud. Antiseptic agents are especially useful for cleaning the surrounding area of the wound. Weak hydrogen peroxide solution can be used as a antiseptic on minor wounds. It will foam white when in contact with the wound and may sting slightly.
5. Underlying structures such as tendons, nerves and blood vessels should be assessed for alterations in function and damage. Changes should be

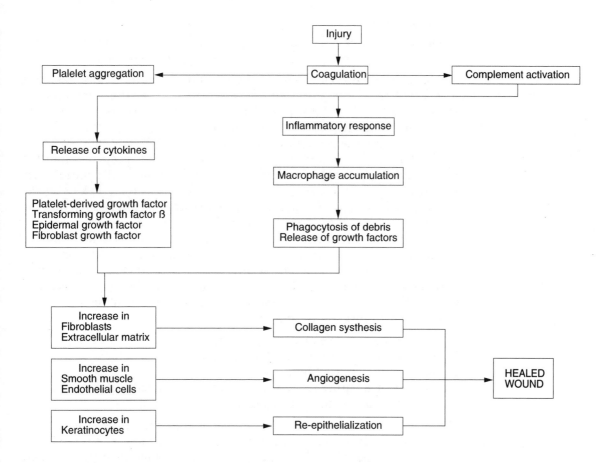

Fig. 3.2 Flow diagram of the wound healing process (from Whitby, 1956).

noted for further reference when the athlete is sent for more specialist attention.

6. For local anaesthesia, 1–2% lignocaine is adequate for minor wounds. Be aware of its administration in toes and fingers when they are affected by cold or Raynaud's phenomenon.

7. Wound closure is through the use of sutures or adhesive strips. Adhesive strips are preferable as they are easy to remove, especially for the athlete. When using adhesive make sure the area is clean and dry. Remove any hair that may be in the way of the strips adhering to the skin. Never cross the strips when applying them. Apply one end of the strip to one side of the wound and gently pull the adhered skin to the non-adhered side to close the wound. Press the free end of the adhesive strip on the other side of the wound. Be careful not to pull the wound edges too close together as this may impede healing. Use gauze to remove excess blood and fluid. Lightly apply a thin layer of antibiotic cream over the strips. If necessary dress the area with a light non-adhesive gauze. Where scalp wounds are concerned, cutting the hair and suturing is usually more appropriate. Alternatively, you can

clean most of the blood from hair and, if the hair is long enough, you can tie the hair together to pull the edges skin around the wound, closing it. Again, apply a thin layer of antibiotic cream.

Abrasions with contusions are more difficult to treat. As has been mentioned above, they heal through a secondary wound healing process. Basically they should be kept dry, and as infection free as possible. The wound and area must be cleaned with cold running water with possibly a very mild soap. Light application of antibiotic cream will help but must not be left on the wound in large amounts as it will keep the area too moist. Make sure the skin is as dry as possible by using sterile gauze to dry the area. If you cannot keep the area open to the air then make sure the dressing is changed every day. Otherwise the scab can interweave with the dressing; also blood and serum may harbour bacteria.

'Turf burns' and other forms of abrasions sustained while participating in sports present a special challenge for professionals who care for athletes; in addition to the usual problems of wound care, these lesions may limit performance in both practice and competition. Hydrocolloid dressings can be used. They allow general abrasion healing, as well as requirements for care of abrasions in athletes, i.e.:

1. good adherence even when sweating;
2. tolerant of clothing and equipment motion;
3. tolerant of increased body motion;
4. tolerant of shearing and collision forces of contact sports;
5. prevent wound exudate transmission to other athletes.

Hydrocolloid dressings debride abrasions through a process termed 'autolysis', which results in a clean wound bed. The dressing provides a moist environment in which the body's own regenerative process may function to debride damaged tissue. Wound exudate interacts with hydroactive particles in the dressing to form a soft, moist gel. This gel functions as an excellent environment for both the skin's own self-debridement process and rapid re-epithelialization. It also permits dressing removal without damage to the newly formed epithelium (Mellion *et al.*, 1988).

Where a wound is sufficient to restrict joint and muscle movement then rehabilitation principles should be applied as if the joint and/or muscle were injured itself. Begin with isometric exercises, progressing to isotonic and weight resistance activities.

Complications

Infections are the most common complications of wound healing. The first step is to take preventive measures, by regularly checking and changing dressings on wounds. Signs and symptoms of infection include those of a continuing inflammatory process, i.e. pain, heat and pain on movement, in addition to tenderness on palpation around the wound site, limb or area oedema, and pus formation. Examine lymph nodes and look for signs of lymphangitis.

Tetanus

This is caused by the organism *Clostridium tetani*, which is a Gram-positive anaerobic bacillus. It may enter the wound by faeces, dust, soil or other objects. This organism releases a powerful exotoxin, called tetano-spasmin. This exotoxin travels up the peripheral nerves interfering with end plate function, and to the spinal cord upsetting inhibitory control of the higher centres on the motor neurones. This leads to the initial clinical features of headache, fever and general unwellness, progressing to 'trimus', which is the classic sign of lockjaw where the mouth becomes hard to close, 'risus sardonicus' in which the facial muscles tighten and the patient looks as if he or she has smelt something horrible, and 'opisthotonus' which affects the extensor muscles, arching the back and extending the neck. At this stage, in extreme cases the patient will contact the bed with only the back of the head and heels. In addition there are blood pressure fluctuations, arrhythmias, dysphagia and respiratory arrest.

Essentially tetanus is a self-limiting disease which needs to be managed. Expert help is vital. Meanwhile it is important to monitor heart rate and blood pressure. The administration of human tetanus immune globulin is the main line to management, as well as antibiotics, and fluid and nutritional advice (in mild cases). Having had tetanus does not confer immunity to further infections. Children are usually immunized in infancy with the 'triple' pertussis, tetanus and diphtheria, inoculation. Booster injections of the tetanus toxoid should be given every 5–10 years if someone is exposed to risks generally, or at the time of incidents.

Cellulitis

This is inflammation of the subcutaneous and connective tissue attributed to *Streptococcus pyogenes*. Signs and symptoms of infection include lymphangitis, enlarged lymph nodes and fever. Further complications of cellulitis are tissue necrosis, abscesses and septicaemia.

Treatment is directed at identifying the bacteria by a swab sample, and then administration of the antibiotics benzylpenicillin and flutoxacilin.

Keloid

This is the development of excessive amounts of dense hyalinized fibrous tissue after a wound. It tends to occur more in negroid groups of athletes.

OMT

The obvious difference between a closed and an open wound is the breaking of the skin. A closed wound can be considered as a soft tissue tear that is oedematous and bleeding internally. The same postural and local soft tissue approach to a closed wound can be applied to an open wound. In weight-bearing structures that lead to postural alteration there will be less muscle pump action and drainage. Aberrant input to the spinal cord should be reduced by OMT to regional joints and soft tissue.

Postural considerations should be assessed in both weight and non-weight-bearing limbs.

PROBLEMS DUE TO HEAT AND COLD

We have little choice with environmental conditions in outdoor sports. We do however have some degree of control over the athlete performing in that environment. Recording environmental conditions, making sure athletes are prophylactically hydrated and conferring with referees and judges will lessen the risk of dehydration and heat illness.

Heat is lost and gained by conduction, convection, radiation and evaporation. These are very basic principles, but it is through the combination of these principles that energy transference or movement occurs.

Conduction is the movement or transfer of heat or cold between two objects that are in contact with each other. The movement of heat is always from the hot to the cold object, i.e from a source of high energy to low energy. For example, swimming in ice cold water will remove heat from the swimmer.

Convection is movement of air that adds heat or takes heat away from the body. Cold air movement on a sunny winter's day will reduce body temperature due to the wind chill factor.

Radiation is reflective heat from an object, which can increase body temperature. For example, artificial turf can radiate heat which can be felt when standing near it on a summer's days.

Evaporation: we have all experienced the loss of sweat from our skin when a breeze of warm air goes past and makes us feel cold. This is important in keeping us cool.

Remember the following points.

1. Sweat is hypotonic. This means that very little salt is lost.
2. Loss of sweat increases the electrolyte concentration in the plasma, making it hypertonic.
3. Therefore, increasing salt intake increases electrolyte concentration in plasma.
4. In activities of long duration in hot environments the addition of hypotonic salt drinks with 6–8% carbohydrate will increase gastric emptying.
5. In the majority of sporting activities, even in the heat, cold water is the best form of fluid replacement.

During vigorous exercise – and particularly during prolonged exercise in the heat – the health and performance of athletes hinge to a significant extent upon adequate fluid replacement. Athletic trainers and athletes should follow established fluid replacement guidelines.

1. Consume 600 ml of cold (about 10°C) water or similar fluid 20–30 minutes prior to exercise.
2. Consume 100–200 ml of fluid every 15 minutes during exercise.

3. Rehydrate without restriction following exercise.
4. Pouring cold fluid on the head or body may provide momentary and invigorating relief but such practices are absolutely inefficient in lowering core temperature or producing favourable cardiovascular changes. Make certain your athletes put more fluid in their stomachs than on their heads.
5. You should be aware of the existing temperature and relative humidity and suggest appropriate adjustments in the athlete's training schedule or competition strategy.
6. In hot weather, athletes should always be encouraged to wear minimal clothing. When clothing is required, light-coloured, loose fitting, porous clothing is best.
7. The athlete's pre- and postexercise body weights should be charted to identify the extent of fluid loss and to assure adequate rehydration prior to the next exercise session.
8. Athletes should avoid alcohol and caffeine ingestion prior to exercise as both are diuretics and can add to dehydration.
9. Be aware of the signs and symptoms of heat illness. These include unusual fatigue, weakness, dizziness, irritability, disorientation and nausea. Exercise should be drastically curtailed or stopped if such symptoms occur.
10. Athletes should make drinking a habit during training. Ensuring adequate fluid consumption only in competitive settings is an unfortunate habit as dehydration can occur just as easily during training. Consuming fluids will allow athletes to train more safely and harder (Murray, 1988).

Certain sports at club level e.g rugby and soccer, are potential risk sports for heat illness. This is especially during pre- and end-of-season training as most athletes think they will not be training as hard as in a game situation. A cooler should be available with mixed ice and water (electrolyte drinks are not necessary). Any games taking place in hot and/ or humid conditions, especially if the players are not accustomed to such weather, should be played in quarters rather than halves if possible.

Fluid replacement is especially important in young athletes, who tend not to drink as much as more experienced athletes. Water breaks should be taken so that they are conditioned to drink. No athlete should be restricted from drinking at any time during a training session. Always have a cooler with ice cold water available for drinking.

The following facts about dehydration should be remembered (Harrison, 1987).

1. Dehydration during exercise is likely above a wet bulb globe temperature (WBGT) index of 18°C, while above a WBGT of 25°C endurance athletes are at risk from heat stroke.
2. The effects of dehydration on performance seem to be mediated by specific changes in thermoregulatory and cardiovascular function.
3. Electrolyte drinks are not necessary; cold water is sufficient in the vast majority of cases (M. H. Harrison, personal communication).

4. It is important to dispel the myth that the environment is the primary source of thermal stress. As Nadel *et al.* (1977) pointed out, environmental heat loads rarely exceed 200 W. Four times this amount of heat is produced by a 60 kg athlete completing a marathon in 2.5 hours by running at 75% of a 4 l/min oxygen uptake (VO_2 max).

5. As the environmental temperature rises and approaches the mean skin temperature, heat losses by convection and radiation decrease, but this is counterbalanced by increased sweat production and evaporation.

6. Information regarding the hazards of dehydration and need for fluid balance does not generally figure prominently in texts devoted to sports science. Rather, and perhaps understandably, fluid balance tends to be discussed in the much broader context of thermal stress as a limiting factor for exercise.

7. The body water lost during sweating, or during dehydration induced by fluid restriction, comes from all the fluid compartments.

8. Thus, very mild dehydration can encroach upon cardiovascular reserve, even though changes in blood volume are minimal at this level of dehydration.

9. Dehydration can influence work capacity independently of its effect on temperature regulation.

Sweat suits

Sweat suits are plastic undergarments that are worn in training sessions to increase weight loss. They are dangerous and should never be worn. Sweat running down the body means that it is not evaporating and therefore the body is not cooling.

Salt tablets

These should be avoided. They are often only partially digested in the gastrointestinal tract. If it is necessary to replace electrolytes, commercial preparations should be used.

Heat-related disorders

The disorders resulting from prolonged exposure to heat and humidity are:

- heat cramps
- heat syncope (tiredness, dizziness)
- heat exhaustion
- heat stroke.

Measures for prevention of these disorders include climatic conditioning, identification of high risk players, changes in the workout plan, changing type of clothing, and most importantly the unlimited availability and use of water.

The replacement of salt and electrolytes is also important, but must be accompanied by plenty of water. If salt tablets are the only source available, at least a pint of water should be drunk with every tablet. Crushed salt dissolved in water is better than the tablet form.

In the USA, from 1964 to 1973 there were 39 deaths related to heat stroke in football; from 1974 to 1984 this was reduced to 15 fatalities.

Heat cramps

Symptoms of heat cramps include large muscle group spasm; gastrocnemius, thigh and hamstring muscles are most often involved. Patients may have a history of regular or recent alcohol intake. This occurs more frequently in certain sports, such as rugby. Treatment consists of rest until spasm stops; ice packs on the affected muscle; application of gentle cross fibre, holding the end point – do not forcibly stretch the muscle, this will only cause more pain; immediate fluid replacement, using cold water in team sports and commercially prepared electrolyte drinks in endurance exercises – in large athletes intravenous administration of dextrose can be used. Heat cramps may be a sign of impending heat exhaustion.

Heat syncope

Otherwise known as fainting, symptoms include weakness, tiredness, dizziness and light headedness. Heat syncope is accompanied by a weak, rapid pulse, and often low blood pressure. Often the athlete is maximally vasodilated, and when they stop the activity, the blood pools; therefore, there is too little venous return to pump adequate blood to the brain. Predisposing factors include ending an activity abruptly without cooling down, dehydration and lack of acclimatization. Treatment involves cessation of activity. The athlete should be moved out of direct sunlight to a cool place. He or she should lie down and elevate the legs. Cool, not cold, towels should be applied to the athlete's body. Get the athlete to drink water. Complications are rare.

Heat exhaustion

Symptoms include profuse sweating, fatigue, weakness, light headedness, delirium (in extreme cases), acute thirst, myalgias and oliguria. Heat exhaustion causes a negative sodium balance over time. It can be due to lack of acclimatization. Body core temperature is significantly elevated, but generally below 39°C. Treatment involves loosening clothing, then rapid cooling of the body with cool towels. Administration of water (or commercial drink) is very important. The feet should be raised, and i.v. saline started, with 1 l over 30–60 minutes. The practitioner should measure the serum sodium; if this is markedly elevated, hydrate cautiously to avoid inducing cerebral oedema. If possible use fans to cool the body; this causes the heat to be drawn out (latent heat of evaporation) and does not drive the heat deeper into the core as can submersion into a cold bath. The athlete may require hospitalization.

Heat stroke

Symptoms of heat stroke include staggering, headache, agitation, seizures, confusion and disorientation. However, the patient will not be sweating; the skin is hot and dry. The back and neck are the best places to feel for lack of sweat. The body core temperature is over 39°C. Progressive central nervous system dysfunction occurs, and progresses towards a collapse of the cardiovascular and central nervous systems. There are multiple electrolyte and metabolic abnormalities: complications extend to all body organs. In the field, immediate external cooling is vital. Remove the athlete's clothes and cover him or her in a single layer of thin wet material. Ice can be used. Keep the airway clear and be prepared to administer CPR. Get the patient to hospital as quickly as possible – this is a medical emergency.

Malignant hyperthermia

Malignant hyperthermia (MH), also known as malignant hyperpyrexia (and porcine stress syndrome in pigs), is a rare muscle physiology disorder. It is an autosomal dominant metabolic disease that can occur in any age group, but is especially dangerous in young, apparently healthy individuals who possess a large muscle mass (Jordan *et al.*, 1979), and it can be fatal. Sufferers are often also sensitive to anaesthetics, especially halothane, enflurane and cyclopropane. The body temperature soars, acidosis ensues, and the heart rhythm becomes irregular (Hunter *et al.*, 1987). As a result of this hypermetabolic response, there is a release of calcium from the sarcoplasmic reticulum leading to initiation of the contraction mechanism. Controversy exists as to whether sympathetic responses are abnormal in MH, and whether they help to initiate MH. The sympathetic nervous system is intimately involved with MH, as evidenced by the following:

1. MH develops in stress-susceptible pigs;
2. the 'fight or flight' reaction can initiate an episode in swine in the absence of triggering anaesthetic agents;
3. typical signs of sympathetic stimulation are observed during active human and porcine MH (Gronet, 1980).

Often these athletes have certain physical characteristics indicating muscle weakness which include strabismus, scoliosis, kyphosis, joint subluxation, ptosis, hernia and clubfoot.

Several factors indicate that an athlete may have MH:

1. an unusually high number of muscle-related complaints;
2. many symptoms that do not occur until the athlete finishes exercising;
3. rectal temperature elevated 10–15 minutes following exercise, e.g. when resting after taking a cool shower (Hunter *et al.*, 1987).

Treatment involves cooling of the patient by any means. Immersion in an ice-and-water bath and exposure to fans is excellent. Refrigerated saline or Ringer's solution administered intravenously is helpful. Cooling can be stopped once the patient's temperature drops below 38°C and resumed if it rises above this level (Jordan *et al.*, 1979).

Acclimatization to training in heat

The following is an example of an acclimatization programme used for American football practice. The longer athletes have to acclimatize themselves the better, but the basics should be covered as soon as possible.

1. Get your athletes out into the heat as soon as possible.
2. Make sure they are protected from the sun with light clothes, and that their necks are protected (this can be done with small towels tucked in baseball caps hanging over the neck).
3. Sun block should be freely available and used.
4. All athletes should be weighed before and after practice. Pretraining weight should be restored by fluid replacement before the athlete resumes training.
5. Workouts should follow this basic plan towards a full practice session over a 5 day period, gradually increasing the amount of clothing and equipment worn.
   - Day 1: train for about an hour at a time, mainly at the beginning and end of the day. Loose fitting, cotton clothing and baseball caps should be worn. Training should be light and tend towards warm-ups, stretching, jogging and general callisthenics. Fluid intake should not be restricted, as on all days.
   - Day 2: increase training session by around 15 minutes. Training should be similar to day 1, with the introduction of short sprints.
   - Day 3: increase to about 1 hour and 40 minutes. Training is as days 1 and 2, with the introduction of anaerobic-type activities. Heavier clothing can be worn.
   - Day 4: training can be performed for up to 2 hours. Anaerobic and aerobic activities can be increased. Use shade to rest if available. Equipment such as helmets can be worn, with a small towel tucked in the back of the helmet hanging down over the player's neck.
   - Day 5: full practice session. It is important to remember water breaks. Certain players may be at greater risk than others, and water intake should be unrestricted.

Table 3.2 shows physiological changes following acclimatization to a hot environment.

Humidity

This is just as dangerous, if not more so, as dry heat. Sweat will not evaporate in an already saturated atmosphere, but the sweat running down the body gives the false impression of losing body heat.

Table 3.2 Physiological (acclimatization) changes due to training in the heat

	Changes
Circulatory system	
Pulse rate	Decreased
Skin blood flow	Time of response increased
	More blood to skin surface
Blood volume	Increased
Blood pressure	Stays regulated
Sweating	
Sweat rate	Increased and quicker response
Evaporation	Increased
Salt loss in sweat	Decreased
Subjective symptoms	
Nausea	Decreased
Syncope (fainting)	Decreased
Dizziness	Decreased
Discomfort	Decreased

Check the weather report for relative humidity. If in doubt, measurement of relative humidity and air temperature should be should be performed, using a sling psychrometer. This measures dry bulb and wet bulb temperature.

Cold injuries

The adaptive process of the body is just as important when it comes to performing in the cold as it is in the heat or humid environment. Adaptation and acclimatization training has to be taken just as seriously in the cold as in the heat.

Heat loss also occurs through a combination of conduction, convection, radiation and evaporation. A body temperature around or below 35°C marks the beginning of reduced metabolic activity. Basically, all metabolic processes slow down. Respiratory rate (hypoventilation), cardiac output (bradycardia) and blood pressure (hypotension) fall, and muscles become functionally shorter and stiffer. Shivering occurs until the temperature drops to around 32°C, when it ceases. Other changes include polyuria (cold diuresis). Continual shivering and the resulting tissue hypoxia leads to increased production of lactic acid and to acidosis. Ventricular fibrillation will develop as the temperature continues to drop. Because of lowered metabolic rate, oxygen requirements are reduced.

Hypothermia

Mild hypothermia (exposure) is probably more common than we think. This may be especially true with supporters at events, who may have to stand in the cold for 90 minutes. Those taking part in winter sports, and sports like hill walking and climbing, may also suffer from hypothermia. The signs and symptoms of hypothermia can be slow and the early stages may go unnoticed. Mood changes, lethargy, lack of concentration, irritability, poor muscular coordination and pessimism are all signs.

Treatment involves getting the athlete under shelter, away from the wind and wet. If the athlete is wet, get him or her dry and into dry clothing as soon as possible. Cover them with blankets, sleeping bags etc. and particularly cover the head (excessive heat is lost through the head). Lie the athlete down until they have warmed up. Do not give hot drinks. Transport to hospital if in any doubt about the seriousness of the athlete's condition. In moderate to severe hypothermia that athlete may stop breathing and/or go into cardiac arrest. Normal CPR should then be performed.

Chilblains (pernio)

These occur usually on the hands and/or feet owing to excessive cold exposure. They consist of reddening, with puritic skin lesions that can become painful. In dark-skinned athletes this is more apparent on the palms of hands and soles of feet. Sudden excessive warming can lead to oedema, blistering, tingling and itching. In extreme cases haemorrhaging and subcutaneous breakdown can occur. Extremities should be allowed to warm gradually. This is best achieved by wrapping the hands and feet in warm material, blankets, gloves etc. Do not rub hands or feet as this accelerates subcutaneous breakdown, which is then a potential site for infection.

Raynaud's syndrome

This is essentially an autonomic spasm of the blood vessels of the fingers and toes, and can occur within minutes. Usually, the athlete knows he or she has this problem. Complications can occur in younger athletes, especially girls. Fingers are the area usually affected and should be protected in even mildly cold weather. Treatment is immediate but slow warming. Do not rub the hands.

Asthma

This can be brought on in the cold owing to a reflexive bronchial narrowing due to the cold air. Get the athlete into the warm and use oral bronchodilators as soon as possible.

Frostbite

This is the actual freezing of body parts, and usually occurs in the extremities or areas of large surface-to-volume ratio like the nose and ears. Exposed areas or areas with minimal clothing will have increased risk of frostbite. The depth and area of the frostbite has to be assessed.

The commonest type of frostbite is superficial with rare occurrences in sport of deep frostbite. Superficial frostbite presents as areas of discoloration; in fair-skinned athletes a white/blue colour while in dark-skinned athletes a light brown anaemic colour is seen.

Treatment is by warming. Care should be taken not to heat the area too fast. Keep the area dry and insulated rather than heated. Transfer to a hospital emergency department.

ATHLETIC TAPING

This is the use of adhesive strapping and bandaging in the protection, prevention and treatment of athletic injuries.

The use of adhesive substances in the care of external lesions goes back to ancient times. The Greek civilization is credited with formulating a healing paste composed of lead oxide, olive oil and water which was used for a variety of skin conditions. This composition was then changed by the addition of resin and yellow bees' wax and, more recently, rubber. Since its inception, adhesive tape has developed into a vital therapeutic adjunct.

Joints that have had moderate or severe ligament tears require protective taping over the following season. A number of factors contribute to reducing joint injury. Of primary importance is the fitness and strength of the player. The muscles and ligaments provide more efficient protection than any taping or brace. After injury, it is extremely important that the musculotendinous and ligamentous units in the injured area are brought back to near normal function. The risk of repeated injury can be reduced by the use of joint or limb power testing, through certain drills or specific demands. Ideally, power should be close or equal to that of the opposite limb. Progressive resistance exercises should be employed through the full range of motion until the two sides are comparable. This should take place before participation sports are allowed.

Taping by adherence to the skin is more efficient than using a brace. It is important to avoid a torniquet effect from a rigid brace. Some athletes do play sports such as football and basketball with braces because they have gross instability in a joint and would otherwise be unable to participate. However, their efficiency is obviously impaired and there is serious doubt that participation is in their long-term interest.

There is a place for adhesive taping in the reinforcement of previous ligament injury. This is particularly true where repair of a tear has been non-surgical, and involving a large part of the ligament. The fibres will lie in a disorganized fashion and a great deal of time must pass before alignment is achieved against the line of stress. During this period, reinforcement is necessary.

Factors in the selection of adhesive tape

Modern adhesive tape has great adaptability for use in athletics because of its uniform adhesive mass, adhering qualities and lightness, as well as the relative strength of the backing material. All of these are of value in holding wound dressings in place and in supporting and protecting injured areas.

A great many types and sizes of adhesive tape are available. The most popular tape in use is the type with a non-yielding backing. However, elastic tape is becoming increasingly popular because it easily conforms to the contour of the body part. Factors to be considered when purchasing tape include cost, grade of backing, quality of adhesive mass and properties of unwinding.

Tape grade

Linen-backed tape is usually graded according to the number of longitudinal and vertical fibres per inch of backing material. The heavier and more costly backing contains 85 or more longitudinal and 65 vertical fibres per inch. The lighter, less expensive grade has 65 longitudinal and 45 vertical fibres.

Adhesive mass

With modern advances in adhesive mass one should expect certain qualities from the tape. It should maintain its adherence despite profuse perspiration and activity, the mass must contain as few skin irritants as possible and must also be able to be easily removed without leaving a mass residue or tearing the superficial skin.

Winding

The winding tension that a tape roll possesses is very important. Athletics, in particular, places a unique demand on the unwinding quality of tape. If tape is to be applied for protection and support, there must be even and constant tension while it is being unwound. In most cases tape needs little additional tension to give sufficient tightness.

Size of tape

A half to one inch (12–25 mm) adhesive tape is used to tape small areas or areas which are difficult to conform to such as fingers, hands, toes and feet.

Purposes and function of tape

In athletics, a very important use of adhesive taping is for protection and support of a previously injured or weakened area, to prevent recurring injury.

The functions of adhesive taping in sports are to prevent undesired mobility of a part, to compress soft tissue and to secure a bandage or equipment piece in place. The osteopath has to learn to match taping techniques to function. These techniques relate to the complete sequence of the practitioner's care of athletic injuries, i.e. injury prevention, first aid, treatment, rehabilitation and protection from reinjury.

First aid

Adhesive taping for first aid care is a temporary measure to protect the athlete from aggravation of an injury, complications and unnecessary discomfort until more specialized attention can be given. First aid taping is usually confined to compression of soft tissue to prevent oedema around the site of the injury or to prevent loss of blood from a laceration. The latter would involve securing an absorbent compress over the wound. First aid taping may also be involved in closing a laceration, as in butterfly tape bandaging.

Treatment

If the athlete must abstain from normal activity as well as athletic participation, adhesive taping relates to restriction of motion and/or tissue compression for assisting the healing process.

Rehabilitation

When the athlete's return to normal activity is anticipated, the protective role of adhesive taping becomes an integral part of the osteopath's tasks. For some athletic injuries, this step may follow first aid care. For others it may follow months of surgical or postsurgical treatment. The purpose is to enable the injured athlete to resume activity that helps him/her to regain flexibility. Each tape is individualized to the limits of activity prescribed, and the taping procedures are employed that best counteract the potentially injurious stresses related to the prescribed activity.

Prevention of reinjury

When the athlete receives clearance for return to full athletic participation, taping becomes related to reinjury prevention instead of rehabilitation. There is a distinct difference between the athlete's return to prescribed activity with reliance on taping for protection (rehabilitation) and the athlete's return to participation with taping utilized as a helpful precaution (reinjury prevention). The risk of reinjury may not be significantly related to the performance demands of the athlete, for example an injury to the left hand of a right-handed quarterback.

Associated with this function of taping is the use of routine preventive taping of body parts where there is no recent history of injury. For example, the opinion of most American team doctors and athletic trainers is that adhesive taping helps support ankles from direct and indirect forces and thus reduces chance of injury. Research on this has been inconclusive.

The purpose of injury-prevention taping in athletics, therefore, is justified if no additional hazards are presented by the application of tape.

Protection of acute, subacute and chronic injuries is extremely important in reducing the athlete's chances of incurring a more handicapping condition. Protection can often be achieved in one of the following two ways:

1. limitation of joint movement by using a predesigned strapping;
2. stabilization by securing protective devices.

Factors which must be considered before tape is applied

1. Contraindications to taping, include skin infections and injury, such as eczema, warts, dermatitis, burns, boils etc. These conditions should be taken care of before taping is considered. Heat, friction and sweating under the tape could significantly irritate the condition. Non-weight-bearing fractures that are stable can be repeatedly taped between rehabilitation visits.
2. The size and shape of the joint or the taper of the limb: unless these factors are taken into account, the osteopath may end up with a mass of wrinkles in the tape job, with resultant loosely adhering strips.
3. The movement, if any, in which the body part is involved. Strapping must protect against injury, but it still must allow the maximum comfort of the body part, such as the joint, so that the athlete will be able to perform the most efficient movements possible.
4. The sport in which the player is engaged. For example, football players as a rule can play quite efficiently despite being heavily taped in several places. The swimmer, on the other hand, would be hampered considerably if his shoulder was taped.
5. The position played in a particular sport; a goalkeeper with his thumb strapped may have limited ability.
6. The seriousness of the injury. In an emergency it is not advisable to tape injuries such as fractures of large and weight-bearing bones, since incorrect handling could precipitate or deepen shock and aggravate the injury.
7. The length of time the tape is to remain on the body. If it is necessary that the tape be kept on the body part for several days, it would be advisable for the osteopath to first cover the part with bandage of some sort. Extended time of strapping can cause the skin to become soft, whitened, wrinkled and easily pulled off when the tape is removed.
8. The degree of oedema expected or present. If the tape is applied immediately on a sprained joint, consideration must be given to the amount of swelling expected so that the pressure can be relieved if it becomes unbearable.
9. The proximity of the subdermal arteries, nerves and bony prominences. The osteopath must know where the pressure points are so as to avoid the possibility of cutting off circulation or nerve transmission, or irritating bony areas. When there is concern, pads and lubricants should be used.

Adhesive tape, if properly applied, will give immediate relief of discomfort and will reduce pain. A thorough knowledge of the anatomic structure is important so that the application of the tape will be of value. It is also important to understand the mechanics of the injured part to be taped, as a purpose of taping is to pull the injured parts to closer approximation and promote repair. If the injury is pulled apart it will be delayed in healing. When the tape is applied incorrectly, pain and discomfort will be evident and, if not corrected, healing will be retarded.

Technique

There are many different techniques of adhesive strapping for knees and ankles. Even the same osteopath may not use an identical strapping method each time he or she straps an ankle. It is important to learn the fundamentals of taping, and adapt them for individual applications. It is a mistake to use a particular type of strapping for everything. All injuries are different, and all require an individual approach to strapping.

Summary

The purposes of adhesive taping can be classified into two groups:

1. injury care;
2. injury protection.

Adhesive tape has a number of roles in the care of injuries:

1. retention of wound dressings in place;
2. stabilization of compression-type bandages that are used to control external and internal haemorrhaging of acute injuries;
3. support of recent injuries to prevent any additional insult that might result from the activities of the athlete.

REFERENCES

Burns, L. (1938) How to keep cool in hot weather. *Journal of Osteopathy*, **ix**(3).

Denegar, C.R. and Saliba, E. (1989) On the field management of the potentially cervical spine injured football player. *Athletic Training*, **24**(2), 108–11.

Dubner, R. and Ruda, M.A. (1992) Activity-dependent neuronal plasticity following tissue injury and inflammation. *Trends in Neuroscience*, **15**(3), 96–103.

Gronet, G.A. (1980) Malignant hyperthermia. *Anesthesiology*, **53**, 395–423.

Harrison, M.H. (1987) Fluid balance as a limiting factor for exercise, in *Exercise: Benefits, Limits and Adaptations* (eds D. Macleod, R. Maughan, M. Nimmo *et al.*), E. & F.N. Spon, London, pp. 367–84.

Cawson, R.A., McCraken, A.W. and Marcus, P.B. (1982) *Pathologic Mechanisms and Human Disease*, Mosby, London, p.193.

Cannon, W.B. (1927) The James-Lange theory of emotions: A critical examination and an alternative theory, *Psychology*, **39**, 106–24.

Hunter, S.L., Rosenberg, H., Tuttle, G.H. *et al.* (1987) Malignant hyperthermia in a college football player. *The Physician and Sports Medicine*, **15**(12), 77.

Jordan, O.M., Wingard, M.D., Barak, A.J. *et al.* (1979) Malignant hyperthermia. A potentially fatal syndrome in orthopaedic patients. *Journal of Bone and Joint Surgery*, **61**, 1064–70.

Kobayashi, H. (1980) *Hormones, Adaptation and Evolution* (eds S. Ishii *et al.*), Japan Sci. Soc Press, Tokyo/Springer-Verlag, Berlin, pp. 15–22.

Leadbetter, W.B. (1993) Basic principles of prevention and care, in *The Encyclopaedia of Sports Medicine* (ed. F.H. Renström), Ch. 23, Blackwell Scientific Publications, Oxford.

Mellion, M.B., Fandel, D.M., Wagner, W.F. and Kwikkel, M.A. (1988) Hydrocolloidal dressing in the treatment of turf burns and other athletic abrasions. *Athletic Training*, **23**(4), 341–6.

Murray, R. (1988) Fluid replacement, gastrointestinal function and exercise. *Athletic Training*, **23**(3), 215–19.

Nadel, E.R., Wenger, C.B., Roberts, M.F., Stolwijk, J.A.J. and Cafarelli, E. (1977) Physiological defences against hyperthermia of exercise. *Annals of the New York Academy of Science*, **301**, 98–109.

Whitby, D.J. (1995) The biology of wound healing. Plastic Surgery. *Surgery, incorporating Scalpel*, **13**(2).

Wolpaw, J.R. and Carp, J.S. (1990) Memory traces in spinal cord. *Trends in Neuroscience*, **13**(14), 137–42.

Woolf, C.J. and Walters, E.T. (1991) Common patterns of plasticity contributing to nociceptive sensitization in mammals and aplysia. *Trends in Neuroscience*, **14**(2), 74–8.

FURTHER READING

Dawson, B., Pyke, F.S. and Morton, A.R. (1989) Improvements in heat tolerance induced by interval running training in the heat and in sweat clothing in cooling conditions. *Journal of Sports Science*, **7**, 189–203.

Hall, G.M. and Lucke, J.N. (1985) Of man and pigs: is malignant hyperthermia a stress-related disorder. Stress and illness. *Stress Medicine*, **1**, 47–53.

Hubbard, R.W. and Armstrong, L.E. (1989) Hyperthermia: new thoughts on an old problem. *The Physician and Sports Medicine*, **17**(6), 97–113.

Raven, P.B. (1989) The body's response to heat. *Sports Training, Medicine and Rehabilitation*, **1**, 145–8.

Rosenberg, H. (1985) Malignant hyperthermia. *Hospital Practice*, 15 March, 139–52.

Sawaka, M.N., Young, A.J., Latzka, W.A. *et al.* (1992) Human tolerance to heat strain during exercise: influence of hydration. *Journal of Applied Physiology*, **73**(1), 368–75.

Tissue dysfunction | 4

When we realize that Dr Still discovered the relationship between the spinal lesion and functional disturbance, and that the correction of said lesion re-established normal health, we may readily understand the profound effect it must have had upon his mind, and why he, then and there, proclaimed that structure determined function.

Martin D. Young, DO

INFLAMMATION

As we have seen in Chapter 3, inflammation is not always present when there is an injury. If it is, there are five cardinal signs of inflammation: heat, redness, swelling, limited joint movement and pain. However, when there is pain, there is not necessarily inflammation. In many clinical presentations of pain and limited joint movement, the injured tissue is in fact colder than surrounding tissue. Due to this finding it may be necessary to reclassify two basic findings. The first is the accepted form of inflammation, i.e. energy production due to the release of heat and accumulation of products (exudates) due to trauma, as a hot injury. And secondly, a basic opposing mechanism occurs presenting a state of active contraction. This leads to poor supply and drainage, leading to an ischaemic-type dysfunction, i.e. a cold injury.

SOMATIC DYSFUNCTION

The musculoskeletal system is the largest system of the body, yet in the performance of its infinite repertoire of motions and postures, it is the most delicately controlled and coordinated. Accordingly, the musculoskeletal system receives most of the efferent outflow from the central nervous system, with the largest portion via the ventral roots of the spinal cord to the muscles, which carry out the motor commands of the CNS.

It is less well appreciated, however, that for related reasons the musculoskeletal system is also the main source of sensory input to the CNS, an input that is also the most widespread, the most continuous and the most variable. This sensory feedback, from many thousands of reporting stations in myofascial and articular components, entering the cord via the dorsal roots, is essential for the moment-to-moment control and fine adjustment of posture and locomotion.

In addition to this influence on the motor pathways, the sensory reporting is selectively routed to various other centres throughout the nervous system, including the cerebral cortex, where it enters into consciousness and the ordering of volitional motor activity. Relevant portions of the reports also reach and are utilized by the autonomic nervous system in the tuning of visceral, circulatory and metabolic activity in response to musculoskeletal demand. Indeed, the sensory input from the musculoskeletal system is so extensive, intensive and unceasing as to be a dominant influence on the CNS and therefore the person as a whole (Korr, 1975).

In this section, 'somatic' is used in its broadest sense to include head, trunk, walls of the body cavity and appendages (Hoag *et al.*, 1969).

Hypertonia

This has been described as a high resting tension within the soft tissues of the body. Musculotendinous hypertonia occurs when the sarcomere length of the muscle is shortened. In maintained tension musculotendinous tissue is working over a reduced range of function, possibly leading to connective tissue accumulation and muscle stiffness (Williams *et al.*, 1988). This resulting reduction in both parallel and serial sarcomere function (see Chapter 2) may not be painful to the athlete, but in the majority of cases leads to complaints of soreness, weakness and feelings of instability during function in other areas. A good example of this is lateral knee, groin and even plantar foot pain, when there is extreme tension of the gluteus medius and tensor fascia latae. Facilitation of the spinal cord will lead to a somatic reflex situation.

It is very common, on deep palpation of areas of sustained hypertonia (possibly accumulative over years), for the athlete to complain of subjective numbness of the tissues in association with the pain, as if the sensory portion of the tissues had been 'switched off'.

Fasciitis

This condition is often ignored in sports medicine, except when it occurs in the hands, legs and feet. Much more common in sports-related presentations than realized, it is often misdiagnosed as 'overuse injury'. Sudden exercise and exertion without proper time for adaptation can lead to illness (see Chapter 2), due to sudden unaccustomed overload which stresses the neuroimmune system. Local fascial presentations of palmar and plantar fasciitis are often due to chronic alcohol abuse and increased training, respectively. Occasionally, the condition has shown to be present all over the body. The most common finding is of a serum eosinophilia, a condition that has been called 'eosinophilic fasciitis'. This has been described as a syndrome characterized by rapid, diffuse swelling and induration of the extremities and/or trunk, with an episode of preceding trauma or physical exertion often reported by the patient (Vengrove and Adelizzi, 1986). The fascia exhibits diffuse as well as perivascular inflammation. Later in the progression of the disease, the skin becomes hidebound, taut and indurated. Flexion curvatures frequently develop. Local fascial tears, stretches and contusions are in reality associated with other soft tissue injuries.

General aches and pains

Many patients present with general aches and pains. Be careful! The myofascioskeletal system is often the first system to express low grade viral and bacterial infections, immunological disturbances (e.g. leukaemia), rheumatological syndromes etc. An athlete who is being prescribed medications repeatedly may be at risk of iatrogenic illnesses (Ketterer and Buckholtz, 1989).

Fibromyalgia

This is a form of chronic, non-articular rheumatic disease characterized by diffuse aches and pains, joint stiffness, sleep disturbance, fatigue and multiple tender areas on physical examination. The term fibrositis was originally used by Gowers in 1904 to describe a condition in which patients presented with multiple tender muscular nodules. Inflammation of the fibrous tissue of the muscle was believed to be responsible for this syndrome. Subsequently, studies failed to substantiate an inflammatory component, however, and the term fibromyalgia, introduced in 1976, was adopted to describe this disorder (Kalik, 1989). This is a common problem presenting in the osteopathic surgery. The athlete may have been told by their allopathic doctor that they have to live with it. The reason for these nodules is not totally understood, but they seem to be areas where connective tissue is layed down within muscular tissue. The symptoms can be precipitated, for example, headaches caused by stress or even when an athlete has missed a meal.

On palpating the tissue it feels 'ropey' and 'dehydrated'. Deep palpation increases discomfort. The muscle may be described as 'fibrotic' with the implication that this is an inappropriate pathological change, but it may be interpreted that the muscle has by an appropriate adaptation transformed into a 'ligament' with its concomitant properties, conforming to the structure–function principle of osteopathy (Collins, 1994).

Osteopathic manipulative therapy (OMT) can be used to treat fibromyalgia. A postural examination is vital. Do not aggravate the area by painfully digging into the soft tissue. 'Rubbing' this tissue condition has limited long-term effects; cross-fibre, functional and strain–counterstrain techniques are preferable. Selective high velocity thrust and articulation to local and general postural restrictions is recommended. As this appears to be a non-inflammatory condition, NSAIDs and aspirin are of limited value. The use of ethylchloride or fluoromenthane vapo-coolants in 'spray and stretch' methods are useful. Other approaches include rehydration, and a reduction in alcohol and nicotine intake. Exercises are self-limiting on their own since they increase local capillary bed circulation in the short term without making any long-term structural change. The joints must be helped to achieve a full range of motion while exercising for it to be beneficial. Psychological factors often precipitate somatic symptoms. Treatment should be carried out at least once a day for a few days, and then based on texture change, joint freedom and feedback from the athlete. Weather sensitivity to chronic somatic problems is a recognized symptom, usually in retired athletes (Shutty *et al.*, 1992).

FRACTURES

The failure of myofascial tissue to withstand physical force generally results in the absorption of energy through to deep (body non-elastic) structures.

Fracture healing

Healing of a fracture (Fig. 4.1) shows similarities with healing of soft tissue from the aspect of proliferation of cells, in secondary wound healing. In the case of bone there is formation of a callus. Due to trauma there is a degree of inflammation and haemorrhaging. Fracture healing can be looked at in two main phases: a bridging phase and remodelling phase.

1. **Bridging phase.** In the majority of fractures there is a degree of splintering and displacement into the surrounding tissues. The broken ends of the bone become necrotic due to torn vascular structures in the

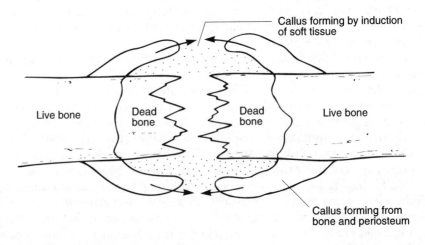

Fig. 4.1 Bone healing.

medullary cavity, periosteum and cortex. At this stage it is important that the ends of the bone are in relation to each other and that movement is stopped. Cells begin to proliferate outside the fracture site. These new cells cover the fracture site with new material forming a bridge of cells around the bone ends. (The immediate ends of the bone are necrotic due to the fracture, so the process of healing does not begin there.) As the process continues, the area around the fracture site mineralizes forming a callus around the dead bone ends. This callus develops an outside layer of fibrous periosteum and external callus over the fracture site. Outside the immediate fracture zone new bone is moving in, while inside the bone, but also outside the fracture zone, there are new trabeculae growing from bone marrow towards the fracture site.

2. **Remodelling phase**. In this second phase the callus bridge is well established and bone begins to fill the zone. This includes the turning into bone of immediate haematoma and soft tissue. The gap between the bone becomes woven or knitted together with bone material. This is different from the external callus above, as the dead bone is now replaced by this woven new bone. Dead bone is replaced by new Haversian systems or osteons and cortical bone. Osteoblasts and osteoclasts contribute to formation of these structures: osteoclasts lead the reintroduction of these structures and osteoblasts produce osteoid and then new bone.

When the fracture is sufficiently healed, the permanent cast can be removed, and replaced by a cast that can be removed for rehabilitation and icing then reapplied afterwards. Some weight-bearing fractures are not fixed with plates and screws or elastic implants, and result in non-union or poor healing with deformity.

Non-union fractures

If bone-to-bone approximation and/or the elimination of motion in the early stages of healing are not adequate, non-union may result. There is formation of dense fibrous tissue (hyaline) which becomes fibrocartilaginous, and can lead to the development of a pseudarthrosis or false joint. The external callus phase may begin, but complete healing is retarded.

Case 1

In January 1993 an 18 year old male soccer player was knocked down while waiting to cross the road. He suffered a complete fracture of his left tibia and fibula. He attended my practice in May 1993 with no cast and using crutches. New X-rays were taken. Physical therapy had been avoided by the doctors he had seen because there was non-union at the fracture sites. He could not put his foot to the floor because he said it felt like 'his shin was going to explode'. My main concern was to get him to walk normally as soon as possible. Osteopathically, it is important to consider the person with the fracture, not just the fracture. The fracture area was in a state of congestion with thickening (hyperplasia) of soft tissue and tight shiny skin. On passive examination his left foot and ankle were so reduced in movement as to be bordering on fusion. His left hip was in a state of extreme hypertonia, as were his low back, thorax and shoulders. Over the past 2 months he had been having tension-related headaches.

The objectives were:

1. *to improve energy-absorbing capacity of the tissues, so that weight bearing was not concentrated at the fracture site;*
2. *to leave the fracture site alone; it is the casualty in this situation not the instigator;*
3. *to improve circulation (supply and drainage) and soft tissue tone to and around the fracture site;*
4. *to get him walking as soon as possible; normal movement (not rehabilitation) is the best way to get normal function;*
5. *to support him around the psychological barriers.*

OMT was applied to the foot, ankle, thigh, hip, back, shoulders and neck. This was a very unspecific approach using articulation, high velocity thrust, and soft tissue to whatever I felt was reduced in function.

When he returned for his second visit 5 days later he was weight bearing, but still limping. After 5 weeks and six treatments he was walking nearly normally. By August 1993 he was participating in non-contact training and jogging. He was back playing with his soccer club just after Christmas that year.

Casting

Not all fractures should be permanently casted, especially stable fractures. Light casts can be applied, and then the cast cut in half using a cast cutter so that it can be reapplied and held with athletic tape and bandage. This allows the athlete to take part in an exercise programme of light weights and resistance activity, as well as being able to ice down any inflammation.

Fitness

It is important to keep the athlete fit while the fracture heals, to maintain cardiorespiratory capacity. Any activity can be performed that does not put the injured area under any undue stress.

Stress fractures

Soft tissues and bones work together, so that when one fails to absorb energy the other increases its capacity. In the majority of cases stress fractures are due to poor energy dissipation and absorption. The osteopath must find the areas of dysfunction that are focusing the energy at the point of bone failure.

JOINT DYSFUNCTION

All joints have primary and accessory movements. Function at these bony junctions is subtle and accommodating to the total need of the organism; a good example is the spine. Reduction of complete range will occur when there is increased motion in another joint or joints. This allows the athlete to continue to perform without any functional restrictions. This process of adaptation has to be slow enough to allow other areas to increase or reduce their motion; if the process occurs over too short a period of time then pain as well as structural damage will develop. This increase in motion of other joints will leave the joint that has reduced function susceptible to injury. It can no longer absorb stress put upon it. Sudden stress on joints that have reduced energy-absorbing capacity will lead to further dysfunction and potential injury. Causes of reduced motion include infections, simple loading of an unaccustomed nature, overloading over time (increased training), and long-term loading of an accustomed nature (adaptive breakdown).

Joint dysfunctions involving changed positions are not often observed. In their simplest form, they may allow what seems to be a full range of motion at a particular joint, while the athlete complains of non-specific symptoms. At worst, alterations in joint position will retard the recovery of a joint and/or soft tissue injury. In either case rehabilitation exercises, due to their linear motions, can reinforce the joint dysfunction causing other structures and joints to 'adapt' leaving the athlete pain free. This does not improve the problem but distributes it, and is a precursor to recurrent injury. Figure 4.2 shows a series of joint dysfunction positions.

How do we detect these joint malpositions? The joint should be palpated and the palpatory findings interpreted in a three-dimensional anatomical manner. Certain questions should be asked before you begin, i.e.:

1. Is what I see normal for this athlete?
2. Is the motion the athlete is performing normal for this athlete?
3. Are there other 'non-complaint' areas that have abnormal motion?
4. Is what I feel normal for this athlete, compared with other tissues?
5. How much of this resting positional alteration is activity related?
6. Are the other joints, local and general, positionally adequate?

What does a malpositioned resting joint feel like? A joint is the meeting point of bones, so in a way joints do not exist, only the structures around them. They are 'housed' within other tissues, so the surrounding tissue is an indicator of resting position of joints. Certain questions should be asked as you put your hands on these joints while they are at rest, i.e.:

1. Is what I am feeling normal soft tissue resting tone?
2. Is what I am feeling just outside the joint area consistent with that inside the joint area?
3. Are opposite joints similar, for this athlete?
4. Are the activity adaptations within an acceptable range?

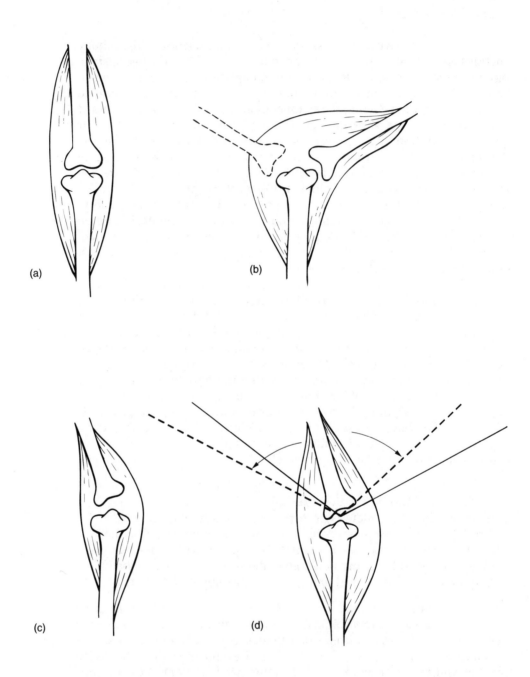

Fig. 4.2 Relation between joint position and range of motion. (a) Normal or neutral position. (b) Normal range of motion. (c) 'Rest' position in somatic dysfunction is displaced from neutral. (d) Range of motion in somatic dysfunction is also displaced, with loss of range toward the side away from the non-neutral rest position as compared with normal. (From van Buskirk, 1990.)

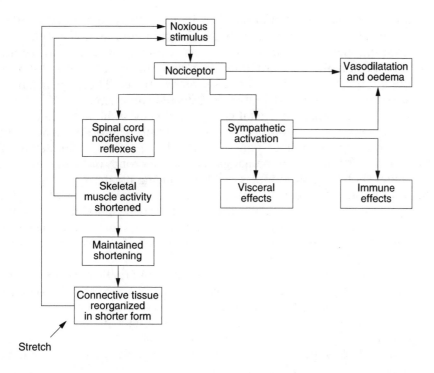

Fig. 4.3 Model of nociceptive origin and maintenance of the somatic dysfunction. (From van Buskirk, 1990.)

5. Do the bones and soft tissue meeting at this joint show continuity as I move my hands from one side of the joint to the other?

It is from this starting point that a three-dimensional static analysis is made. What positions can these alterations present? There are no rules, just trends based on anatomical limitations and functional adaptation. A joint can rest in any of the following positions or combinations thereof: flexion, extension, medial and lateral rotation, medial and lateral shift, anterior and posterior shift, compression, distraction, elevation, depression.

The points below present part of a model that should be the basis of thought for any osteopath in the field of sports medicine and it should be remembered and built upon.

The following model examines in a stepwise fashion how nociceptors might create the rich fabric of the somatic dysfunction (Fig. 4.3).

1. Minor trauma activates nociceptors in muscle, but probably not involving the whole muscle. Note that disease or trauma in any somatic or visceral structure will also produce nociceptor activation.
2. Nociceptor activation sends impulses to other axon branches of the same nociceptor and into the spinal cord.
3. Impulses in the axon branches release peptide transmitters producing vasodilatation, extravasation of fluid, and attrition of immune cells in

and near the site of trauma. The immune cells then release other chemicals, reinforcing local vasodilatation and extravasation and lowering the local threshold for nociception. Because nociceptor branches involve the initiating organ and other organs at a distance, the latter may also show the axon reflex effects. Thus, for instance, skeletal and heart muscle may be affected simultaneously.

4. Impulses entering the spinal cord synaptically stimulate spinal neurones. These spinal neurones can send impulses into the higher CNS for the appreciation of pain, or into the spinal interomediolateral system to stimulate the preganglionic autoneurones or finally, into the spinal skeletal muscle motor pool, producing nocifensive reflexes.

5. The pain, if perceived, may be poorly localized owing to the convergence of multiple sources on to the same spinal neurones and to the divergence of signals along neighbouring segments of the spinal cord. None the less, any pain and most reflex effects will be maximal in the segment of origin.

6. Most nociautonomic reflexes involve the sympathetic nervous system, with responses as diverse as cardiopressor, vasopressor or vasodilator effects; gastrointestinal stasis; or brochodilatation. The specific response will be based on the sympathetic effect in the segmentally targeted organ. Maintenance of sympathetic drive tends to be detrimental to the normal function of the organ(s) involved. Immune function will be diminished.

7. Nociceptive reflexes involve both specific segmental responses and often multisegmental attempts to minimize the noxious input by removing stress from the affected nociceptors. In some cases, the injured muscle will be shortened by action of its synergists or those fibres within the muscle that are not traumatized. In other cases, overlying muscle will contract to guard the underlying damaged structure. In general, the final determinant of muscle contraction in a nocifensive reflex is whatever will minimize the noxious drive at the spinal level.

8. Axon reflex and sympathetic vasodilatation effects engorge the affected muscles, producing direct mechanical restriction of motion. This occurs whether the muscles were the original source of injury or were involved secondarily, as in a viscerosomatic reflex. Tissue engorgement also stimulates local nociceptors, as do the tissue injury chemicals like serotonin, histamine, bradykinin and potassium chloride.

9. Now, any attempt to restretch the affected muscles to their normal (non-stretched) position will restress the original nociceptors and trigger activity in any others with lowered threshold. This positive feedback effect reinforces the guarding nocifensive reflexes. Keep in mind that the position best minimizing nociception in the case of a nociceptive reflex is not likely to be at the maximally shortened position for a muscle around a joint. This is true primarily because maintenance of such an extreme will inevitably increase the stress on other structures in the body, including both the antagonist muscles and any muscles needed to stabilize the severely out-of-balance body.

Thus, it is much more likely that titration of a noxious input will produce a new musculoskeletal relationship that is no longer in a neutral position, but not at the maximum range.

10. Continuing contraction of those muscles actively maintaining the shortened position will produce products of fatigue that also activate the nociceptors. This process will tend to recruit additional reinforcement for the abnormal position.

11. If the abnormal position of the joint is maintained by nocifensive reflexes for a period of time (probably measured in hours to a few days), the somatic dysfunction changes from acute to chronic. The significant indicator of this change is the onset of connective tissue reorganized by the tissue fibrocytes. In the shortened muscle, the connective tissue fibres will become more random in orientation and, therefore, less able to take stress along the ordinary lines of force. In the lengthened muscles, creep will elongate the connective tissue, producing slack without stressing the lengthened muscles. Now maintenance of the joint in the non-neutral position dictated by both the nocifensive reflexes and the connective tissue changes no longer requires continuous muscle activity. Active contraction would occur only whenever the system is stressed, reactivating nociceptors. However, because the adjusted position at the joint is neither gravitationally, positionally nor functionally balanced, such stresses will be chronic and recurrent, making it easier to produce nociceptor activation and possible perception of pain.

12. The somatic dysfunction is now in a state that includes significant resistance to motion in a direction counter to the original shortening (decrease range of motion), a chronic nociceptor activation that may or may not be perceived as pain, and continuous autonomic activation, producing visceral and immune deficits (Van Buskirk, 1990).

NEURAL DYSFUNCTION

Facilitated segment

Of central importance to the osteopathic principle is the concept of the 'facilitated segment'. However, this concept has become confused over the years. Many practitioners talk of vertebral levels that are tender and or oedematous as being facilitated. This is not true.

A facilitated segment is an area in the spinal cord which is subjected to a more or less continuous bombardment of afferent impulses which 'facilitates' or subliminally excites the motor neurone in that area of the spinal cord (Rumney, 1963). Acute lesions occurring in joints which are freely movable and subject to normal movement in many directions rarely persist long enough to become chronic; usually they are corrected by the normal movements of the joint. The science in which structural relations are recognized as being of chief importance in the aetiology of disease is called **osteopathic pathology** (Burns, 1933). Not all restricted joints are associated with the athlete's problem.

Trophic function

This is a topic that is vital to the furthering of the osteopathic concept, yet it is an area to which little attention has been paid, both physiologically and clinically.

In embryonic development, when the advancing axon tip of a peripheral neurone reaches and joins the cells it is to innervate, an intercellular partnership – a functional unit – is formed which endures for the life of the organism. The complete differentiation and continued growth and development of these cells and of organs they form are dependent upon the establishment and maintenance of the innervation. This has been demonstrated for skeletal muscles, various glands, sensory organs and viscera. When the neurone and the cells it supplies are separated, e.g. by cutting or crushing the nerve, changes begin in the denervated cells which may progress over periods of many days, or even months. These progressive changes may result in profoundly altered functional and morphologic characteristics; in impaired capacity for growth, healing and regeneration; and in altered enzyme activity, mitotic activity, metabolism and chemical composition (Korr, 1967).

We are taught that the nervous system innervates structures for movement and sensation. The word 'trophic' means that the nervous system 'feeds' the tissues at the end of its supply, i.e. viscera and skin. The nervous system is vital for the supply of nutrients to tissue for building after cell breakdown. Limiting these trophic effects can present as clinical changes, either acutely or chronically. Acute trophic affects are rare due to the fact that cell turnover is not immediate, but examples are Sudeck's atrophy and shoulder–arm–hand syndrome. Chronic changes due to trophic disturbance are seen far more in a clinical environment. These present as dryness, peeling and loss of elasticity of skin. This kind of condition is common on the back, hands and feet. Dryness is a consequence of skin breakdown and bleeding as the athlete scratches the dry, itchy skin. The usual approach is antibiotic and hydrocortisone cream. This condition can be very distressing for the athlete.

Case 2

A 26 year old woman, a local ice dancer, presented having developed itchy hands and feet. After a few months the skin was dry, bleeding and blistering. She had been prescribed antibiotics and hydrocortisone and told she had eczema due to walking a lot and putting her hands repeatedly in hot and cold water in the kitchen. She did not smoke and drank very little alcohol.

On examination of her spine she had extremely hypertonic paravertebral musculature from her occiput to her sacrum. However, she did not complain of back or neck pain. The skin on her back showed patches of dryness which she said she was always putting moisturing cream on. Passive ranges of spinal movement were good but the quality of movement was poor. Areas of particular attention were C1–C4, T1–T7 and T11–L3.

Her posterior hip musculature was also hypertonic. She also had erratic menstrual periods that were heavy when they occurred.

Treatment was directed at improving muscular tone and joint quality movement. Techniques chosen were cervical and lumbar traction, and HVT to upper cervicals, upper thoracic and upper lumbar region. Soft tissue treatment was cross-fibre stretch of very short duration, so as not to irritate the tissues. The objective was to reduce soft tissue tone and improve motion of joints. In this type of condition it is important to treat little and often so as not to 'give' the athlete back pain. The skin showed signs of healing and the itching had stopped within 24 hours.

If this kind of condition can happen in a clinically visual manner, then it may also occur non-visually, e.g. involving internal organs.

VASCULAR DYSFUNCTION

For a basic understanding of vascular dysfunction, I refer to Dr Harry M. Wright, DO, from Kirksville College of Osteopathy and Surgery, who wrote the following in 1956, in the *Journal of the American Osteopathic Association,* titled 'The Origins and Manifestation of Local Vasomotor Disturbance and their Clinical Significance'.

> Appreciation for the importance of 'lowered resistance' or functional impairment of a tissue resulting from an alteration in its circulation in the pathogenesis of infectious diseases is found in this statement of more than 30 years ago (1936) by Nedzel:
>
> In the modern trend of medical bateriology we are coming more and more to the concept that the mere presence of bacteria or their increased virulency is not always sufficient to cause an infection. Often it is necessary to have another factor, the so-called lowered resistance . . . no matter what its cause. This latter factor, first, permits the localisation of bacteria, and second, favors their activities, which are then accompanied with proper pathological changes in tissues of lowered resistance.
>
> How may local vascular disturbances act as a pathogenic mechanism?
>
> 1. By reduction in the functional reserve of an organ or tissue, that is, impairment of its capacity to respond to increased physiological demands. This is dramatically illustrated in a patient with coronary heart disease. The signs and symptoms of increased functional demands on an ischaemic myocardium are known only too well to both the patient and the physician to need enumeration here.
> 2. By lowering resistance to infection by bacteria or secondary invaders. Or, as Dubos expressed it, '. . . only when something happens which upsets the equilibrium between host and parasite does infection evolve into disease'. In this manner, local

vasomotor disturbances may play an important role in the pathogenesis of acute and chronic infectious diseases.

3. By alteration in the response of a tissue or viscus to normal nervous and hormonal influences. Such alterations in tissue response may mislead the physician because diagnostic signs and symptoms may be masked. For example, ischaemia of the stomach or duodenum may so alter response to the normal parasympathetic influence on secretion and motility that the symptoms may appear to be that of parasympathetic hyper-activity. This concept has previously been discussed by Korr.

4. By local vascular disturbances in any of the endocrine glands, which might conceivably act as a pathogenic mechanism producing widespread effects which might obscure their local origin. For example, an alteration in the circulation of the thyroid gland might directly influence its activity and thereby the metabolic activity of every cell in the body. An analogous situation might be cited for any of the endocrines.

5. By vascular disturbance in nervous tissue itself. An altered circulation through local areas of the brain, spinal cord, or the peripheral nerves may produce many, diverse, often remote, and diffuse effects.

LYMPHATIC DYSFUNCTION

This system should be considered on its own as the majority of system disturbances, from the common cold to cancer, involve the lymphatic system. No injury or infection, however small and insignificant, should be assessed without consideration of the lymphatic system. Just for a moment separate, in your mind, this system from the vascular and see how complete it is: the part the lymphatic system plays due to its close relationship to the tissues in nourishment, assimilation, secretion and elimination or purification; the entrance of this system into the infective areas and the immediate activities of the nodes and channels whether a finger is cut or a heel bruised; the long-tinted lines on the arm when blood is poisoned has started through an infected hand abrasion, the checking up and collecting of septic materials that help to prevent sudden poisoning; and greatest of all, the necessity of perfect vascular normality to assist the lymphatics functioning under stress (Millard, 1921).

OBJECTIVES OF OMT

The general indications for manipulative treatment are as follows.

1. For moving body fluids, especially to open arterial and neural channels and to promote better venous and lymphatic drainage.

2. For modification of somatosomatic reflex patterns, e.g. when a vertebral restriction results in muscle spasm about the area.

3. For modification of somatovisceral reflex patterns, illustrated by the vertebral restriction which creates excessive efferent flow over the autonomic nervous system and thus disturbs visceral function.
4. For modification of viscerosomatic reflex patterns in which afferents from a viscus activate the anterior horn cells to produce a somatic response in the paravertebral tissues.
5. For a tonic or bracing effect on circulation and general body function in the postoperative, acutely infectious or debilitated patient.
6. For maintenance care when somatic dysfunction is recurrent because of circumstances that cannot be eliminated. Palliative measures, usually at regular intervals, are required to prevent escalation of demands on the patient's accommodation mechanisms and to de-escalate them temporarily (Kimberly, 1980).

GENERAL AND SKIN INFECTIONS

The presentation of an infection is the result of a breakdown in the homeostatic balance between infection or invasion of the microorganism and facilitation of the individual to suit the conditions for invasion (see Vascular dysfunctions, p. 195). The majority of athletes have an efficient immune system that enables them to live with air-borne, food-borne, and water-borne microorganisms. Once a diagnosis is made, the osteopath must formulate the prescription of treatment and the various approaches it should take, e.g. nutrition, medication, hygiene, manipulation.

Prevention

The general avenues of infection are:

- the athletic environment
- athlete–athlete contact
- equipment–athlete contact
- nutrition
- infection within the athlete.

The athletic environment

Some simple precautions will reduce the risk of infection in the changing showering environment. Disinfect the changing and showering rooms and connecting passages before and after the game. The medical room should also be cleaned, in the morning, at lunch time and before closing for the day (or as required). Athletes will walk around barefooted in the medical room, skin is exposed, and unwell athletes may be more susceptible to air-borne microbes. Neither of these cleaning procedures has to be a major undertaking on a daily basis. A plastic refillable spray bottle should be filled with disinfectant and warm water. (Do not forget to write on the bottle that it is disinfectant, so that it is not mistaken for anything else.)

You can then move around fairly quickly spraying and wiping surfaces, including the floor. It is advisable that the floor is not carpet but lino or some other easily cleaned surface.

Changing rooms, and also rooms where indoor sports are performed, should always have some form of ventilation. Dance studios are notably poor regarding ventilation.

Playing fields where there is public access present a potential hazard when dogs are walked and allowed to defecate.

Athlete–athlete contact

Methods of cross-infection between athletes are usually indirect, via air, dust, water and skin-to-skin contact.

Air-borne infection is usually transmitted by droplets. The method of transmission is by small droplets of protein-covered microbes that are small enough to be carried by air currents, while larger protein-covered microbes settle on surfaces, clothing and nutrients. Dust-borne infection includes *Staphylococcus aureus* which may lie in dust for some time. Poor quality water is a health risk. Physical contact may transmit warts for example, which can be just by shaking hands.

Equipment–athlete contact

Sharing equipment is common, and can spread infection. This is known as transmission by fomites, i.e. by inanimate objects. Transmission by used towels is one of the most usual; others include footwear, shorts, 'athletic supports', socks, water bottles, etc. Sharing of drinking vessels is another method of cross-infection; a way to prevent this is to have water bottles that have pull-out spouts, so that the athlete can jet the fluid into his or her mouth without contact with the container.

Nutrition

Food, milk and water that are not cooked properly or stored incorrectly are a nutritional hygiene risk. Food preparation should be overseen by the medical staff, especially when food is being cooked under non-hotel conditions (although some hotels also need to be looked at). Someone from the medical team should check the kitchens, subtly, when travelling, especially abroad. Storage of milk is especially important; if in doubt throw it away.

Infection within the athlete

Where an athlete has contracted an infection, further transmission within the athlete can occur, e.g. *Staph. aureus* infection can be transmitted by the bloodstream leading to an infective endocarditis.

Skin infections

Let us briefly look at the most common skin infections and some of the
treatment approaches.

Viral infections

- Ultra-microscopic organisms.
- Reside as parasites within systems.
- Main types: herpes, warts and molluscum contagiosum.

1. Herpes simplex – cold sores:
   - initiated from herpes virus strain;
   - most common on back, nose, ears, mouth and genitals;
   - yellowish, itchy, crust-like lesions;
   - pain and lymph gland swelling possible;
   - always present – resistance low – herpes;
   - treatment: camphor, alum, alcohol, silver nitrate, over-the-counter
     preparations.
2. Verruca vulgeria – warts:
   - raised, rough surfaces, contagious;
   - several types, seed warts, small black dots;
   - subject to bacterial disorders;
   - treatment: removal by a physician – should be left alone during
     season.
3. Verruca plantaris – plantar warts:
   - sole of foot, palm of hand;
   - fallen metatarsal arch or bruise to foot;
   - corn-like appearance – painful, hard, point tenderness with long
     roots;
   - treatment: surgical removal.
4. Venereal warts:
   - form on genitals;
   - foul, yellowish smell;
   - not as a result of sexual contact;
   - treatment: surgical removal.
5. Molluscum contagiosum:
   - forms on skin, especially hands and face;
   - small papules or beads that have a dimple in the centre;
   - may appear along a scratch, Koebner's lines;
   - treatment: there are many over-the-counter preparations

Bacterial infections

- Single celled, plant-like microorganisms.
- For example staphylococci or streptococci.

1. Impetigo:
   - initiated by both staphylococci and streptococci;
   - skin infection, common in swimming and wrestling;

- small pustules form yellowish crust lesions;
- highly contagious:
- treatment:
  - thorough cleansing, 4–5 ×/day;
  - warm water/vinegar;
  - boric acid;
  - dry area completely;
  - antibiotic cream.

2. Furuncle – boils:
   - occur from hair follicle irritations;
   - staphylococci strain forms pustules;
   - back and neck common areas;
   - red, hard, enlarged;
   - mature and rupture spontaneously – pus (yellow);
   - highly contagious;
   - treatment: should not be squeezed, use hot towels, treat like an open wound.

3. Carbuncle – multiple boils:
   - also staphylococci;
   - larger and deeper with several openings;
   - may produce fever;
   - treatment: surgical drainage and antibiotics.

4. Folliculitis – hair follicle:
   - ingrown hair, beards, infects hair follicle;
   - 'barber's' itch;
   - more prevelant in black athletes;
   - treatment: use chemical hair remover, not razor blades.

5. Acne – pimples:
   - acute adolescent problem;
   - combination of blackheads, pustules and cystis;
   - precipitating factors include diet, emotion etc.;
   - emotional problems may develop;
   - treatment: keep clean and medicate.

6. Hordeolum – sty:
   - eyelash follicle;
   - usually staphylococci;
   - starts with redness of eyelash;
   - pustules in a few days;
   - treatment:
     - hot towels and 1% yellow oxide of mercury;
     - chronic – consult physician.

Fungal infections (trichophyton or epidermophyton)

- Grow in warm, dark, moist areas, unsanitary.
- Common name ringworm or tinae.
- Named after area of body.

- Superficial skin – highly contagious.
- Chronic fungal infection use Whitfield's Ointment (benzoic acid compound).

1. Tinae pedis – 'athelete's foot':
   - trichophyton tubrum fungus;
   - contagious – also depends on athelete's susceptibility;
   - extreme itching on the soles of the feet, between the toes;
   - rash with small pimples – yellowish serum;
   - treatment:
     - keep dry and cool;
     - mild hydrogen peroxide – antifungal – or salicylic acid in isopropal alcohol;
     - standard antifungal spray – Tinactin etc.;
     - standard antifungal powder – Micil etc.;
     - best action is prevention;
     - never wear same shoes every day, keep in cool place (storage);
     - treatment regimen may take around 21 days.
2. Tinae capitis – head:
   - common in young;
   - starts on scalp and spreads;
   - from contaminated animals, barber's clippers, combs;
   - treatment: best treated systemically by a physician.
3. Tinae corporis – upper extremities (ringworm):
   - ring-shaped, reddish vesicular areas;
   - may be scaly and crusty;
   - excessive perspiration – susceptibility;
   - treatment: Whitfield's Ointment.
4. Tinae ungulum – toenails:
   - particularly in water sports athletes;
   - like chronic athlete's foot;
   - nail thickens and separates from base;
   - treatment: mild hydrogen peroxide, Whitfield's Ointment etc.
5. Tinae cruris – 'jock rash or itch':
   - unilateral or bilateral in groin area;
   - brownish, reddish lesion;
   - itching mild to moderate;
   - must be treated until cured;
   - treatment:
     - Tinactin – OTC medications;
     - powder for groin area;
     - prevention is best method;
     - keep area dry and clean.

Parasitic infections

1. Mites:
   - ticks, suck blood from system;

- bury in skin;
- can spread encephalitis;
- treatment: OTC and prescribed medications, e.g. malathion lotion.

2. Lice – head and body:
   - can be contracted anywhere;
   - dark, warm areas – clothing;
   - treatment: Kwell shampoo, day 1 and day 7 and malathion lotion, normal hygiene in between.

REFERENCES

Burns, L. (1933) Principles of therapy dependent on the osteopathic pathology of sprains and strains. *Journal of the American Osteopathic Association*, **July**, 100–2.

Collins, M. (1994) Towards a physiology of the myofacsial system. *Journal of Osteopathic Education*, **4**(2), 108–12.

Hoag, J.M., Cole, W.V. and Bradford, S.G. (1969) *Osteopathic Medicine*, McGraw-Hill, New York.

Kalik, J.R. (1989) Fibromyalgia: diagnosis and treatment of an important rheumatologic condition. *Journal of Osteopathic Medicine*, **3** (2) 10–19.

Ketterer, M.W. and Buckholt, C.D. (1989) Somatization disorder. *Journal of the American Osteopathic Association*, **89**(4), 489–99.

Kimberly, P.E. (1980) Formulating a prescription for osteopathic manipulative treatment. *Journal of the American Osteopathic Association*, **79**(8), 506/43–513/50.

Korr, I.M. (1967) The nature and basis of the trophic function of nerves: outline of a research program. Axonal transport and trophic studies. *The Collected Papers of I.M. Korr*, American Academy of Osteopathy.

Korr, I.M. (1975) Proprioceptors and somatic dysfunction. *Journal of the American Osteopathic Association*, **74**, 638–50.

Millard, F.P. (1921) Applied anatomy of the lymphatics. *Journal of the American Osteopathic Association*, **May**, 489–91.

Rumney, I.C. (1963) Structural diagnosis and manipulative therapy. *Journal of Osteopathy*, **January**, 21–33.

Shutty, M.S., Cundiff, G. and DeGood, D.E. (1992) Pain complaint and the weather: weather sensitivity and symptom complaints in chronic pain patients. *Pain*, **49**, 199–204.

Van Buskirk, R.L. (1990) Nociceptive reflexes and the somatic dysfunction: a model. *Journal of the American Osteopathic Association*, **90**(9), 792–809.

Vengrove, M.A. and Adelizzi, R.A. (1986) Eosinophilic fasciitis. *Journal of the American Osteopathic Association*, **86** (8), 508/81–510/83.

Williams, P.E., Catanese, T., Lucey, E.G. and Goldspink, G. (1988) The importance of stretch and contractile activity in the prevention of connective tissue accumulation in muscle. *Journal of Anatomy*, **158**, 109–14.

5 | History and clinical evaluation

HISTORY TAKING

Perhaps the most fundamental difference between medieval and modern medicine is that the former was primarily based on pure empiricism directed by mysticism and intuition, whereas the latter attempts to understand the mechanisms of disease – through an objective scientific analysis – and to treat it by influencing well-defined points along the pathways of its development. Up to the present time, the greatest progress that has been made along these lines has resulted in specific therapeutic procedures that are designed to eliminate in each case the particular primary cause – the eliciting pathogen of a disease . . .

By contrast, throughout the centuries, we have learned virtually nothing about rational, scientifically well-defined procedures that would help the body in its own natural efforts to maintain health quite apart from the attacks on the pathogen . . . Let us remember that it is not the microbe, the poison or the allergen, but our reaction to these agents that we experience as disease.

(Selye, 1955)

Screening and medical records

This is possibly the most important part of the care of athletes. Case histories and previous medical examination results should be available for all athletes, rather than waiting for an injury and then attempting to obtain the information. It is not uncommon for a young athlete to come to me with one problem, e.g. an ankle sprain, and I have then found, through a case history, that they have chronic chest problems that are not being treated. A young athlete with a chronic chest problem tires easily, making them potential victims of accidents. The job of the team osteopath should be to promote health and make a contribution to the future of the athlete. The team osteopath should not only look for disqualifying conditions, but conditions that can be improved upon, enhancing the athletic potential of the young athlete.

The preparticipation examination should be general.

1. General case history. Does the athlete look well?
2. Orthopaedic assessment.

(a) Joint, bone or soft tissue injuries?

(b) Ranges of joint movement – start with the axial skeleton and move out. This should be broken down into active, passive and active resisted. You are looking for joint range and especially quality of motion.

(c) Palpate areas of soft tissue that may seem to limit quality of motion; there may be an old injury that the athlete forgot to tell you about.

(d) Flexibility tests will help you to advise the athlete on what should be stretched.

3. Cardiovascular assessment.

(a) Infections and illnesses that could affect heart function (see Thorax, p. 294).

(b) Upper limits of blood pressure not requiring evaluation (Strong, 1979): 130/75 mmHg for children 11 years and younger; 140/85 mmHg for children 12 years and older.

(c) Children and adolescents with mild elevation of blood pressure should be re-evaluated every week to establish a range of values. They should also be exercise stress tested with mild or moderate hypertension (Silver *et al.*, 1983).

3. Neurologic assessment.

(a) Past cranial and spinal trauma.

(b) Concussions depend on the amount of time unconscious and the number of concussions (see Chapter 6).

(c) Cranial and spinal operations (postsurgical).

(d) Depending on the type of operation, they should refrain from all activity until cleared by a neurologist.

(e) Extremity examination.

Disqualifying conditions

Following any examination that reveals a disqualifying condition there is nearly always some degree of compromise that can be made with the athlete. This ranges from reducing activity to changing activity. It is important that if you advise an athlete to give up an activity you spend time to explain why. Always tell them that it is your opinion and that you would be happy for them to get a second opinion. Psychologically, it can be devastating and can easily send the athlete into a state of depression. Advice about not taking part in any particular sport naturally depends on the presenting condition and the sport; for example, an athlete with an enlarged liver should not be involved in contact/collision sports, an athlete with one ovary need not be disqualified from anything, and an athlete with a heart defect will have to be individually assessed.

Female athletes

Certain questions can be asked specifically of female athletes. Parents or guardians should be in attendance if they are under 18 years of age.

1. How old were you when you had your first menstrual period?
2. How often do you have a period?
3. How long do your periods last?
4. How many periods have you had in the last 12 months?
5. When was your last period?
6. Do you ever have trouble with heavy bleeding?
7. Do you have questions about tampon use?
8. Do you ever experience cramps during your period? If so, how do you treat them?
9. Do you take birth control pills or hormones?
10. Do you have any unusual discharge from your vagina?
11. When was your last pelvic examination?
12. Have you ever had an abnormal PAP smear?
13. How many urinary tract infections (bladder or kidney) have you had?
14. Have you ever been treated for anaemia?
15. How many meals do you eat each day? How many snacks?
16. What have you eaten in the last 24 hours?
17. Are there certain food groups you refuse to eat (e.g. meat, bread)?
18. Have you ever been on a diet?
19. What is your present weight?
20. Are you happy with this weight? If not, what would you like to weigh?
21. Have you ever tried to control your weight by vomiting? Using laxatives? Diuretics? Diet pills?
22. Have you ever been diagnosed as having an eating disorder?
23. Do you have questions about healthy ways to control weight?
24. Do you have any questions about any aspect of your health or training?

(Adapted from Johnson, 1992.)

It is very important when looking after a group of athletes to have a certain amount of medical history before they participate in any activity. This is especially relevant when travelling abroad. From these medical records provision can be made in advance with regard to possible risk factors, dietary and medication needs, blood type, and in the case of children a disclaimer, so that a decision can be made in the absence of communication with a parent or guardian.

An example of a general medical history sheet to be filled out before participation is shown on pages 207–8.

All histories should be directed to an evaluation of the patient's general health first and then to their specific complaint. The osteopath should always consider the psychological status, autonomic nervous system and clinical presentation when taking a case history.

When taking a history in an athletic environment it is important that you are not disturbed and the initial consultation is in a one-on-one situation. It should be in complete confidence with no other players or

British American Football Association
Junior Great Britain National Team
Medical History

For us to take care of you properly it is important that you fill in this form as accurately as possible. Please write clearly (capital letters) and in black or blue ink.

- -

Full name:..
Date of Birth: (D) ... (M) ... (Y) ... Telephone number: ....
Address: ....
....
....

- -

General Health
Please read this carefully, before answering the questions.
Have you or do you suffer from any of the following conditions recently or regularly or for any period of time in the past. Only tick the line if the answer is yes.
Headaches and/or migraines ... Blindness ... Deafness ... Loss of smell ... Sore throats ... Asthma ... Bronchitis ... Chest infections ... Heart conditions ... Blood pressure ... Diabetes ... Glandular fever ... Eczema ... Skin infections (acne) ... Athlete's foot ... Constipation ... Diarrhoea ... Kidney injury ... Kidney infections ...

- -

Medications (if any), name and dose
....
....
Blood type (if known): ...
Have you ever been told that you should not participate in contact sports, for any medical reasons? ...
If yes, please give details ....
....

- -

Have you ever had any injury to the following that you have had to visit hospital or have treatment for?

1. Head: History of injury NO ... YES ...
2. Neck and spine: History of injury NO ... YES ...

- -

Do you have any medical needs that could be arranged for you ahead of time or when we arrive at our destination?
....
....
....

Are there any specific foods or drinks that you specifically do not like or are allergic to?

....

....

....

- -

Next of kin (parent or guardian)

Name: ....

Address: ....

....

Telephone: Day .... Night .... Weekends ....

Address: ....

....

Signature: ....

Date: ....

Walter Llewellyn McKone, DO, MRO   30 July 1991

Below is an example of a daily treatment session record sheet. This is filled in by the practitioner every time there is a treatment and/or examination session, for your own records.

British Youth
American Football Association

Injury Report Sheet No ......

Date .... Time ....

Weather .... Temp ....

Name	Injury/Area	TTT/Medication

....

....

....

....

....

Below is an example of a daily report sheet. This is filled in after morning and/or evening treatment and/or examination sessions and handed to coaching staff for their information.

British Youth
American Football Association

Daily Injury Report

Date .... AM/PM.

Name	Injury/Area	Go/No Go/Limited Practice

....

....

....

....

....

coaching staff within earshot. If you are called to review an athlete's status this should be in the presence of the initial therapist. Here you can:

1. review the initial history;
2. listen to the athlete's story,
3. listen to the therapist's story.

Listen to the athlete to help make things clear. Do not put words into their mouths, but at the same time it is important to shape an image of what has happened that you both agree on. It is just as important to understand the athlete as it is for the athlete to understand your approach. This is where a vocabulary of training techniques and playing methods is invaluable.

Observation and conversation

On meeting your patient for the first time it is important to observe the following:

- style, state and type of clothes worn;
- personal hygiene and grooming;
- posture;
- ease of movement;
- hair and skin condition;
- does the patient look you in face when talking? Too little or too much?

First impressions are important as an immediate yard stick which may influence your later assessment of the patient. Even before you formally take the case history you may like to take note of how well the patient converses in small talk.

Basic information

This should include age, sex, height, weight and address. A description of the illness, injury or training problems in the athlete's own words is important. They should be allowed to speak freely as this will allow you to assess their emotional status in connection with their problem. Control of the conversation after a few minutes is important as this will allow you to form a model of the needs of the athlete, thus enabling you to make the appropriate first steps. It is important that you do not form an opinion too early. A degree of indecision allows for flexibility. Develop your history along the following structure.

Present complaint

It is useful to begin the history with, 'what can I do for you?' Again it is important to let the athlete speak for at least a minute before you interupt, unless they are have problems describing their complaint. Then try and control the conversation, especially if there is more than one problem. Make them show you (indicate) where the pain, ache or discomfort is. Get them to describe how it feels: gnawing, gripping, sharp etc. Information regarding the intensity, radiation and duration will help to come to an area and related tissue diagnosis.

Onset

This is a description of the beginning of the symptoms and/or signs of the condition. Within the course of history taking try to elicit the mechanism of injury. This may be a specific event or less specific repeated minor trauma. Repeated minor trauma events are rarely the same actions; but they are actions that affect the same tissue. This makes it even more difficult for the athlete to remember what happened.

Often the athlete will not recognize the relevance of the repeated action. Get the athlete to indicate where the problem is while you are taking the history. What the patient calls the coccyx may be the lower lumbars to you. Was the onset of symptoms sudden or gradual?

Times of the day

Patterns of the signs and symptoms in a 24 hour period should be sought, if there are any. Does the athlete sweat at any time, day or night? If so when is this worst?

Activity relations

What actions aggravate, relieve or do not aggravate the signs and symptoms? The length of time the situation is made worse, the recovery pattern (e.g. immediately or gradually) and what actions the athlete takes to control the situation should also be asked.

Daily pattern

Daily patterns in pain and discomfort should be noted. For example, is it worse in the morning, afternoon or evening? This information can be combined to give a weekly trend in symptoms, especially temperature variations. Chronic spinal or limb pain may be a function (past or present) of movement patterns.

Past medical history

This is important, especially in musculoskeletal pain. Past history of events as far back as childhood are vital in forming a picture of possibilities. Many non-sports events will present themselves as sports-related incidents many months or years later. This is why a general history is vital before becoming specific. These events include trauma, illness, systemic complications (CVS, respiratory etc.), allergies, operations etc.

Family history

How is the health of the rest of the athlete's family? Are his or her parents, brothers and sisters well? Are there any disorders that run in the family?

Past treatments, tests and medications

Has the complaint been treated before, if so by whom and what tests were performed? Treatments could have been by qualified or unqualified practitioners. What drugs have been administered by the therapist? Have any drugs been self-administered? Previous tests should be noted, e.g. X-rays and blood screens, and how long ago they were performed.

Socioeconomic status

Athletes will probably come from different socioeconomic backgrounds, especially in amateur team sports.

Nutritional status

Is the athlete manipulating his or her diet too much in an attempt to control weight? Are they keeping to basic healthy principles or trying out some new fad? Many athletes do not understand the significance of fluid replacement. Alcohol and tobacco intakes (including chewing) should be assessed.

Important: Always take the athlete's general state of health into consideration first, after they have described their signs and symptoms. Make sure that the signs and symptoms are not expressions of general or specific infections. Make sure that the signs and symptoms are not expressions of individual or combined systemic dysfunctions, e.g. thrombosis or otitis media. Ask questions along these lines before forming any opinion of the athlete's problems. Stay open minded, observe the facts, and form a mental model of the athlete's problem. Stay mentally agile. The osteopathic sieve (Fig. 5.1) will help to think in a structured approach. **Remember**, it is very rare that one structure is the cause of the patient's symptoms. All structures and emotional levels make a contribution to the athlete's presentation. An injury happens to an area of the athlete, not to one structure. All the structures in and travelling through that area will be affected.

Does the athlete seem physically and physiologically suited to their particular activities? It is important that the osteopath puts him or herself in the best possible position to treat the athlete. Do not assume that they know how to do things properly. The majority of athletes, amateur and professional, believe they are doing the best for themselves; however, they get most of their information from other athletes.

Ask about the following preventive measures:

- Hydration: water is important as we have seen.
- Dehydration: ingestion of diuretic fluids is counterproductive.

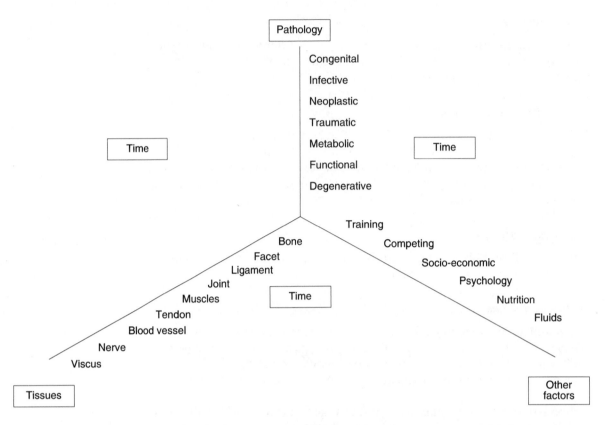

Fig. 5.1 Theoretical three-dimensional axis of a 'sieve' for factors and their combinations considered in diagnosis. (Adapted from Smith, 1984.)

- Flexibility: many athletes believe that they are doing enough stretching and in the right way.
- Strength training: many strength programmes are poorly worked out, and can even disrupt athletic potential.
- Type of anaerobic and aerobic training: ask for a brief description of their routine and the number of times carried out per week. For example, half an hour a week of anaerobic exercise without aerobic exercising is potentially dangerous.

Aetiology

This means the cause of the problem. As Edward J. Stieglitz, distinguished geriatrist, stated, 'The concept of specific aetiology, so finely phrased by Koch in his postulates and blindly followed by generations of bacteriologists and clinicians, has retarded progress in aetiologic analysis for many years.' In the allopathic view, disease is equated with pathogenic agents – disease is produced by the action of a given pathogenic agent and is characteristic of that agent. In short, there are as many diseases or kinds of diseases as there are 'aetiologies'. From this viewpoint it is natural that the therapeutic attention of the physician should be focused on the aetiological agent or its effects. He has essentially only two therapeutic alternatives: first, if possible, remove the pathogenic agent or block its action and trust that with the aid of supportive measures, the effects of that agent will somehow be reversed; second, if failing to identify or remove the pathogenic agent, then apply other agents or measures which tend to produce opposite effects. Indeed the true meaning of the word 'allopathy' is other or opposite effect or affection (Korr, 1962).

'Things do not just jump out and grab you. You have to help by altering the environment for the pathogen' (Haynes, 1980).

Provisional diagnosis

It is always useful to make a few provisional diagnoses. This does not mean you deviate from your examination procedure, but allows you to build your protocols for being able to make educated judgements. If further examination proves you wrong then find out why. If your judgement was correct then find out why.

EXAMINATION AND EVALUATION

Clinical procedures: General systems examination, e.g. cardiorespiratory, neural etc. Structural procedures:

- Standing – landmarks, symmetry, tone, movement.
- Sitting – changes from standing, activity and passive exam.
- Lying – active and passive exam.
- Considering the sports and psychological status of the athlete.
- Use of case histories as examples.
- Aetiology and predisposing factors.
- Prescribing OMT, medications, rehabilitation etc., based on an understanding of altered physiology. Treatment modalities.
- All first time consultations should include a general systems examination.
- Examination procedures of the unwell athlete.

On numerous occasions you will be told by an athlete that they just feel a little under the weather. After you have asked them about their general health it is important to have a system of examination that you always use. Try the following general steps.

1. Observation. Look at the athlete generally. Is the light-skinned athlete pale/yellow; is the dark-skinned athlete musky/ashen looking? These are extremes, so it is important to practise observations in this skin spectrum. Check temperature of forehead with back of hand. Listen to their speech, to detect any changes.

2. Eyes. Check the colour of the eyes, the conjunctivae for anaemia and the sclera for jaundice. Palpate eyes for equal ocular pressure. Check pupillary reflexes, speed of light responses (symmetry) and fundus.

3. Ears. Look for external signs of ear infection, e.g. weeping, crusty skin as in otitis externa. Check drum and canal for obstructions and infection.

4. Mouth and tongue. Look at the tongue for signs of smooth, cyanotic, furring, fissuring and fungal plaques. Look in the mouth and throat for swelling, paleness, fungal plaques and ulcers.

5. Shake and put a clinical thermometer in the athlete's mouth.

6. Starting at the fingertips, check the nails by looking at their structure, press the nails to blanch them and see how quickly they return to their original colour. Hold both hands and gently squeeze and palpate them. Watch the patient's face. Assess the skin of the palms for sweating, contracture, blanching in spots, breaks in the skin and paronychia. Are the fingers exceptionally long or clubbed? Are the fingers and joints very flexible on passive motion examination? Check the pulse for rate and rhythm in synchronization with the rate of breathing. Palpate and observe the upper extremities for tenderness (soft tissue and bone), palpatory tissue quality, breaks in the skin, temperature extremes, lumbs and bumps. Check passive and active joint motions and reflexes.

7. Examine the neck. Observe asymmetry in trachea, oedema, distension and tracheal movement on swallowing, check lymph nodes (submandibular, neck, axillary, occipital) and the neck (goitre).

8. Remove thermometer and read temperature.

9. Check blood pressure.

10. Begin a broad cardiovascular system and respiratory exam. Sit athlete at 45° (jugular venous pressure), assess character of carotid pulse. Palpate root of neck, thorax for parasternal heaves and thrills, symmetry expansion/recoil of rib cage. Auscultate thorax and carotids. Check lung sounds (diaphragm), percussion, heart apex (bell) and carotids (diaphragm).

11. Discuss and examine breast tissue.

12. Observe, palpate and auscultate abdomen and groin. Observe oedema, distension, pulsations and continuity. Compare both sides of the groin. Palpate for tenderness, lymph glands, pulses, hardness and gaps in tissue. Auscultate for sounds.

13. Examine lower extremities starting with a general observation. Check for oedema, loss of definition, colour changes, vascularity, deformity, sweating and breaks in the skin. Palpate for tenderness, pulses, extremes in temperature change, soft tissue tone and lymph glands. Check for signs of infection, especially between the toes (athlete's foot) and nails (ingrown toenails). Hold and squeeze the feet (metatarsalgia). Carry out passive and active joint examination and check reflexes.

14. Spinal and paravertebral structures. Have patient lying prone. Observe skin for colour and signs of infection, oedema (thoracic to

sacrum), symmetry and hair. Palpate for sweating, oedema and tenderness of soft tissue tone and spinous processes, and spasms.

15. Have patient stand. Check posture, gait, balance (eyes closed index finger to nose, lifting leg into air) and active spinal, neck and shoulder movements.
16. Test urine sample and blood erythrocyte sedimentation rate.
17. Follow up any areas where you feel further investigation is warranted.

Structural examination

The structural examination begins with the athlete undressed down to their underwear or shorts. The structural examination covers observation, palpation, active movements, passive movements and active resisted movements.

1. Examination should begin with a standing exam. The athlete should be observed standing in four positions: posterior, anterior and both lateral aspects. The most common mistake by the osteopathic student is standing too close to the athlete, so that an overall impression cannot be achieved.
2. Observation: note skin colour, acne, moles, hair distribution, weight bearing, muscle tone, fascial drag, bony landmarks, shoulder and pelvic levels and rotation, limb rotation, spinal curves.
3. Palpation: note sweating, skin tone, fascial tone, muscle tone etc.
4. Active movements: spinal and neck movements are generally looked at first, followed by limb movements.
5. Sitting: while in the sitting position changes in pelvic, shoulder, spinal and muscular elements should be noted. All accessible tissue should be palpated for tone changes and enlargements, auscultated, percussed, hammered and looked into. Active, passive and active resisted movements should be reviewed, especially for examination of the thorax, neck (and spine), head and upper extremity.
6. Lying: supine examinations are carried out for the upper and lower extremities, face, neck, thorax, abdomen, pelvis and lower extremities; prone examinations are for the shoulders, spine, pelvis, lower extremities. All should follow the same procedures.

REFERENCES

Haynes, R.W. (1980) Personal communication, British School of Osteopathy.

Johnson, M.D. (1992) Tailoring the preparticipation examination to female athletes. *The Physician and Sports Medicine*, **20**(7), 61–72.

Korr, I.M. (1962) The somatic approach to the disease process. *Journal of Osteopathy*, **January**, 16–24.

Selye, H. (1955) Stress and disease. *Science*, **122**, 625–31.

Silver, H.K., Kempe, C.H. and Bruyn, H.B. (1983) *Handbook of Pediatrics*, 14th edn. Lange, California.

Smith, A.E. (1984) *Osteopathic Diagnosis*. British School of Osteopathy, London.

Strong, W.B. (1979) Hypertension in sports. *Pediatrics*, **64**, 693.

Regional trauma, dysfunction and treatment

6

. . . there is probably no better experimental or research laboratory
for human trauma in the world than the football fields of of our
nation.

R.C. Schnider, Head and Neck Injuries in Football,
University of Michigan

INTRODUCTION

Football is responsible for more injury and trauma than most other
contact sports. The large number of players and psychological extremes
add to this. Injuries to the head, neck and other areas are often seen. Under
these circumstances it is important to develop a systematic approach to the
injured athlete. This chapter is a basic overview of what I consider to be
some of the important factors in a basic understanding and approach to
injury and dysfunction. This is based on osteopathic principles and
approaches taught to me by members of the National Athletic Trainers'
Association from the National Football League, to whom I am in debt.

Anatomy is vital in osteopathy, where one of the basic principles is the
structure–function relationship. Each of the following sections on the
different anatomical regions begins with a review of anatomy, which
should not be bypassed.

THE HEAD

Anatomy

Bones

Bones of the head are divided into the cranial (eight bones), facial (14
bones) and miscellaneous (seven bones) portions.

- Cranial: occiput, sphenoid, ethmoid, frontal, temporals (2) and
  parietals (2).

- Facial: vomer, mandible, maxillae (2), palatines (2), zygomatics (2), lacrimals (2), nasals (2) and inferior conchae (2).
- Miscellaneous: ossicles (6) and hyoid.

Ossification of cranial bones

Occiput This ossifies in two main parts. First, the squamous part is formed from fibrous membrane, which is made from an upper (interparietal) and a lower (supra-occipital) portion separated by an interparietal line, coming in laterally to medially from both sides. Ossification centres appear one on either side of the median line in the second month of intra-uterine life. The interparietal line fuses about the third month of intra-uterine life, but may persist throughout life. Second, the rest of the occiput ossifies in cartilage.

Sphenoid The body, lesser wings, root of the greater wing (including its down growth) and the lateral pterygoid lamina develop in cartilage. The rest of the greater wing and the medical pterygoid lamina develop in membrane. At birth the sphenoid consists of three sections: the central body and lesser wings, and two lateral sections made up of the greater wings and pterygoid processes. In the first year the greater wings and the body unite; the lesser wings meet above the body forming an elongated smooth surface. The process of ossification of the sphenoid is complete by about the 25th year.

Ethmoid Ossification is in cartilage from three centres, one for the perpendicular plate and one from each labyrinth. About the fourth and fifth months of intra-uterine life the centres of each appear. At birth the two labyrinths are partially ossified while the rest of the bone is cartilaginous. The perpendicular plate and the crista galli begin to ossify from a single centre in the first year after birth. They then fuse with the labyrinths during the beginning of the second year.

Frontals Ossified from fibrous membranous tissue from two centres appearing about the eighth week of intra-uterine life. At birth the bone is separated by a metopic suture which begins to unite about the second year, fusing by about the eight year.

Temporals These form from four independent centres. The squamous part ossifies in membranous condensed mesenchyme, about the seventh to eighth week of intra-uterine life. The petromastoid part forms from several centres appearing in the cartilaginous otic capsule, about the fifth month of intra-uterine life. The tympanic part forms in collagenous fibrous tissue, about the third month of intra-uterine life. At birth this is present as an incomplete tympanic ring. The styloid process ossifies from the cranial end of the cartilage of the hyoid arch.

Parietals Each bone ossifies from two centres about the seventh week of intra-uterine life in fibrous, condensed mesenchyme. These centres unite early, while ossification radiates towards the margins of the bone. The angles of the bones are the last parts to ossify, thus forming the fontanelles at birth.

Ossification of facial bones

Vomer Early in intra-uterine life the nasal area consists of a plate of cartilage. It forms the antero-inferior part of this cartilage, in a strata of connective tissue that the vomer ossifies. Around the eighth week two ossification centres appear, one on each side of the median plane. About the 12th week the centres unite forming the cartilage septum of the nose. At about puberty the lamella are completely united.

Mandible This is the second bone of the body to begin to ossify (sixth intra-uterine week) in dense fibrous cartilage. Both halves of the jaw have their own single centres of ossification. These centres appear in the membrane overlying the anterior half of Meckle's cartilage (the cartilage of the mandibular arch), near the mental foremen about the sixth week of intra-uterine life. The mandible is in two halves at birth, and is united in the median plane by fibrous tissue, the symphasis.

Maxillae This paired bone develops from a single sheet of mesenchymal tissue, from a single centre. There are two or more premaxillary centres.

Palatines These ossify in membranous connective tissue from one centre of ossification. The centre appears during the eighth week of intra-uterine life. The palatine bones are made up of a horizontal plate, perpendicular plate, orbital process and a sphenoidal process.

Zygomatics Each zygomatic (cheek) bone ossifies from one centre, from a fibrous tissue precursor about the eighth week of intra-uterine life.

Lacrimals These ossify from one centre, appearing about the twelfth week of intra-uterine life in mesenchymal tissue.

Nasals The entire septum of the nose originates from a cartilaginous plate. About the eighth week of intra-uterine life two centres of ossification appear, one on each side of the median plane. These centres unite about the twelfth week. Around the age of puberty the developing lamellae are nearly united.

Inferior conchae Each ossifies from its own centre about the fifth week of intra-uterine life.

The cranial sutures

These are areas where the bones of the skull meet and articulate, separated only by a zone of connective tissue, the sutural ligament or membrane.

The sutural ligament is not simple, displaying regions of differentiation concerned in the growth and binding together of the apposed bone surfaces. This site of active bone growth is at the same time a firm bond of union between the neighbouring bones, which nevertheless allows a little movement (Prichard *et al.*, 1956). Prichard then goes on to say, 'Sutural fusion does not even commence until the late twenties, proceeding slowly thereafter; yet it is clearly necessary that sutures should cease to function as mobile joints as rapidly as possible after birth.' (*Gray's Anatomy*, 35th edn, 1973). It does not refer to the following sentence from the same paper. Why?

At the suture the periosteum splits into two layers. The outer layer continues on to the other bone. The inner layer continues into the suture forming the fibrous capsule over the edge of the bone. This inner layer of periosteum is continuous with the dura mater. With its weak fibre bundles running in all directions and its sinusoidal blood vessels, it could well allow some slight movement of one bone against the other and so could be regarded as analogous to a synovial joint cavity (Prichard *et al.*, 1956).

The types of suture can be generally grouped into the following:

- serrate – saw-like, e.g. saggital;
- denticulate – tooth-like projections, e.g. lambdoid suture;
- squamous – one bone overlaps with its neighbour, e.g. between the temporal and parietal bones;
- plane – simple apposition of contiguous surfaces, e.g. between the maxillae;
- gomphosis – peg and socket, e.g. the greater wing of the sphenoid and the body.

The bones of the cranium consist of an inner and outer table separated by cancellous bone, the diploe. These bones are covered with a periosteum that travels through the sutures and is continuous on the inside of the cranium, being renamed the dura. On the inner aspect of the cranium is a fibrous membrane, the endocranium, which is the outer layer of the dura mater. The base (norma basalis) of the skull is irregular in nature and has been split into three sections. Anteriorly, it consists of the bony plate; the middle part is posterior to the bony plate but anterior to the foreamen magnum. Finally, the posterior aspect consists of the remaining inferior aspect of the skull.

Covering the brain and spinal cord are the meninges. The meninges consist of three layers, the dura mater, arachnoid and pia mater. Of the three layers, the dural layer is the thickest and is attached throughout the interior of the skull. This dural layer is less coherent at the dorso-lateral aspect of the brain. Epi- or extradural haemorrhages occur between the bone and membrane, where the latter is more loosely attached and, therefore, more easily separated (*Gray's Anatomy*, 35th edn, 1973).

Within the head there are four dural specializations, as follows.

1. Falx cerebri: vertically placed between the cerebral hemispheres, origin from the straight sinus and insertion the crita gallae. Its free margin lies immediately above the corpus callosum.

2. Tentorium cerebelli: horizontally placed, it lies between the under-surface of the occipital lobe and the upper surface of the cerebellum. Its upper surface is attached posteriorly to the falx cerebri.
3. Falx cerebelli: this is small and vertically placed, extending downwards from under the surface of the tentorium, between the cerebellar hemispheres.
4. Diaphragma sella: this is attached to the clinoid processes forming the roof of the pituitary fossa. It is perforated by an opening for the transmission of the infundibulum, as it passes from the outer cinereum to the pituitary gland.

The cranial nerves

The motor or efferent sections of the cranial nerves originate from within the brain from nerve cell groups called nuclei of origin. Connections between these nuclei and the cerebral cortex is made by the corticonuclear fibres. Nuclei of cranial nerves do not begin in space.

The sensory or afferent sections of the cranial nerves originate from outside the brain. These nerve cells may be grouped together forming ganglia or they may be situated in peripheral sensory organs such as the eye or ear. These cells run into the brain ending as groups of nerve cells forming nuclei of termination of pure sensory input.

The olfactory nerve (1)
Supplying the sense of smell, these unmyelinated, sensory nerves originate from the mucous membrane of the nasal cavity. They traverse the cribriform plate of the ethmoid bone ending in the glomeruli of the olfactory bulb. Each bulb has a tubular sheath of dura mater and pia-arachnoid.

The optic nerve (2)
This nerve should be considered as a extension of the brain substance rather than an ordinary cranial nerve. Fibres of this nerve are mostly afferent forming the innermost layer of the retina, converging on the optic disc. As these fibres exit the intraorbital cavity they receive their myelin sheaths, traverse the lamina cribrosa forming the optic nerve. Within this intraorbital cavity the optic nerve is closely surrounded by four recti and a quantity of fat (corpus adiposum orbitae), supporting the ciliary vessels and nerves. Within the optic canal the nerve is in close relation to the ophthalmic artery and the nasociliary nerve and is separated from the sphenoidal and ethmoidal sinuses by a thin lamina of bone. An important factor is that intracranially the optic nerve is enclosed in three sheaths, which are continuous with the membranes of the brain: the outer sheath, derived from dura mater, the intermediate sheath, derived from arachnoid mater, and the inner sheath, from pia mater which is vascular and invests the nerve closely. This pial plexus houses branches of the superior hypophyseal and the opthalmic artery intracranially, the recurrent branches of the ophthalmic artery in the optic canal and from the

posterior ciliary arteries and the extraneural part of the central retinal artery in the orbit. Venous drainage is via the central vein of the retina. These sheaths (meninges) are the same as the meninges elsewhere. The majority of the optic nerves terminate in the lateral geniculate body; a small proportion go to the pretectal nucleus and superior colliculus.

The optic chiasma is the optic pathway intersection, which inferiorly rests on the diaphragma sella. Again, the chiasma is supplied arterially through the vessels investing the pia mater. Venous drainage is into the basal veins and the anterior cerebral vein.

After the optic chiasma the optic nerves continue as the optic tract. The tract continues posterolaterally to the two lateral geniculate bodies, here dividing into medial and lateral 'roots'. A large number of these nerve fibres pass through the lateral geniculate body, while the medial fibres pass on below the medial geniculate body to the superior colliculi. Here, they establish optic reflex pathways. The optic radiation, a broad bundle of fibres, begins from the lateral geniculate body. They then 'fan out' towards the calcarine fissure on the medial surface of the cortex of the occipital lobe of the cerebrum.

The oculomotor nerve (3)

This nerve supplies all the extraocular muscles of the eye, except the oblequus superior and the rectus lateralis. This is the somatomotor portion of the nerve. Through its connection with the ciliary ganglion it supplies the sphincter pupillae and the ciliaris, which are intraocular structures. This is the visceromotor portion of the nerve.

Fibres of the oculomotor nerve originate from the floor of the interpeduncular fossa at the medial margin of the cerebral peduncle. When it emerges from the brain the nerve is invested in pia mater and lies in the subarachnoid space. Running between the superior and posterior cerebral arteries it continues on to the lateral side of the posterior communicating artery. It perforates the arachnoid and lies in the triangular interval between the free and attached borders of the tentorium cerebelli. Continuing on the lateral side of the posterior clinoid process it descends into the lateral wall of the cavernus sinus, lying above the trochlear nerve. Here it enters the orbit through the superior orbital fissure. It then divides into a superior branch, supplying the levator palpebrae superioris muscle and the superior rectus muscle, and an inferior branch supplying the medial rectus muscle and the inferior oblique muscle. These somatomotor fibres arise from a complex of nuclei, in the oculomotor nucleus, lying in the midbrain beneath the aqueduct about the level of the superior colliculi.

The visceromotor fibres are preganglionic parasympathetic fibres arising from the Edinger–Westphal nucleus. They pass to the ciliary ganglion, travelling through the short ciliary nerves to supply the sphincter pupillae and ciliaris. This motor pathway is much more concerned with focusing than with the light reflex. It has a sympathetic root from a branch of the internal carotid. This consists of postganglionic fibres from the superior cervical ganglion traversing the ciliary ganglion emerging in the short ciliary nerves. They supply the blood vessels of the eyeball and may include fibres which supply the dilator pupillae. The sensory root is formed by a ramus communicans to the nasociliary nerve which contains sensory fibres from the eyeball. It reaches the ganglion in the short ciliary nerves passing through it without being interrupted.

The trochlear nerve (4)
This is a pure somatomotor nerve which supplies the superior oblique muscle. Its fibres arise from the large multipolar neurones from the trochlear nucleus situated in the floor of the cerebral aqueduct. After leaving the nucleus the fibres run downwards and laterally, decussating with its opposite fibres before leaving the midbrain at the lower level of the inferior colliculi. It is the only cranial nerve to leave the brain stem dorsally. It continues to descend to the base of the skull where it pierces the dura stratum at the margin of the tentorium cerebelli. It travels forwards to the lateral wall of the cavernus sinus where it communicates with the internal carotid sympathetic plexus, travelling on to enter the superior orbital fissure. In the orbit it inclines medially, above the origin of the levator palpebrae superioris, to enter the orbital face of the superior oblique.

The trigeminal nerve (5)
The terminal nuclei are chiefly sensory, dealing with touch, the mesencephalic with proprioception, and the spinal with pain and temperature. These nuclei lie in the pons, midbrain and medulla/upper cervical cord, respectively. Here the nerve contains both sensory and motor fibres. The sensory fibres are for the skin and mucous membrane of the face and the motor fibres for the muscles of mastication and probably the extraocular muscles. The trigeminal nerve has three divisions: ophthalmic, maxillary and mandibular. The motor nucleus is in the upper pons.

The abducent nerve (6)
This is a somatomotor nerve that supplies the lateral rectus muscle. The nucleus of the abducens nerve lies in the pons in the floor of the rhomboid fossa. After leaving the brain stem anteriorly, at the lower margin of the pons between the pyramid and the olive, it pierces the dura mater, runs intradurally and continues forwards over the superior border of the petrous temporal bone. Passing through the lateral wall of the cavernous sinus it then leaves the intracranial cavity, entering the orbital cavity through the medial end of the superior orbital fissure, innervating the lateral rectus muscle.

The facial nerve (7)
The seventh cranial nerve has both a motor and sensory root. The motor root supplies the muscles of the face, scalp and auricle, the buccinator, platysma, stapedius, stylohyoid and the posterior belly of the digastric. The sensory root receives input from the corda tympani gustatory fibres from the presulcal area of the tongue and, from the palatine and greater petrosal nerves, taste fibres from the soft palate; it also carries the

preganglionic parasympathetic (secretomotor) innervation of the submandibular and sublingual salivary glands, lacrimal glands and glands of the nasal and palatine mucosae.

The facial nerve can be thought of as having two nuclei, one for the motor fibres (facial nucleus) and the other for the preganglionic secretory fibres (superior salivatory nucleus). The two roots travel through the internal acoustic meatus where at its lateral end they enter the facial canal as a single trunk, here giving off branches to the superficial petrosal nerve, stapedius nerve and the corda tympani (taste fibres to the anterior two-thirds of the tongue and, as above, the preganglionic fibres to the mandibular and sublingual glands). At the bend with the petrous bone there is a swelling known as the geniculate ganglion. The nerve continues to run in the medial wall of the tympanic cavity and turns caudally to emerge from the skull through the stylomastoid foramen; it then runs forward in the parotid gland. Here, it divides with the parotid gland, forming the parotid plexus, distributing to the facial muscles.

The arterial supply to the facial nerve comes intracranially from the anterior inferior cerebellar artery, in its canal from the superficial petrosal branch of the middle meningeal artery, and the posterior auricular or occipital arteries, and extracranially from the stylomastoid, posterior auricular, occipital, superficial temporal and transverse facial arteries. Venous drainage is into the venae comitantes of the superficial petrosal and stylomastoid arteries.

The vestibulocochlear nerve (8)
The eighth cranial nerve can be considered as two afferent nerves, the vestibular and cochlear nerves from the ear. The vestibular is concerned with equilibrium and the cochlear with hearing.

The vestibular nerve arises from the vestibular ganglion in the internal acoustic meatus. The nerve processes terminate on the sensory epithelium of the semicircular ducts, the sacculus and the utriculus. They then converge to form the vestibular nerve, dividing into ascending and descending branches, to then terminate in the vestibular nuclei in the floor of the rhomboid fossa. There are four nuclei, superior, medial, lateral and inferior. Some of the fibres pass to the cerebellum, nuclei of nerves of the eye muscles and into the vestibulospinal tract in the spinal cord.

The cochlear nerve arises from the spiral ganglion, from which the peripheral processes of the nerve cells are connected to the hairs of the organ of Corti. These nerves converge together on the floor of the internal acoustic meatus continuing on into the cranial cavity with the vestibular nerve. On reaching the brain stem the cochlear nerve lies lateral to the vestibular nerve, being separated again by the inferior cerebellar peduncle. The fibres terminate in the ventral and dorsal cochlear nuclei. Some fibres form connections with the lateral lemniscus.

The glossopharyngeal nerve (9)
The ninth cranial nerve supplies sensory innervation to the middle ear, parts of the tongue and pharynx, parasympathetic secretomotor fibres to

the parotid gland and motor fibres to the muscles of the pharynx. Therefore, it contains motor, visceromotor and taste fibres.

The nerve arises as three or four rootlets from the medulla oblongata, leaving the skull through the jugular foramen with the vagus nerve. Before it actually passes through the foramen it forms the superior ganglion, which is small and considered to be a detached part of the inferior ganglion. After it leaves the foramen it forms an inferior ganglion which is larger and has branches that convey gustatory and tactile signals from the mucosa of the tongue (posterior third) and sensory signals from the oropharynx, soft palate and fauces. The inferior ganglion is also connected to the superior cervical sympathetic ganglion. It continues lateral to the internal carotid artery and the pharynx while it arches towards the tongue; here it begins to divide into a number of terminal branches. These branches are the tympanic, carotid, pharyngeal, muscular, tonsillar and lingual.

The vagus nerve (10)
The tenth cranial nerve supplies not only the head, but also the thorax and the abdomen, where it divides into a plexus. Here we have the largest vegetative nerve of the parasympathetic system containing both motor and sensory fibres. It arises as eight to ten rootlets from the medulla oblongata; leaving just behind the olive they form the nerve before exiting the skull through the jugular foramen. It forms two ganglia, like the glossopharyngeal nerve: the superior ganglion before the jugular foramen and the inferior ganglion after its exit. The superior ganglion is joined to the sympathetic trunk by a filament from the superior cervical ganglion and is concerned with general somatic sensations mediated by the auricular branch of the vagus. The inferior ganglion is connected to the hypoglossal nerve, superior cervical sympathetic ganglion and a loop between the first and second cervical spinal nerves. The sensory nerve cells of this ganglion have some involvement with visceral sensibility (taste) from the epiglottis and vallecula, and to some degree with general visceral afferent information from the larynx, pharynx, heart, lungs, oesophagus, stomach, small intestine and part of the colon.

The vagus nerve then continues down the neck in the carotid sheath; here it lies between the internal carotid vein and the internal carotid artery. It continues downwards with its relation to the internal carotid vein exchanging the internal carotid artery relation for that of the common carotid artery to the root of the neck. Remember that the common carotid artery gives rise to the internal carotid artery. After the root of the neck the vagus nerve course differs on either side of the body.

On the right the nerve continues downwards posterior to the internal jugular vein and crosses the first part of the subclavian artery. Entering the thorax it continues down through the superior mediastinum, lying first behind the right brachiocephalic vein, then right of the trachea and posteromedial to the right brachiocephalic vein and the superior venae cava. The nerve continues on behind the right principle bronchus to reach the posterior aspect of the root of the right lung, and there breaks up into posterior bronchial branches, here joining with fibres from the second, third and fourth thoracic sympathetic ganglia to form the right posterior pulmonary plexus. Two or three branches from the caudal part of the plexus continue down to the dorsal part of the oesophagus where, with a branch from the left vagus, they form the posterior oesophageal plexus. Within the abdomen the posterior vagal trunk divides into a small gastric branch, supplying the stomach, and a large coeliac branch, ending in the coeliac plexus.

On the left it enters the thorax between the left common carotid and the left subclavian arteries, and behind the left brachiocephalic vein. Continuing down through the superior mediastinum, it crosses the left side of the aortic arch, passing behind the root of the left lung. Behind the root of the lung it divides into the posterior bronchial branches, joining with fibres from the second, third and fourth sympathetic ganglia forming the left posterior pulmonary plexus. Two branches from this plexus combine with a twig from the right posterior pulmonary plexus on the front of the oesophagus to form the anterior oesophageal plexus. A trunk from this plexus, containing fibres from both vagus nerves, continues down in front of the oesophagus entering the abdomen through the oesophageal opening of the diaphragm.

Within the abdomen the anterior vagal trunk supplies fibres to the cardiac antrum, dividing into right and left branches. The left branch supplies the anterosuperior surface of this viscus. The right branch consists of three main parts. The first part continues to divide into an upper branch which enters the porta hepatis and lower rami, which principally supply the pyloric canal, the pylorus, the superior and the descending parts of the duodenum, and the head of the pancreas. The second part supplies the anterosuperior surface of the stomach and the third branch follows the lesser curvature of the stomach as far as the angular notch.

The branches of the vagus nerve are as follows:

in the jugular fossa:

- meningeal
- auricular

in the neck:

- pharyngeal
- branches to the carotid body
- superior laryngeal
- recurrent laryngeal (right)
- cardiac

in the thorax:

- cardiac
- recurrent laryngeal (left)
- pulmonary
- oesophageal

in the abdomen:

- gastric
- coeliac
- hepatic.

The accessory nerve (11)

The 11th cranial nerve is initially formed from both cranial and spinal roots, known as the internal and external rami, respectively. However, the cranial section should be considered as part of the vagus nerve as it distributes its branches through it.

The cranial root is smaller than the spinal root and cells arise from the nucleus ambiguus and probably from the dorsal vagal nucleus. The cranial root fibres emerge from the medulla oblongata, running laterally to the jugular foramen. Passing through the jugular foramen it separates from the spinal portion and continues over the inferior vagal ganglion to which it adheres. Its distributions are primarily in the pharyngeal and recurrent laryngeal portions of the vagus nerve. It may be the source of motor fibres supplying the muscles of the soft palate. The spinal root begins from a column of motor neurones, the spinal nucleus, as low as the fifth cervical segment. They emerge between the ventral and dorsal nerve roots of the upper cervical nerves, uniting to form a trunk ascending the ligamentum denticulum and the dorsal roots of the spinal nerves. It then enters the skull through the foramen magnum, behind the vertebral artery. It continues upward and laterally to the jugular foramen. On exiting the jugular foramen it runs laterally and backwards posterior to the internal jugular vein in about two-thirds of subjects, and anterior in about one-third of subjects. The accessory nerve can continue on to cross the transverse process of the atlas, descending obliquely, medially to the styloid process, the stylohyoid and the belly of the digastric. It continues on to the upper part of the sternocleidomastoid, supplying it and joining with branches of the second cervical nerve. The nerve emerges on the posterior aspect of the sternocleidomastoid, just above the middle of the muscle, then continuing on to cross the posterior triangle of the neck lying on the levator scapulae. It is separated from the levator scapulae by the prevertebral layer of deep cervical fascia and adipose tissue occupying the triangle. In this superficial position it has relations to the cervical lymph nodes and receives communications from the second and third cervical nerves. Eventually, the accessory nerve passes under the anterior border of the trapezius, about 5 cm above the clavicle. At this point, together with branches from the third and fourth cervical nerves, a plexus is formed deep to the surface of the trapezius. It is from this plexus that the trapezius receives its innervation.

The hypoglossal nerve (12)

The 12th cranial nerve is the motor nerve to the tongue. The hypoglossal nucleus lays in the floor of the fourth ventricle in the medulla. It passes out of the anterolateral surface of the medulla between the olive and the pyramid. Passing posterior to the vertebral artery and running through the hypoglossal canal it continues out of the canal anteriorly, lateral to the occiput, internal carotid and lingual arteries. It then passes over the apex of the greater cornu of the hyoid bone. Continuing on it runs anteriorly, looping over the hypoglossus, deep to the mylohyoid, to end in the terminal branches underneath the submandibular gland.

Arteries to the brain

These consist of the internal carotid and vertebral arteries.

Internal carotid artery

Travels through the dura, medial to the anterior clinoid process. It immediately gives off the ophthalmic and posterior communicating arteries. Ascending between the optic nerve and optic tract it ends as the anterior and middle cerebral arteries. The anterior cerebral artery runs medially above the optic nerve, joining its parallel artery via the anterior communicating artery. The middle cerebral artery travels laterally in the stem of the lateral cerebral sulcus.

Vertebral artery

Travels through the dura behind the occipital condyle and lies in a groove on the margin of the foramen magnum. It lies between the hypoglossal nerve and the first cranial nerve. It travels forward between these two nerves to the lower border of the pons where it merges with its parallel artery forming one basilar artery. The posterior inferior artery travels to the cerebellum and is the largest branch of the vertebral artery. The basilar artery ascends from the lower border of the pons to the upper border where it bifurcates forming a 'T' shape. These are the right and left posterior cerebral arteries. Three large, paired arteries branch from the basilar cerebral artery. These are from posterior to anterior: the posterior cerebral arteries, the superior arteries and the anterior inferior cerebral artery.

Venous drainage

Veins of the head and neck can be divided into the following:

1. veins of the exterior of the head and face;
2. veins of the neck;
3. the diploic veins, the meningeal veins, the veins of the brain and the venous sinuses of the dura. We shall refer here only to the veins of the head and face.

   The external veins of the head and face are the following.

Supratrochlear vein

Starts from the forehead, joins the supraorbital vein, forming the anterior facial vein.

Supraorbital vein
Starts around the zygomatic process of the frontal bone, joins with the supratrochlear vein to form the facial vein.

Facial vein
This is formed by the combination of the supratrochlear and the supraorbital veins at a point medial to the eye and lateral to the upper part of the nose. It travels downwards and laterally across the front of the face, lateral to the mouth, towards the angle of the jaw. It is joined by the retromandibular vein just before it terminates in the internal jugular vein. This vein does not have any valves, so facial muscular movement is important and it is connected to the cavernous sinus.

Superficial temporal vein
This drains a broad area over the scalp's temporal region. This vein continues downwards anterior to the ear, joining with the maxillary vein, to form the retromandibular vein as it continues down.

Pterygoid plexus
This is located between the temporalis and lateral pterygoid, and partly between the two pterygoids. It is also connected to the cavernous sinus.

Maxillary vein
A short vein formed by veins from the pterygoid plexus, uniting with the superior temporal to form the retromandibular vein.

Retromandibular vein
Otherwise known as the posterior facial vein, this vein is located in the parotid gland and divides as it descends into two branches. These are an anterior branch passing forward and joining the facial vein and a posterior branch passing backward and joining the posterior auricular vein to form the external jugular vein.

Posterior auricular vein
This vein is located behind the ear and receives blood from the occipital and superficial temporal veins. It continues down to join the posterior branch retromandibular vein in or just below the parotid gland.

Occipital vein
Begins in the network at the back of the head. As it descends over the occipital region it pierces the trapezius, at its cranial attachment. It then continues deep through the suboccipital region joining the deep cervical and vertebral veins.

Lymphatics

All the lymph vessels of the head and neck drain into the deep cervical group of lymph nodes. These give rise to the jugular trunk, and from here the right and left sides of the body differ. On the right, the jugular trunk can end in the junction of the internal jugular and subclavian veins or may join the right lymphatic duct. On the left, it enters the thoracic duct; occasionally it may enter the internal jugular or subclavian vein.

The deep cervical group of lymph nodes are divided into superior and inferior.

1. Superior deep cervical lymph nodes – the majority are deep to the sternocleidomastoid, usually consisting of a group of one large and many smaller nodes, known as the jugulodigastric group. These drain from the tongue. Efferents from the upper deep cervical lymph nodes pass to the lower deep cervical group and direct to the jugular trunk.
2. Inferior deep cervical lymph nodes – partially deep to the lower part of the sternocleidomastoid, extending to the subclavian triangle, being closely related to the brachial plexus. One particular node lies just above or on the omohyoid muscle; this is called the jugulo-omohyoid lymph node. The efferents from the lower deep cervical lymph nodes join the jugular trunk.

The lymphatics of the head and neck can be separated into drainage of superficial tissues and drainage of deep structures, including the viscera. The superficial tissues of the head and neck include the following:

in the head:

- occipital
- retro-auricular (mastoid)
- parotid
- buccal (facial)

in the neck:

- submandibular
- submental
- anterior cervical
- superficial cervical.

The deep tissues of the head and neck include the following:

in the head:

- nasal cavity
- nasopharynx
- middle ear
- mouth
- teeth
- tonsils
- tongue

in the neck:

- pharynx
- cervical part of the oesophagus

- larynx
- trachea
- thyroid gland.

Muscles and fascia of the head and neck

Scalp (epicranius)
The epicranius consists of the occipitofrontalis and the temporoparietalis.

Superficial fascia
This is adherent to the skin and the underlying epicranius and its aponeurosis, the galea aponeurotica. It is continuous with the superficial fascia of the back of the neck; laterally, it is prolonged into the temporal region, where it is looser in texture.

Occipitofrontalis
Broad, musculofibrous layer, which covers the skull from the nuchal lines to the eyebrows. It has four parts, two occipital and two frontal, connected by the galea aponeurotica.

Temporoparietalis
A sheet of muscle that lies between the frontal part of the occipitofrontalis and the anterior and superior auricular muscles.

Galea aponeurotica (epicranial aponeurosis)
This covers the upper part of the cranium and forms with the epicranius a continuous fibromuscular sheet extending from the nuchal lines to the eyebrows. It is united to the skin by the firm, fibrous superficial fascia. Nerve supply to the occipital part is by the posterior auricular branch, and the frontal part is supplied by the temporal branches of the facial nerve. Occipital slips draw the scalp backwards; frontal slips raise the eyebrows and skin over the root of the nose.

Muscles of the eyelids

Orbicularis oculi
This muscle surrounds the circumference of the orbit and consists of orbital, palpebral and lacrimal parts. The fibres of the orbital part form an uninterrupted ellipse of the eye of which the circumference covers the outer limit of the eye where the fibres of the palpebral part form the eyelid. The lacrimal part lies behind the lacrimal sac. It is attached to the lacrimal fascia, to the upper part of the crest of the lacrimal bone, and the adjacent part of the lateral surface of the lacrimal bone. Nerve supply is by the temporal and zygomatic branches of the facial nerve. The orbicularis oculi is the sphincter muscle of the eyelids. The palpebral portion can act under voluntary control, or reflexly, closing the lids gently.

The lacrimal part of the orbicularis oculi draws the eyelids and the lacrimal papillae medially; at the same time it exerts traction on the lacrimal fascia and is said to dilate the lacrimal sac.

Corrugator supercilli

This is a small pyramidal muscle, at the medial end of the eyebrow, deep to the frontal part of occipitofrontalis and the orbicularis oculi. It is innervated by temporal branches of the facial nerve. It draws the eyebrow medially and downwards, producing the vertical wrinkles of the forehead.

Muscles of mastication

It is osteopathically important to remember that a strong layer of fascia, derived from the deep cervical fascia and named the parotid fascia, covers the masseter and is firmly connected to it. Even more importantly, it is attached to the lower border of the zygomatic arch, and invests the parotid gland.

Masseter

This muscle is quadrilateral and has three superimposed layers: the superficial, middle and deep layers. Origin (O) of the superficial layer: by a thick aponeurosis from the zygomatic process of the maxilla, anterior two-thirds of the lower border of the zygomatic arch; insertion (I): the angle and lower half of the lateral surface of the ramus of the mandible. The middle layer: O: deep surface of the anterior two-thirds of the zygomatic arch and from the lower border of the posterior third; I: middle of the ramus of the mandible. The deep layer: O: the deep surface of the zygomatic arch; I: upper part of the ramus of the mandible and into the coronoid process. Nerve supply (N): branch of the anterior trunk of the mandibular nerve.

Temporal fascia

This covers the temporalis. It is covered laterally by auriculares anterior and superior, the galea aponeurotica and part of orbicularis oculi. Osteopathically, it is important to remember that the superficial temporal vessels and the auriculotemporal nerve cross it upwards.

Temporalis

O: from the temporal fossa and deep surface of the temporal fascia. I: in the medial surface, apex, anterior and posterior borders of the coronoid process, and the anterior border of the ramus of the mandible. N: deep temporal branches of the anterior trunk of the mandibular nerve. Action (A): elevates the mandible and approximates the teeth. To perform this action properly it relies on the anterior fibres to pull the mandible upwards and the posterior fibres to pull the jaw backwards. This is clinically important.

Lateral pterygoid
This muscle has two heads, upper and lower. O: upper head from the infratemporal surface and infratemporal crest of the greater wing of the sphenoid bone; lower head, from the lateral surface of the lateral pterygoid plate. I: into the depression on the front of the neck of the mandible, and into the articular capsule and disc of the temporomandibular articulation. N: supplied from a branch of the anterior trunk of the mandibular nerve. A: assists in opening the mouth, pulling forward the condylar process of the mandible and the articular disc, while the head of the mandible rotates on the articular disc. Closure, the reverse movement, causes backward gliding of the articular disc and condyle of the mandible and is controlled by the slow relaxation of the lateral pterygoid, while the masseter and temporalis restore the jaw to the occlusal position.

Medial pterygoid
O: attached to the medial surface of the lateral pterygoid plate and the grooved surface of the pyramidal process of the palatine bone. I: passes downwards, laterally and backwards being attached by a strong tendinous lamina, to the lower and back part of the medial surfaces of the ramus and angle of the mandible. N: branch from the mandibular nerve. A: assists in elevating the mandible. It acts with the lateral pterygoids, protruding the mandible. When two pterygoid muscles on one side contract the mandible is swung forwards and to the opposite side.

The eye

The eyeball or globe sits in fat in the orbit of the skull. The clear membrane slightly bulging on the anterior surface is the transparent cornea, through which light initially enters the eye. Immediately behind the cornea is the first of three chambers, the anterior chamber, which contains a watery fluid, the aqueous humour. Through the posterior wall of the anterior chamber can be seen the coloured ring of the eye, the iris. The pupil, the space formed by the inner ring of the iris, is filled posteriorly by the middle of the lens. A second chamber, the posterior chamber, is behind the iris forming a ring around the lens; this also contains aqueous humour. The main chamber of the eye contains a jelly-like substance, the vitreous humour, which again consists mostly of water.

The body of the eye is a wall made up from three basic layers: the sclera, the uvea and the retina. The outside of the globe is made from the sclera, which is a dense connective tissue. This tissue combined with the intraocular pressure maintains the shape of the eye. In the uvea, the next layer, are contained the vascular structures. Anteriorly, the uvea forms the iris and the ciliary body, from which the fibres (suspensory ligaments) of the lens attach. Posteriorly, the uvea is otherwise known as the choroid layer. The innermost layer is the retina, which contains the light-sensitive cells.

Figure 6.1 is a schematic diagram showing the visual light reflex pathway; Fig. 6.2 shows the autonomic nervous supply to the eye.

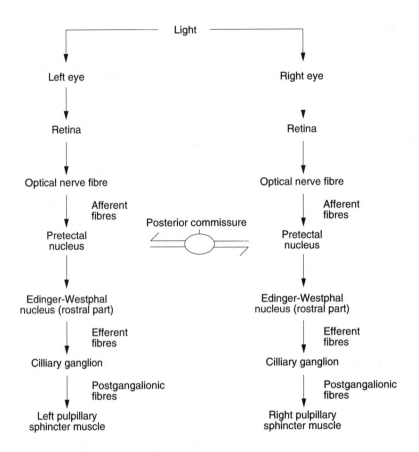

Fig. 6.1 Visual light reflex pathway.

The ear

The ear consists of the external ear, the middle ear and the internal ear.

The external ear is the auricle (lobe) and the external acoustic meatus. An elastic structure makes up the auricle. This elastic cartilage is a combination of depressions and elevations which differ from athlete to athlete, being genetically determined. These depressions and elevations consist of the following:

- the helix, or outer rim of the ear;
- the antihelix, or inner rim of the ear;
- the scapha, or upper third, between the outer and inner rim;
- the concha, inside the inner rim;
- the tragus, which overhangs the entrance to the ear;
- the antitragus, above the lobe.

The external acoustic meatus is an S-shaped tubular structure communicating between the inside and outside of the ear. It is directed, from outside to inside, medially, anteriorly and slightly superiorly. As it continues medially it directs medially, anteriorly and slightly inferiorly. It

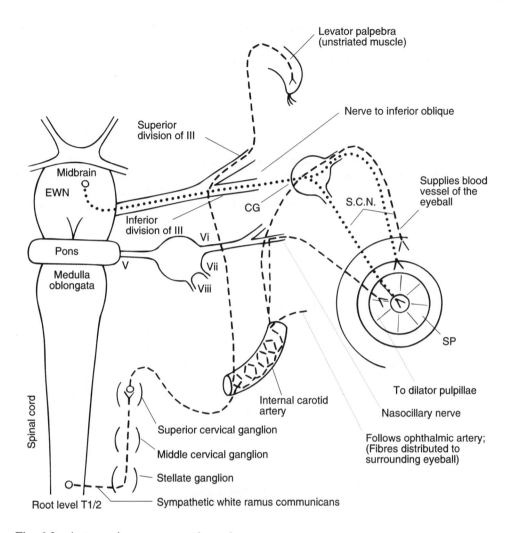

Fig. 6.2 Autonomic nervous supply to the eye.

is a cartilaginous tube covered in connective tissue. It ends with the ear drum or tympanic membrane. There are glands beneath the epidermis, the ceruminous glands. The ear drum is the partition between the external ear and the middle ear. It is a grey, glistening membrane, not visible from the outside.

The middle ear consists of the tympanic cavity and the auditory tube. The tympanic cavity is an air-filled cavity that contains three small bones or ossicles: the malleus, incus and stapes. The auditory tube travels from the base of the tympanic cavity obliquely downward and forward and opens on the lateral pharyngeal wall. This allows for equalization of pressure in the middle ear. This is osteopathically important, for directing OMT during glue ear and hearing disturbance involving the auditory tube. There is a small muscle in the ear known as the tensor tympani, which lies in a superior canal in the tympanic cavity.

The internal ear is within the petrous bone forming the bony osseous labyrinth, which is practically full adult size at birth. Within the osseous labyrinth is the membranous labyrinth. Between this osseous and membranous structure is the perilymph. The internal ear is supplied by the eighth cranial nerve.

The mouth

The mouth consists of squamous epithelium and is bordered by a roof, inner lips, inner cheeks, throat and floor in which lies the tongue. This is a sensitive and delicate structure supplied by the trigeminal nerve: above by the second division (maxillary) and below by the third division (mandibular).

The cranio-spinal (suboccipital) junction

This area has also been termed the occipito-atlanto-axoid area or the suboccipital triangle. Reflex lesions are frequent here, traumatic lesions relatively less so. Cathie reports:

> 'I used the term "cranio-spinal junction" because it calls to mind the two regions involved, the cranium and the spine, and includes the occiput, atlas and axis, which bones surround the spinal cord where the cord is continuous with the brain. The area is in close relation with the superior cervical ganglia. The combined motions here total those of a ball-and-socket joint.'
>
> Observations made on the Halladay teaching spine show that owing to the shape of the articular facets and differences in the flexibility of the ligaments, motion between the occiput and atlas is not as free as motion between the atlas and axis. This explains why mobilization between the occiput and atlas is at times difficult to secure while comparatively easy to secure between the atlas and axis.
>
> The fact that the strong superficial muscles of the shoulders and spine have no attachments to the atlas or axis bones, but pass completely over them to their attachments on the occipital bone, is one of the reasons why the area is so open to traumatic lesion. For instance, the trapezius passes clear of the atlas and axis to exert varying pulls upon the occiput above. In the four-footed animal this would be of little consequence; in the 'erect' human being it demands consideration.
>
> (Cathie, 1974a)

Suboccipital muscles
- Rectus capitis posterior major – O: spine of the axis; I: lateral part of the inferior nuchal line; A: extends the head and rotates head to the same side as the muscle.
- Rectus capitis posterior minor – O: posterior arch of the atlas; I: medial part of the inferior nuchal line; A: extends the head.

- Obliquus capitis inferior – O: spinous process of axis; I: transverse process of atlas; A: turns face to the same side.
- Obliquus capitis superior – O: transverse process of the atlas; I: into occipital bone above and lateral to rectus capitis posterior major; A: bends the head backwards and to the same side.

Nerve Supply By the dorsal ramus of the first spinal (suboccipital) nerve (C1).

Drainage

Occipital vein – see above.

The occipital lymph nodes are located where vessels and nerves pass through the nuchal fascia, superficial to the attachment of the trapezius. This an important point osteopathically as the hypertonia of the cervico-occipital fascia can lead to enlarged nodes due to poor drainage.

Head stabilization and visual tracking

Head stabilization and visual tracking are two of the basic necessities in sport. These are motor skills learned through practice and good coaching. Understanding this system is important, as any upset in the autonomic and/or cerebellar control mechanisms will present with subclinical and clinical signs that may be seen in the early stages of the dysfunctional or pathological sequence. Here we will look at the basics of this system. The interrelationships involved in this mechanism are extremely complicated, and the space available in this book may not do it full justice.

Head stabilization is seen for example in cricket, where the head is kept still at the crease while the batsman watches the bowler 'running in' to deliver the ball. The sprinter running 100 m is trained to keep his or her head still while running down the track. Similarly, if we watch slow motion film of a tiger going in for the kill we see that the eyes are locked on the prey and the head is locked with the body. This relationship between head, neck and body in motion or tracking moving objects is natural to the tiger, but athletes must be trained.

The mechanism of stabilization is based on a series of interacting reflexes feeding information from the environment and from within the structures themselves (Fig. 6.3). The eyes are stabilized within their sockets by reflexes controlling the eye muscles and the balance centres, i.e. the vestibulo-ocular reflexes (VOR). The VOR is the principle mechanism that keeps visual images stable on the retina as we move our heads (Lisberger, 1988). The hair cells of the semicircular canals and otoliths of the inner ear are exquisitely sensitive mechanoreceptors that provide this input to the brain. Otolithic macular hair cells are sensitive to the actual position of the head in relation to earth, and also vertical and linear accelerations (as in a car moving off from stationary).

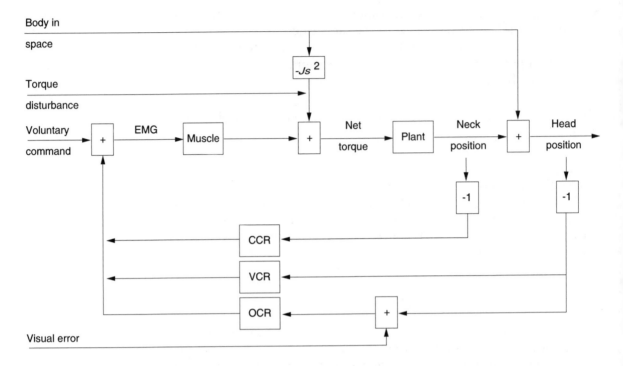

Fig. 6.3 Block diagram of the head control system. Experimental and physiological inputs are on the left; the outputs of head and neck position are on the right. The feedback loops include the cervico-collic reflex (CCR), the vestibulo-collic reflex (VCR) and an optico-collic reflex (OCR). The moment of inertia of the head, J, produces a torque on the neck during angular acceleration (s^2). (From Peterson and Richmond, 1988.)

Movement of the head discharges semicircular canal afferents transmitting information to the second-order brain stem vestibular nuclei (Fig. 6.4). Information is projected monosynaptically to the motor neurones that innervate the extra-ocular muscles, giving rise to a short-latency reflex pathway, a 'three (tri)-neurone arc', that mediates the VOR. Head stability naturally stabilizes the visual field, but importantly it ensures a stable 'reference' against which the hair cells, located within the head, can measure further stimuli. If the eyes move with the head, the visual image on the retina also moves, giving rise to a powerful 'retinal slip' signal. This visual stimulus evokes the opticokinetic reflex (OKR) which, although it has a longer latency than the VOR, also produces compensatory movements of the eyes that tend to stabilize the retinal image. Therefore, head movements stimulate both VOR and OKR in a synergistic fashion (Dutia, 1989). However, fast, smooth and coordinated movements cannot be realized by feedback control alone because, in biological motor control systems, the delays associated with feedback loops are long and the feedback gains are low. Thus, internal predictive models of the motor apparatus need to be utilized in the course of these computations. The internal models in the brain must be acquired through motor learning in

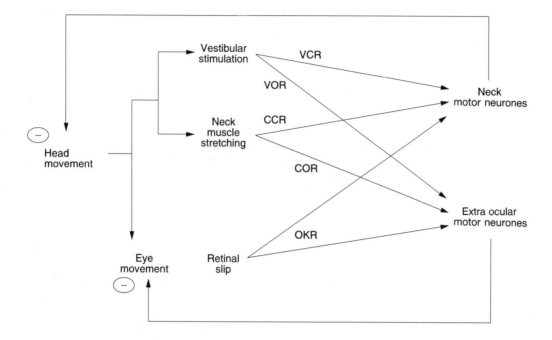

Fig. 6.4 Schematic diagram of reflex systems activated by head movement. VCR, vestibulo-collic reflex; VOR, vestibulo-ocular reflex; COR, cervico-ocular reflex; CCR, cervico-ocular reflex; OKR, opticokinetic reflex. (From Dutia, 1989.)

order to accommodate the changes that occur with the growth of controlled objects such as hands, legs and torso, as well as with the unpredictable variability of the external world (Kawato and Gomi, 1992).

The cerebellum appears to act as a metasystem whose main task is not to mediate any reflex *per se*, but to optimize its parameters. It is responsible for adjusting the directions, gains and time relations of these reflexes to optimize them for current conditions. Thus, the cerebellum mediates both short- and long-term adjustments of reflexes so as to adapt them to the particular needs of the movement. Thus it is relatively difficult to discern much effect of the cerebellum on the 'normal' behaviour of any reflex (Stein and Glickstein, 1992).

Movement of the head is by the action of the neck musculature. Afferent information from the muscle spindles of the neck muscles accompanies that of the VOR and OKR in the form of the cervico-ocular reflex (COR). The neck is very important in mediating the relative displacements between the head and the trunk. All these reflexes appear to have inter-neurone circuitry. In addition, the cervico-collic reflex (CCR) is where information from neck afferents is transmitted to neck motor neurones (Dutia, 1989).

The vestibulo-collic reflex (VCR) is the name given to the set of reflexes acting on the muscles of the neck that arise from stimulation of vestibular receptors in the labyrinth. The reflexes activate the neck muscles in such a

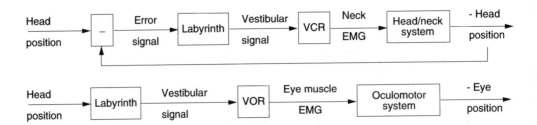

Fig. 6.5 Block diagrams of the vestibulo-collic reflex (top), a 'closed loop' system. This is an overdamped servosystem. The vestibulo-ocular reflex (bottom) is an 'open loop' system that is underdamped. (From Peterson and Richmond, 1988.)

manner as to counteract any head movement sensed by the vestibular apparatus; this activation helps to maintain head stability in space. Its task is similar to that of the better studied VOR which stabilizes the eye position in space when the head moves.

The VCR operates as a closed-loop negative feedback system (Fig. 6.5): its output, compensatory (−) head position, opposes (and partly cancels) the input driving signal. The output of the VOR, compensatory eye position, has no direct influence on the head position signal: the VOR operates as an 'open-loop' system (Fig. 6.5). For ideal operation, an open-loop reflex such as the VOR should have a gain of 1; this causes the output (eye movement) to exactly compensate for the input (head movement), so that the eye is fixed in space. For closed-loop systems such as the VCR, it becomes slightly more difficult to compute the gain of the reflex. Although the reflex gain is still the ratio of the output to the input signal, the closed nature of the loop implies that the signal that gets transformed by the system is the difference between the input and output, an 'error' signal that shows how far the reflex is from its desired goal (keeping the head fixed in space). Motor disturbances are sometimes observed in human patients who have suffered damage to the neck. Case studies in the clinical literature describe the syndrome, known as 'cervical vertigo' or 'cervical nystagmus', characterized by symptoms of gait disturbance, dizziness and nystagmus. In these patients, symptoms often followed an episode of neck muscle strain, and could be relieved by injecting local anaesthetic into neck muscles or applying a cervical collar. It is apparent osteopathically that there does not even have to be the clinical presentation of pain or strain. Deep hypertonic cervical or even upper thoracic soft tissue can contribute to the same problems (Peterson and Richmond, 1988).

Head injury

Injury to the head is relatively uncommon. When head injuries do occur, this should initiate a systematic response from the practitioner for assessment and transportation of the athlete. Injury to the head should never be taken lightly. It should always be assessed in a quite, calm environment, if possible, although in a field situation this may be impossible. Head injuries occur more in contact and collision sports.

Sequelae of head injury

Head injury can result in hypercapnia ($PCO_2 > 40$ mmHg) and hypoxaemia ($PO_2 < 70$ mmHg). Both these situations can lead to cerebral oedema and increased intracranial pressure. Under these circumstances arterial blood gas measurements are important as they are the best way of giving an overall indication of the efficiency of the airway and ventilation. These measurements should be repeated at regular intervals.

Causes of imparied O_2 and CO_2 exchange

1. Hemispheric and/or basal ganglia lesions may cause Cheyne–Stokes respiration.
2. Indirect injury to brain stem due to pressure from intracranial clot may cause uncal herniation.
3. Injury to upper brain stem may result in rapid, shallow breathing (central neurogenic hyperventilation).
4. Injury to medulla often results in very irregular respiration (ataxic).
5. Impaired blood supply to the brain due to shock (hypovolaemic or neurogenic) or arterial injury.
6. Airway obstruction by blood, mucus, vomitus, foreign body (avulsed teeth) or impacted tongue impairs respiratory exchange.
7. Chest injury (fractured ribs, flail chest, sucking wounds, pneumothorax, haemothorax) impairs breathing.
8. Delayed complications (pulmonary embolus, fat embolus, disseminated intravascular coagulation).
9. Metabolic factors that may further alter respiration include ketoacidosis, uraemia, salicylism, hepatic encephalopathy and poisoning.

Hypoxia and acidosis of neurones

Hypoxia and acidosis, as a consequence of head injury, result in rapidly deteriorating neuronal function.

Increased intracranial pressure

The state of hypercapnia increases cerebral blood volume, leading to additional increases in intracranial pressure, which further embarrasses respiration in a cycle of deterioration (Fig. 6.6).

Definitions

A minor head injury is defined as when there is no loss of consciousness, the athlete responds with normal conversation, answers questions and returns to normal function within about a minute. The most common of these is the concussion and laceration. Minor head injuries occur more commonly in games such as football and rugby.

Table 6.1 shows a head injury grading scale.

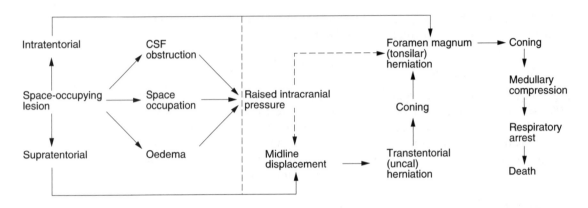

Fig. 6.6 Sequence of events that may lead to and follow raised intracranial pressure. (Adapted from Sharr, 1984)

Table 6.1 Severity of concussion

Grade	Feature	Duration
1 (mild)	PTA	<3 min
	LOC	None
2 (moderate)	PTA	>30 min
	LOC	<5 min
3 (severe)	PTA	>24 hours
	LOC	>5 min

PTA, post-traumatic amnesia; LOC, loss of consciousness.
(From: Canto, R.C. and Micheli, L.V. (1991) *ACSM's Guidelines for the Team Physician*.)

Assessing head injury

The following guidelines should enable you to superficially assess the individual and determine his or her need for further investigation. Positive findings in any one of the following areas is enough to warrant further attention.

1. Unconsciousness ('knocked-out'). This can vary from transitory fleeting loss to prolonged loss of consciousness. Any athlete who is rendered unconscious should undergo further investigation.
2. Mental confusion. The individual is confused as to what is going on. This can vary from slight to complete disorientation. It can also be momentary to prolonged. Any athlete who is mentally confused as a result of trauma is the responsibility of the osteopath until in the hands of paramedics or the emergency department.
3. Memory loss. Storage and recall of information is a high level neurological process. Memory loss is a common symptom, seen with or without loss of consciousness. This amnesia comes in two main types: **anterograde**, i.e. loss of memory concerning events after the

trauma, and **retrograde**, i.e. loss of memory of events prior to trauma. A third type is **automatism**, where the athlete has no memory of what he is doing. In this state a player may continue to play without knowing he has a head injury.

4. Tinnitus. This may be present as a short-lived symptom after a head-to-head collision, and is known as 'having your bell rung' in football. If this condition persists then further investigation is needed.
5. Loss of vision. This can be transient, lasting a couple of seconds to minutes. If the player experiences even a momentary loss of vision he or she should not return to the game. They should have a check-up by a neurologist before being allowed to continue in further games. Make sure you talk to the specialist, to make sure they have attended.
6. Inequality of pupils. This is due to unilateral third nerve palsy from uncal herniation, which characteristically causes early dilatation of the ipsilateral pupil and a poor response to light (Hutchinson's pupil) (Friedman, 1983).
7. Nystagmus ('dancing eyes').
8. Nausea and vomiting. This may occur immediately or up to hours later.
9. Headache. If headache persists for more than 10 minutes then the player should not return to the game. If it is actually getting worse in this time period then the athlete should be sent for further examination.
10. Reduced coordination. There may be a decrease in the ability to perform simple tasks, e.g. standing on one foot, touching index finger to nose with eyes shut, lying on his or her back and placing heel of foot on opposite knee etc. Give the athlete a few minutes to recover after these tests and then repeat them.
11. Irregular breathing pattern (Cheyne–Stokes breathing).
12. Fluid from ears (otorrhae) and/or nose (rhinorrhea). This may be blood or cerebrospinal fluid or both.

The following signs may be an indication of an expanding lesion.

1. A deteriorating level of consciousness: increased confusion, increased irritability, more emotional, unresponsive and less aware, drowsy, wants to be left alone.
2. Eyes: a fixed stare, does not track, i.e. follow finger, pupils unequal, dancing eyes (nystagmus).
3. Cardiovascular system: slow, weakening pulse.
4. Bilateral strength comparison: unequal strength of arms, legs etc; no strength on one side of the body.
5. Coordination, as above.
6. Clear fluid and/or blood from nose and/or ears.

Signs of severe head injury include prolonged loss of consciousness and the patient only responding to painful stimuli. Some useful terminology are:

- **closed head injury**, where there is no breaking of skin on scalp or face;
- **open head injury**, where there is a break in skin of the head or face;

Table 6.2 The Glasgow Coma Scale

Eye opening (E)	
Spontaneous	4
To speech	3
To pain	2
Nil (no response)	1
Motor response (M)	
Obeys	6
Localizes	5
Withdraws	4
Abnormal flexion	3
Extensor response	2
Nil	1
Verbal response (V)	
Oriented	5
Confused conversation	4
Inappropriate words	3
Incomprehensible sounds	2
Sounds	2
Nil	1
Glasgow Coma Score (E + M = V) = to 15	

- **coma**, where there is no response to even the most powerful stimuli;
- **unconsconscious state**, where the athlete is not consciously responding to external stimuli. There may be reflex actions.

The most common method of assessing head injury is with the use of the Glasgow Coma Scale (Table 6.2).

Skull fractures

Fractures of the skull can range from simple outer table fractures to severe fractures that lacerate the brain tissue. These fractures can be described generally as follows:

- linear (like a line)
- comminuted (multiple pieces)
- depressed (in towards the brain).

Fractures that combine with a skull laceration, damage to a sinus or the middle ear are called compound fractures. Any fracture that is located at the base of the skull is termed a basilar fracture.

In a field situation, especially where a headguard is not worn, a fracture is sometimes accompanied by a scalp laceration. It is important to take time examining the laceration site. This site may be numb on gentle palpation. Other sites can be checked by general scalp palpation and questioning. Also enquire about neck pain. Blunt head trauma, which is the most common type of head trauma, is generally associated with some degree of neck, or even upper extremity, symptoms.

Skull fractures may predispose to intracranial haematoma or a meningeal infection. Close attention should be paid to bleeding and/or fluid from the ears, nose and eyes. There may be multiple injury sites. Altered function of the senses, i.e. hearing, smell and sight, and neurological signs (facial paralysis, numbness etc.) may indicate a deterioration in the player's condition.

Treatment
In the case of closed skull fractures, observation of the player's neurological status, i.e. making sure they stay within normal parameters, may be all that is required. Compound fractures require debridement in a sterile environment. Compound depressed skull fractures need even more attention with the main objective being both debridement and decompression or elevation of bone. Prophylactic administration of antibiotics and anticonvulsants may be used for depressed fractures. Any scalp injuries that may be accompanied by fractures, any neurological signs, or blood or clear fluid from ears or nose require plain X-rays and if possible magnetic resonance imaging (MRI) scans.

Scalp injuries

These are fairly common in contact sports and generally of a minor nature. They often present as lacerations and abrasions. These include cuts and abrasions from glancing impacts and may present as subdermal haematomas and crushed soft tissue from direct impacts, which may also have subdural haematomas. If the impact on the scalp, or head as a whole, is strong enough to cause further damage, there may be significant bleeding in the subgleal or subperiosteal space. Accumulation of blood may be seen behind the ear (Battle's sign), around the eyes in the periorbital tissues (panda bear or raccoon sign), external ear canal and behind the ear drum (haemotympanum).

Treatment
The general approach to lacerations and abrasions is cleaning followed by application of gauze, hydrogen peroxide, ice compression and topical antibiotics. If the player's hair is long enough, strands may be draw out and tied to act as sutures; otherwise use a regular suture.

Maxillofacial fractures, lacerations and abrasions

The maxillofacial structures cover the face, including the lips, nose, eyes, mouth, teeth and jaw. In any maxillofacial injury the primary concern is maintaining an open airway. Excessive haemorrhaging may make it difficult to breathe, especially if the mouth/lips are affected. This is compounded if the athlete is unconscious. The conscious athlete must be kept calm while action to control the haemorrhaging takes place. It is very easy for an athlete to breathe in blood and/or broken teeth. Once haemorrhaging is under control a careful neurological assessment should be performed. If you are outside in the cold it is best to move the athlete inside. They may get showered and changed if the injury is not too bad, but they must be accompanied all the time until they reach an accident and emergency department. If the injury is more serious they should be sent immediately to the accident and emergency department.

1. Airway. Make sure the athlete is breathing. Leaning the head forwards reduces the risk of blood clotting and/or teeth causing airway obstruction.
2. Haemorrhaging. Try to control haemorrhaging by compression with sterile gauze and an ice bag.
3. Spinal injuries. The majority of maxillofacial injuries are a form of blunt trauma, which means there is a risk of cervical spine or upper extremity involvement.

Fractures

Fractures of the maxillofacial region include the Le Fort fractures, named after the French surgeon who in 1901 described these midface fracture lines. They are generally catagorized into types I, II and III (Fig. 6.7).

- Le Fort I – in this level of fracture the maxilla is separated from the face on a horizontal plane, under the nose, extending the width of

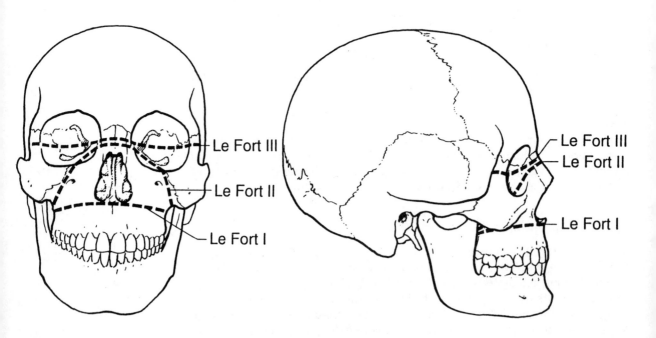

Fig. 6.7 The three types of Le Fort fracture.

the face. This plane passes through the base of the antrum, separating the maxilla from the nasal floor, stopping at the inferior end of the pterygoid plates.

- Le Fort II – in this type of fracture the plane separates the maxilla and nasal bones from the orbit. Here the plane line starts from under (for example) the right cheek, travelling medially and ascending between the nose and the orbit, continuing over the nose then descending between the orbit and the nasal bones finishing under the left cheek. The fracture plane is through the upper half of the pterygoid plates, through the infraorbital region and across the lachrymal bones.
- Le Fort III – this is the most extreme of the fractures. Here, the horizontal fracture plane separates the facial bones from the cranium. The line is through the zygomatic arches, the posterior orbit and the ethmoidal sinus.

Remember these fractures are usually symmetrical but are rarely 'textbook' examples.

Other fractures include the following.

- Fracture of the malar complex, consisting of the zygomatic arch, the malar bone and part of the lateral and inferior orbital walls. Here, it is possible to have a 'blowout' fracture at the weakest point of the orbital floor due to direct impact, i.e. a sudden increase in intraorbital pressure. This may be caused by direct or indirect violence, due to soft tissue impact increasing pressure from an object. The zygomatic arch can be depressed through direct impact. Presentation may include, in a severe form, epitaxis, facial numbness, painful eye movement, possibly an alteration in the level of consciousness, and possibly a visible change in the shape of the face, all on the side of the impact. Treatment involves decompression, by levering the bone out and repositioning it surgically. Like all fractures these may be stable or unstable. Covering the area with gauze and icing will help to control pain. If the athlete is in pain because of eye movement, cover both eyes.
- Fracture of the nasal complex, including the cartilaginous part, the upper bony part and the septum. Impacts can be frontal, lateral or combinations thereof. The obvious presentations are epitaxis and deformity. Ideally, these deformities are corrected under anaesthesia. Bleeding should be stopped and the nose iced.

Mandibular fractures

The most common sites of mandibular fracture are:

- neck of the condyle with or without temporomandibular joint (TMJ) dislocation;
- angle of the mandible;
- the body of the mandible;
- at the symphysis.

Again, like all fractures they may be stable or unstable. Presentation includes malocclusion, bitten tongue, difficulty in speaking and palpable or visual deformity. In cases where headguards are worn, releasing the chin strap may not be a good idea in severe cases. If in doubt leave the chin strap in place until X-ray films show the extent of the damage. Where chin straps are not worn, the usual first aid approach is adequate. Make sure they are not swallowing blood and they have a clear airway. Ice helps to control pain and bleeding until arrival at the hospital emergency department.

Post-trauma care

These fractures have to be reduced and immobilized, for at least 4 weeks. The process of immobilization can involve wiring with splints externally or internally. Cranial and facial movement can be directed to reduce the amount of scarring, increasing vascular, neural and lymphatic integrity to the area.

Damage to teeth and fillings

These may be made unstable at their roots (luxed), fractured partially or fully, or impacted. The danger of a dislodged (avulsed) tooth is aspiration into the airway. Bleeding can be stemmed by placing cotton wool in the mouth.

If the tooth is avulsed one of the following procedures can be followed.

1. If you replant the avulsed tooth immediately:
    (a) Wash the tooth with a pH-balanced cell preserving solution.
    (b) If none is available, use sterile saline. **Do not use water**.
    (c) Do not attempt to sterilize the tooth.
    (d) Do not wipe or scrape the root of the tooth.
    (e) Replant the tooth in the correct alignment.
    (f) Have the athlete bite gently on a gauze to hold the tooth in place.
    (g) Take the athlete to a dentist immediately.
2. If you do not replant the tooth immediately:
    (a) Place the avulsed tooth in a small, clean container, e.g. a contact lens case.
    (b) If you do not have a container, place the tooth in paper or cloth that has been soaked in cold fresh milk.
    (c) If no milk is available use sterile saline or saliva.
    (d) Do not attempt to clean the tooth.
    (e) Do not cover or wrap the tooth in anything dry.
    (f) Do not put the tooth in water, alcohol, juice or powdered milk.

The loss of a filling can be very painful, but the pain may not be immediate. If there is deep pain, oil of cloves provides adequate anaesthesia until the athlete reaches a dentist. If there is going to be some time before the athlete gets to a dentist, a temporary filling can be used.

Intracranial haematoma

This is a collection of blood due to bleeding anywhere within the cranial contents, and includes subdural, epidural, subarachnoid and intracerebral haematomas. These are classified as space-occupying lesions. All these intracranial haematomas can occur due to the shearing forces of collision or contact. Some may present well after the event, up to days or weeks later. Any athlete who complains of a headache, stiff neck or any symptom that may be associated with the brain or contents should be thoroughly examined. The slow bleeding of intracranial haemorrhages is life threatening, and time is vital.

Intracranial haemotomas have the following signs and symptoms.

1. Headache. This is a common symptom. A full examination should be carried out in any patient presenting with this symptom.
2. Vomiting. Typical cerebral or intracranial vomiting is rarely preceded by nausea and is projectile in character. Vomiting associated with raised intracranial pressure is rarely similar to this cerebral type where nausea is more common. It should be remembered that vomiting is often a late sign of raised intracranial pressure, so that athletes may arrive at the surgery complaining of severe headache and vomiting days or weeks after the traumatic event.
3. Papilloedema. This is the most important sign of raised intracranial pressure. It is diagnosed with an ophthalmoscope, and it is important to know the normal variations of the optic disc. It does not present immediately after the event and may take days or weeks to present.
4. Visual and pupil disturbances. Due to the nature of the injury there may be a homonymous hemianopsia from thrombosis of the posterior cerebral artery in a uncal herniation. An abnormality in the gaze secondary to brain stem injury may be present, and is more likely in children. There may be ipsilateral pupillary dilatation due to the effect on the third cranial nerve.
5. Mental and mood changes. This has also been mentioned before. It may be more noticeable by the individual's family or close friends. Changes may be subtle and difficult or impossible to diagnose in the surgery.
6. Epilepsy or fits. These tend to be a sign of a chronic presentation.
7. Heart rate. Slowing of the heart rate (bradycardia) is due to effects on the vagal centres in the medulla. This is an important sign.
8. Breathing. As with the heart rate, the respiratory centres in the medulla can be affected. This will cause alterations in the breathing pattern, such as Cheyne–Stokes breathing.

Epidural haematoma

This occurs when a dural artery is ruptured, approximately 85% occurring due to injury of the middle meningeal artery. It can also occur as a result of damage to the meningeal vein or dural sinus. The haematoma is between the skull and the dura mater, and is usually associated with a skull fracture. They tend to bleed fairly quickly. The head injury is often classified as mild, with a short period of unconsciousness. The time period between the injury and the athlete losing consciousness can be from minutes to hours. This is due to the high pressure arterial system, compared with the lower pressure venous system of the subdural haematoma.

Subdural haematoma

This usually occurs when the cortical bridging veins between the brain and dura are torn, on the opposite side to the impact. 'Cerebral twisting' within the cranium is the most common cause of this presentation, especially in contact/collision sports. It is usually due to the low pressure venous system, but can result from damage to the arterial system. In its more acute form this event includes cerebral or brain stem contusion or both, and a rapidly declining neurological status. Due to this low pressure system damage a slow bleed is common. Neurological deterioration may occur over 2 or more weeks due to the chronic bleed.

Intracerebral haematoma

This is bleeding within the brain itself. Again this may be a sequela of a brain contusion. This tends to follow a similar path to that of a brain contusion, but is much more dangerous.

Headache

Headache should never be assumed to be of a simple origin. A full clinical history should always be completed, including all psychological and somatic systems.

The athlete with a headache should be asked the following questions.

1. Is the headache recent or chronic?
2. What is the location and distribution of the headache?
3. Is there a history, recent or past, of trauma or infection?
4. Does the headache have any pattern, e.g. daily, occupational, training-related, sexual activity, nutrition and hunger, medication, reading, writing, menses, or when resting?
5. Are there any associated signs or symptoms? These could include sweating at night, general low grade fever, stiffness in the neck, photophobia, sinus problems, respiratory disorders, constipation, diarrhoea, and past injuries or disorders.

The following are some of the most common causes of headache and their usual signs and symptoms.

1. Subarachnoid haemorrhage. The signs and symptoms may include dizziness, vertigo, insomnia and mood changes, especially depression.
2. Cerebrovascular accident (CVA). The headache tends to be non-throbbing and there may be contralateral paraesthesia, anaesthesia and facial weakness.
3. Meningitis. Symptoms are progressive nuchal rigidity, lethargy, fever and altered consciousness. Symptoms are increased by head shaking,

jugular vein compression or any action that increases intracranial pressure, e.g. coughing and sneezing.

4. Post-traumatic headache. Common in contact and collision sports participants. This may suggest a subdural haematoma. Any of the signs and symptoms in 1 above may develop.

5. Trigeminal neuralgia (tic douloreux). This is a stabbing form of facial/ head pain, lasting from seconds to minutes, that covers the second or third division of the trigeminal nerve, i.e. the maxillary and mandibular regions. Exacerbation is usually through cold, wind, touch and chewing. There is a tendency towards chronic presentation; however fortunately, in a large number of cases, it is osteopathically treatable.

6. Space-occupying lesion. This is difficult to assess and may be a combination of all the above. Any enlarging mass in the intracranial cavity will show signs and symptoms based on the function it is disrupting. The clinical assessment should be effective enough to know that something is wrong, and the athlete referred to a specialist.

7. Benign intracranial hypertension. Women are more frequently affected than men. There are again signs of increased intracranial pressure. Specific diagnosis needs hospitalization.

8. Temporal arteritis. This condition appears to affect more women than men, especially around the age of 50. Non-specific signs and symptoms are the general trend, including weight loss, arthralgia, fever, malaise and lethargy. Wearing a hat, combing hair and chewing cause increased pain, as the temporal artery is irritated by these actions. Palpatory findings are focal tenderness, modulation, decreased pulsation and thickening of the temporal artery. Blood tests show an increased erythrocyte sedimentation rate (≥ 100 mm/h). Corticosteroid treatment is effective and NSAIDS may reduce symptoms.

9. Tension headache. These make up the aetiological bulk of headaches. Causes range from emotional stress to the stress of events. In extreme cases they may be associated with vomiting and diarrhoea. The location of pain in the head can vary, but tends to cover an area from the subocciput to the area covered by the trapezius. On a local level, due to the reduction in movement of the suboccipital joints and muscle, structural changes occur leading to the headache. Restriction of motion, characterized by muscular tightness that is often accompanied by increased localized metabolic activity, can be provoked by hyperexcitability in the neuromuscular reflex feedback loop, by vasoconstriction and constriction of the lymphatics, and by an increase or reorganization of connective tissue within the muscle. Irreversible atrophic changes resulting in destruction of individual muscle fibres can also occur and are characterized by replacement of the skeletal muscle with a fatty type of tissue. Fatty planes of tissue can be readily distinguished from skeletal muscle by MRI performed with a standard spin-echo pulse protocol (Hallgren et al., 1994). Neurological examination is unremarkable. Osteopathic manipulative therapy (OMT) tends to relieve the immediate discomfort.

10. Migraine. This is generally classified as 'classic' or 'common' migraine, with a spectrum of presentation between the two. A spasm is followed by dilatation of the external carotid arteries. Auras and visual disturbances accompany the classic presentation. These include hemianopic field disturbances, scotomas and scintillations that enlarge, spreading peripherally. Common presentations are less dramatic. Treatment consists of the administration of ergot preparations, narcotic analgesics and OMT. There are numerous factors that may set the condition off.

11. Cluster headache. This is also known as Horton's histaminic cephalgia, and is considered to be a migraine variant. Presentations tend to be periocular, unilateral, non-throbbing and lasting from minutes to hours. The attack may be accompanied by a Horner's syndrome, nasal stuffiness and tears. Treatment is the same as for migraine.

12. Hypertension. These headaches accompany increased intracranial pressure following subarachnoid haemorrhaging. They are usually mild and bilateral, with pain decreasing towards the end of the day.

13. Occipital neuralgia. This is an occipital headache that may be felt slightly periorbitally. There may be slight oedema and tenderness in the region of the suboccipital muscles. Pain results from irritation of the suboccipital nervous tissue. Treatment includes OMT and NSAIDs.

14. Postherpitic neuralgia. Headache tends to follow the dermatome of the affected nerve. Signs and symptoms include burning and sharp pains that may range from severe and constant to mild and activity related. This type of headache responds very well to OMT. Narcotics, non-narcotics and NSAIDs are indicated.

15. Somaticoskeletal dysfunction. This area is vast. Specific lesions as far down as the pelvis and even postural dysfunction and gastrointestinal tract problems can ultimately lead to headache. Neural, vascular and lymphatic tissue rely on soft tissue tension range for their health. Maintained tension can precipitate alteration in the VOR and VCR, as we have seen (p. 238).

Mouth injuries

The most common problems found in the mouth (tongue, gums and cheeks) are white lesions that are sore, named leukoplakia. These mostly reflect the athlete's general health, unless they have specific aetiologies. History, including medications and dietary habits, should be taken, and the athlete's general well-being assessed.

Ulceration
This is usually circular in appearance, white, with a red centre. The athlete tends to avoid acid or irritants such as spices, due to the extreme soreness and stinging nature of this lesion. Commonest locations are inside the lips, outside the gums and on the lateral borders of the tongue.

Tobacco smoker's keratosis
The lining of the mouth shows an even, white appearance, especially on the inside of the lip where the cigarette is always placed. This area of white patching becomes thickened, but there is no dysplasia. It is reversible once the athlete stops smoking.

Smokeless tobacco
This includes dry snuff, sachet of moist tobacco like a tea bag, and chewing tobaccos which are loose-leaf (shredded tobacco leaves), plug (compressed tobacco) and twist (twisted leaves) looking like liquorice. Again, habitual use leads to leukoplakia in a patch form especially at the site where the tobacco is habitually placed. Constant use leads to a receding of the gums leading to increased risk of bone and tooth loss. Three to six per cent of leukoplakia lesions have the potential to convert to cancer (Glover *et al.*, 1990).

Frictional keratosis
This is usually caused by the rubbing of material on the gums or lining of the mouth. A common factor is an ill-fitting gum shield where the rubbing produces a non-dysplastic epithelial change. The gum should be kept clean with regular mild mouthwash until healed.

Thrush
Commonly appears as white scattered plaques. These are spores and hypae of *Candida*. Can be easily wiped away.

Candidosis
In the early onset form in childhood, unlike thrush this cannot be wiped away. There will tend to be extraoral signs of *Candida* infection on the nails or skin. There may be a history of respiratory infections which may be a reflection of general dysfunction of the immune system (especially T-cell). In the late onset (adult) form, lesions are seen as a more speckled/nodular form of leukoplakia, anywhere in the oral cavity. Smoking and oral irritation are predisposing factors. These lesions, as in the early onset form, are not a precursor to malignancy.

Oral cancer
The speed of the plaque presentation and its rapid growth as a very white, well-defined lesion with a less white discoloration in the immediate area are the signs of oral cancer. It tends to be a squamous cell carcinoma on biopsy. If in doubt refer immediately to a specialist.

Gum shields (mouthguards)
It cannot be emphasized enough how important a well-fitting, good quality gum shield is. It will prevent many cases of injury. This is not only because of the obvious reduction in risk of concussion but also because poor occlusion, especially in contact and collision sports, weakens the body as a whole. Temporomandibular joint (TMJ) function can be

Table 6.3 Types of oral injuries seen in female athletes

Sport	Lip laceration	Chin/ tongue laceration	Chipped tooth	Broken tooth	Displaced tooth	Lost tooth	Jaw fracture	TMJ (sprain)
Basketball	207	78	57	10	24	3	0	7
Soccer	51	39	8	1	0	0	0	0
Lacrosse	22	11	7	1	0	0	2	0
Field hockey	39	20	4	7	5	1	3	0
Volleyball	30	31	8	1	0	0	0	0
Softball	26	20	8	2	4	0	5	0

(Source: Morrow and Bonci, 1989.)

compromised and the power of the whole body reduced. Have you ever tried to lift something heavy with your mouth open or your jaw deviated to one side? It is argued that many sports, e.g. soccer, should encourage the wearing of gum shields, which help dissipate the force of heading the ball. The amount of soft tissue injury protection provided by a gum shield is debatable, but there are indications that there is less dental injury (Morrow and Bonci, 1989).

Table 6.3 gives details of the types of oral injuries seen in female athletes in different sports.

Injury of the ears

Trauma to the ears mostly affects the external ear. This trauma may be associated with signs of skull fractures, at sites of the middle ear, mastoid process, TMJ (and jaw) and the basilar or temporal region. Lacerations to the ear that are haemorrhaging externally could be masking the leakage of cerebrospinal fluid. As well as external traumatic presentations, an athlete may suffer from middle or internal ear infections or dysfunctions.

Lacerations to the auricle
Lacerations occur most frequently at the creases where the auricle meets the head, behind the auricle, at the top, and where the lobule meets the head. Occasionally, a vertical laceration can occur in front of the tragus. Lacerations other than that in front of the tragus are a little more difficult to treat.

Once the area and skull have been examined, the area should be cleaned, an antibiotic applied and the ear kept as close to the head as possible by compression, using ice. The extent of the injury will determine whether further medical intervention is needed. Where the laceration is in front of the tragus, compression and ice are used to stop the bleeding and butterfly sutures can be used to close the laceration; these generally heal very well.

Cauliflower ear (haematoma auris)
This is the formation of a haematoma in the scaphoid fossa or antihelix of the external ear. Bleeding occurs between the skin and the cartilage due

to grinding or friction; this is common in rugby. If this injury is allowed to 'organize' itself it may form a thickening of disrupted tissue known as a keloid.

In its acute phase it may be possible to drain the haematoma by aspiration in a sterile environment. NSAIDs and ice packs should be used to control the bleeding and inflammation. Antibiotics can be used as a preventive measure.

Perichondritis

This is inflammation of the covering of the auricle cartilage, the perichondrium. It may be a sequela of a haematoma. It will be swollen, hot and painful. The usual treatment is with broad-spectrum antibiotics. Keeping the ear cool with a cold compress and NSAIDs will help the inflammation and pain.

Otitis externa

This infection usually involves the skin of the whole external canal, and occasionally also the tympanic membrane. It may be caused by inserting cotton buds, hairpins, matchsticks etc. into the ear. Organisms that may be found include haemolytic streptococci, *Staphylococcus aureus* and *Pseudomonas pyocyaneus*. The acute presentation involves inflammation, tenderness and weeping. In the less acute presentation there is tenderness, swelling and redness, with a crust edge to the infection. The glands in front of the tragus will be slightly swollen. This infection can affect the tympanic membrane and deafness may be present, but is usually slight. This condition can occur in both ears. This may also be signs and symptoms of failing general health, e.g. this may be associated with leukaemia.

Both topical and systemic treatments are useful. A topical antibiotic cream, neomycin based, can be applied with a cotton bud to the visible part of the infection. A strip of gauze, soaked with ichthyol in glycerin, may be used to pack the ear. With more chronic forms ear drops can be used to loosen any debris in the canal.

Otomycosis

As the name suggests, this is a fungal infection that may be a complication of otitis externa. The colour of the meatus can range from white to brown or black. Organisms usually present are *Aspergillus albicans* or *A. niger*. This infection must be cleaned regularly and carefully. A powder can be used that contains nystatin. Treatment should continue for a few weeks after the infection seems to have cleared as the fungus may be still present.

Impacted ceruman (wax in the ears)

This is fairly common in athletes. It may result from the combination of moisture and heat in showering. Excessive wax may accumulate blocking hearing or giving a feeling of fullness in the canal. Occasionally, it may cause tinnitus if the wax is pressing on the ear drum.

Treatment is by removal of the wax. Check the ear first to assess the extent of the blockage, and make sure the drum is intact (if you can see it) and there are no other foreign bodies present. One of the most common methods of wax removal is syringing the ear. Water used should be at body temperature. A little hydrogen peroxide can be added to the water as a mild disinfectant. With a receptacle under the ear, hold the lobule of the ear and draw it gently down and backwards. Water from the syringe should be directed upwards and backwards along the posterior wall of the meatus. It is important to keep the pressure constant; too much force is dangerous and it is possible to rupture the ear drum. If this method is not successful after two attempts, ear drops should be used. These can be over-the-counter preparations or warm olive oil, and are used over a period of 24 hours to loosen the wax. After wax has been removed, examine the external meatus again.

Otitis media
This can present acutely or chronically, and involves inflammation of the lining membrane in the middle ear cleft. The range of presentations are from a simple inflammation to pus formation. Bacteria such as streptococci, staphylococci and *Haemophilus* are usually present. The main route of infection seems to be along the Eustachian tube. It may develop as sequela from infections of the nasopharynx, sinuses, oropharynx or tonsils. Otitis media is especially common in children due to the frequency of upper respiratory chest infections. Infected secretions may be forced up the Eustachian tube by pressure changes caused, for example, by swimming (underwater) and excessive nose-blowing. This condition can be extremely painful, often described as a sharp lancing pain deep in the ear. There is some degree of deafness, more so in the later stages, due to an accumulation of fluid in the middle ear, where the ossicles and associated membranes are under some pressure. Purulent discharge indicates perforation of the ear drum, with less pain due to a release in the pressure. Tinnitus and vertigo can also accompany this condition. Other symptoms include a general feeling of being unwell, high temperature, pulse rate, slight headache and a furred tongue.

In the early stages of this condition diagnosis is primarily based on the appearance of the ear drum. This loses its lustre and changes from grey to greyish pink, to pink and bright red. In the later stages the drum appears as a doubled roll with a dimple in the middle, the dimple being the point of attachment of the malleus. In the final stages of the acute form the drum is very red and appears with a yellowish nipple. The mastoid bone will be tender and the condition may be confused with mastoiditis.

A tuning fork is the best method of testing the ear for deafness. Useful hearing tests include Rinne's test, which may be positive in the early stages, and Weber's test in cases of bilateral inflammation. Hearing tests should be performed in a quiet room.

Rinne's test This is a test for conductive deafness; the object is to see if bone conduction is better than air conduction. Make sure the external canal is clear. Sound the fork and hold it in line with the external acoustic meatus in front of the ear. Ask the athlete repeatedly if they hear the fork. The moment they stop hearing the fork place the base on the mastoid process. Repeat the process the other way around. If the athlete continues to hear the fork in the air after bone conduction then the test is positive. This is normal. If he or she hears the fork better on bone conduction then the test is negative. Sometimes the athlete may hear the fork in the other ear which, in chronic infection, may have a more acute sense of hearing.

Weber's test The object of this test is to see if both inner ears are normal, i.e. this test bypasses the normal route through the middle ears. It detects sensori-neural deafness. If there is a disturbance of the inner ear, the sensation of the vibrations will be impaired. The tuning fork is struck and placed on the midline of the head (vertex). The patient will point to the ear in which there is conductive deafness, because they can hear the vibrations in the inner ear more clearly. When both ears are affected the patient will indicate the ear that is most affected, because the inner ear has become more sensitive. In cases of sensori-neural deafness the sound will be heard in the more intact cochlea and nerves, but the middle ear has to be normal.

Schwabach's test Here, the fork is struck and placed on the athlete's mastoid process. As soon as the sound is no longer heard it is quickly transferred to the examiner's mastoid process. If the examiner continues to hear the fork then the Schwabach test on the athlete is said to be shortened. This depends on the examiner's conductive capability.

Compression changes
When travelling by air, pressure changes, especially when landing, can cause poor pressure readjustment in the ear and can be extremely painful and distressing. A predisposing factor is overproduction of mucus due to upper respiratory tract infection. The Eustachian tubes will be difficult to unblock. Damage to the drums may be seen as redness on examination.

Ear drops can sooth the problem and reduce the risk of infection. The athlete should not travel in pressure situations until the discomfort has gone. Repeated insult will be more painful and may lead to permanent damage. OMT is directed at decompressing the Eustachian tube.

Eye injuries

Every athlete should have 6/6 to 6/9 vision, good accommodation and smooth ocular movements.

Visual acuity is tested with the Snellen test chart. Each eye is tested separately. If an athlete standing 6 metres from the chart can only read the type that should be read 18 metres away, then the visual acuity is said to be 6/18. Successful reading of the 6 metre line means the athlete has 6/6 vision, i.e. perfect vision. Any athlete who has less than perfect eyesight should undergo further assessment by an opthalmologist.

General eye examination
The following basic areas should be covered:

- history
- general examination
- general function
- opthalmic examination.

History This is carried out in the same way as general history taking. Establish the site of discomfort (injury), a description of the pain, the mechanism of injury, and any aggravating, relieving and non-aggravating factors. Establish whether eye protection was being worn, and contact lenses or glasses. Obtain past history of eye, face, head or spinal trauma or infection. Observation and description of the athlete's condition is also important, including redness of the eye (subconjunctival haemorrhage), visual disturbances, infection of the small glands or hair follicles around the base of the eyelashes (stye), or diplopia.

General examination Both eyes should be looked at for overall symmetry and asymmetry. Asymmetrical eyes are very rare. Slight facial deformity and a past injury may lead to eye pain. Looking at the eyes in the following order may be useful.

1. Orbital rim and cheek: this area should be examined for symmetry and palpated for tenderness. A periorbital contusion (black eye) may begin around the orbital rim (over the eyebrow) and track down over the upper eyelid. Deviation of the nasal bones should also be examined.
2. Eyelids: ptosis, haemorrhage, lacerations and ecchymosis of the upper lid should be looked far.
3. Orbit: look for subconjunctival haemorrhage (red eye), pooling in the lower part of the anterior chamber after injury (hyphaema), abrasions, lacerations and foreign bodies. Intraorbital pressure can be compared with the athlete's eyes shut and gentle pressure applied with the fingers.
4. Cornea and sclera: integrity of these structures, colour and no signs of damage or inflammation, are normal.

General function This includes accommodation, movements, pupil reflex etc.

Ophthalmic examination Includes examination of the optic disc, looking for anteroventral nipping, patches on the retinal wall etc.

Orbital blowout fracture
This is a fracture of the orbital floor as a result of impact, e.g. with a tennis or squash ball, to the eye; the resulting sudden increase in intraorbital

pressure 'blows out' the orbital floor into the maxillary sinus. As well as severe pain, other common signs and symptoms include:

- unilateral epitaxis;
- inability to follow examiner's finger when moved or look around;
- diplopia;
- enophthalmos;
- subconjunctival haemorrhage (red eye) and ecchymosis;
- periorbital oedema, ecchymosis or emphysema;
- unequal pupil height compared with opposite side.

Movement of the eye will greatly increase the pain. Cover both eyes with eye pads to stop the athlete looking about, and explain why you are doing this as it may be very alarming. A mixed ice and water bag over the pad, covering the injured side of the face, may be of some help. However, cold is dangerous to the eyeball and should not be applied for more than 5 min at a time.

X-rays (Water's view) may be useful; tomograms may provide more information.

Periorbital contusion

This is also known as a 'black eye', in its bruised or ecchymotic presentation. In the majority of cases the player will recover without much intervention by the osteopath. However, it is important to run through a basic examination of the eye, its movements, integrity of the surrounding bony structures and neurological status. Treatment is with an ice and water bag, which should not be held on the area for more than 5 min at a time.

Hyphaema

This is the accumulation of blood in the anterior chamber of the eye. It may be so minor that it is missed on examination. There is usually a history of trauma to the eye, or the orbit from a fracture, resulting in disruption of the vascular integrity of the eye. With these presentations there is a risk of rebleeds, sometimes called 'eight-ball haemorrhages'. The common presentation is a semicircular pool of blood covering the lower half of the iris, just below the pupil. The athlete should refrain from any physical activity, which might precipitate rebleeding; if rebleeding occurs it is most commonly within the first week. Anti-fibrinolytic drugs should be considered. Ice over the occiput or neck may be useful. Prognosis is generally good, especially if there is no rebleed, no further eye damage and the blood clears rapidly.

Detached retina

This is where the retina detaches from the underlying retinal pigment epithelium inside the eye. It may occur weeks, months or even years after a trauma. Trauma may take the form of blunt eye injury or repeated minor trauma (e.g. in boxing, rugby or football). Forms of retinal detachment include vitreous body degeneration, liquification and traction. The athlete may complain of a 'curtain' or 'veil' or a blind spot (positive scotoma) of darkness interfering with sight. The condition may progress to the point where the athlete complains about 'flashes of light', which is due to physical stimulation of the retina as the scotoma progresses. Normal ophthalmoscope examination may be useful. As the area of detachment is elevated from the retinal pigment, it loses its transparency, and the normal vascular architecture is disrupted. With continuing elevation a convex (plus) lens should be added to the viewing port of the ophthalmoscope. This will allow you to focus sharply on the internal surface of the detachment. Treatment is by laser surgery, cryosurgery or OMT, depending on the cause. A good history is important.

Eyeball contusion
This is due, mainly, to blunt trauma and results in hyphaema. Treat as any eye contusion.

Corneal abrasion
This is usually caused by foreign bodies in the eye, resulting in loss of the surface epithelium. Symptoms include a feeling of something in the eye, even if nothing is seen on examination, pain and tears (epiphora). Examination should be performed using fluorescein sodium (Minims® or Opulets®) and rose bengal (Minims®) solutions which stain the cornea allowing you to clearly see any denuded or devitalized areas. In cases of extreme pain a topical anaesthetic can be used. Always check for additional eye injury. Treatment is generally minimal. The pain and discomfort should be managed with restriction of movement of the eyelid. A patch over the eye can be used. Large abrasions may need some topical medication. An eyewash may bring some relief. Cover both eyes if pain is too much due to movement. Prognosis, if uncomplicated, is very good. Healing should be under way within 24–48 hours. Do not continually use topical medication as this can interfere with healing, especially topical anaesthetics.

Foreign bodies
These are usually in the form of mud, grit or soil, or occasionally an eyelash. The risk of corneal abrasion is greater with soil and negligible with eyelashes. Signs, symptoms, treatment and prognosis are the same as for corneal abrasion. A tissue cottonbud can be useful in the removal of objects from the eye.

Corneal laceration
This may occur with blunt trauma as well as sharp objects. Any laceration of the eye should be taken very seriously. Shattering of eye protectors or foreign bodies are the commonest presentation. Lacerations can affect both the eye globe and the eyelid (upper and lower). The eyelid will show pain, swelling, haemorrhage and external laceration. Trauma to the eyelid

can affect the globe if it is deep enough. Injury to the globe presents with pain, decreased vision, distortion or displacement of the pupil, and possibly loss of the fundus red reflex.

Examination of the eyelids and eye globe should always be performed together.

Eyelids:

- normal anatomical relationship and symmetry with other side;
- opening and closing the eyelids;
- there may be damage to supportive functional structure, e.g. the lacrimal system.

The globe:

- haemorrage, especially subconjunctival bleeding;
- pupil symmetry, i.e. round, central and symmetrical – make sure there is no displacement of the pupil, which may indicate deep laceration;
- scleral laceration: this may also displace the pupil;
- prolapsed uveal tissue, usually presents as a dark brown or black mass;
- intraocular bleeding, may cause loss of the fundus red reflex.

If there is any hint of the above tissue damage the athlete should be sent to an ophthalmologist or accident department as soon as possible. Cover both eyes as this will reduce eye movement. Reassure the athlete that this is just a precautionary measure. Prognosis depends on the speed of treatment, location and severity of the injury.

Conjunctivitis
The usual presentation is irritability and redness of the eye, occasionally with swelling of the eyelid. An example is 'swimmer's eyes', resulting from chlorine irritation. Likely pathogens include *Staphylococcus aureus* and adenovirus. Cross-infection may occur by droplet infection, and especially by sharing towels. Treatment is generally with broad-spectrum antibiotics, e.g. chloramphenicol and neomycin ointment and drops. Where the infection is viral, antibiotics are prescribed to prevent secondary infection. OMT is directed at the superior cervical ganglia, cervical joints, soft tissue, upper thorax, especially the ribs, and the soft tissues.

Stye
This is an infection of the root of the eyelash. It generally occurs on the rim of the bottom eyelid and presents as a red/white pimple that is sore and hot. Treat with hot compress to improve blood supply to the area. Topical antibiotic cream may be used to reduce the risk of further infection.

Contact lenses
More athletes are wearing contacts lenses than ever before. There are generally two types, hard and soft. Hard lenses are more likely to cause eye irritation and abrasion than soft. If a contact lens is accidentally removed from the eye, it should be wetted with a sterile lens solution

before being reinserted. Saliva or non-sterile liquid should not be used to moisten the lens as this may lead to infection.

Injuries of the nose

Epitaxis

Nose bleeds (epitaxis) are fairly common occurrences in contact sports such as rugby and boxing. Fortunately, they are rarely serious. Signs and symptoms are blood leaking from one of the nasal passages; rarely both are affected. Usually there is a history of recent trauma. Some presentations can be alarming, especially if the blood has already started to clot and stopped bleeding for a while and then the clot is dislodged. A nose bleed with no history of recent trauma, i.e. in the past few days, may indicate a more serious problem, especially if it is accompanied by other signs and symptoms such as headache, visual disturbance and mood and memory changes.

Do not let the athlete pinch the nose and tip the head back, as the respiratory passage will begin to fill up with blood. Apply cold to the occipital region, around the neck (ice in a towel) and/or over the nose. Pinching the nose and leaning forwards is acceptable with cold applied. If bleeding continues, packing the nose with gauze or cotton wool and pinching it will stem the flow. The athlete should not blow the nose for a few hours, and even then very gently. The inside of the nose may begin to itch as the vessels begin to heal. In cases where bleeding does not stop vessels may have to be cauterized; in this case the athlete should be sent to the hospital emergency department. Prognosis is good in the majority of cases. Players can usually return to play immediately as most nose bleeds will stop in a few seconds. If it takes a few minutes, the player should sit out until the bleeding has stopped, for 5–10 min.

Deviated septum

This usually accompanies a nose bleed. Check for deformity of the nose, remembering that the athlete may have broken his or her nose before. There will be swelling and deviation of the nose from the midline which suggests a nasal fracture. To assess visually, stand behind the athlete while they are seated and look over their forehead; also, ask the athlete to look at themselves in the mirror to see if there is any deviation. Check for further facial fractures with gentle but firm pressure around the area. As with epitaxis, a cold pack helps to reduce the pain and control any bleeding. If you are concerned about the extent of the damage send them to the hospital emergency department. Prognosis is usually good.

Important note: do not forget that a player who has a nose bleed may also be concussed, have a broken nose or other fractures. Do not be distracted by the bleeding.

Foreign bodies

Players may breathe in debris or insects, especially aphids. On rare occasions an athlete may be stung in the nose by an insect. An attempt to remove the foreign body should be made by blowing the nose gently but firmly. In the case of a sting, applying cold to the outside may reduce the discomfort. If the insect is still in the nose, tweezers can used with a flashlight to help vision, however this can push the insect or object further in. Get the player to mouth breathe to reduce the risk of inhalation and send them to the emergency department.

The temporomandibular joint, mandible and maxillar

Examination of the TMJ, mandible and maxillar should be performed in the order:

1. observation
2. palpation
3. active motion
4. passive motion

Observation

Deviations in the symmetry of the mandible are highly relevant, and should be looked for in the initial examination of the jaw. The athlete should be sitting, with at least 1 metre distance between you, and should be viewed from the front. Begin by looking at the edge of the skull and face in relation to the jaw. Continue to look at the jaw in relation to the orbits, cheek bones, nasal bones, throat and ear levels. Look for discrepancies in facial contours due to oedema, abrasions and change in skin tone.

Palpation

In palpation we are again looking for alterations from normal in quality of tissue texture, temperature, deformity, mass, numbness and tone. In addition palpate inside the external meatus with your little finger for any fullness.

Active motion

The athlete should try and move the jaw, as slowly as possible and with caution. Look for deviation in the movement of the jaw, from the midline, while it is opening and closing. If this is not too bad then the athlete should try lateral, i.e. side-to-side, motion. Both the up-and-down and side-to-side motion may have to be repeated a few times.

Passive motion

The athlete lies supine and the practitioner sits on the couch beside the athlete facing him or her. The practitioner's thumbs are placed on either side of the midline, on the point of the jaw, while the middle and index fingers are placed below and above the angle of the jaw, respectively. Passive up-and-down and side-to-side movements can be carried out on the athlete.

With injuries or dysfunctions to the mandible or maxillar look for the following changes:

- malocclusion (change in bite);
- stability of bony structures;
- pressure point pain and tenderness;
- restriction in opening, closing and chewing;
- neurological changes;
- motion deviation.

Important note: as with all injuries to the head, screen for a neurological baseline.

TMJ sprain/strain

This is an injury to the capsuloligamentous and/or musculotendinous apparatus. It is caused by a blow to the jaw, usually from the side, which stretches the structures on the side of the impact, and compresses the TMJ on the contralateral side. The following may result from trauma to the jaw:

- haemarthrosis
- capsulitis
- meniscal displacement
- subluxation
- dislocation
- fracture.

Treatment depends on the extent of the sprain/strain complex and the contribution made by the other injury factors above. The basic treatment is the same as all other joint dysfunctions. Special consideration is made here for the meniscus within the joint.

TMJ dislocation

This is not a very common presentation. It may be confused with a subluxation. In this dislocation/subluxed state the mouth tends to be held open and the point of the jaw is slightly forward. TMJ dislocation may be associated with a fracture. Perform the examination procedure as quickly as possible as time is vital in a dislocation. X-ray should be performed, and the athlete sent to an emergency department if reduction is not possible. The athlete will have the mouth open all the time if transportation to hospital is necessary. This is an uncomfortable position and the tendency is to try and close the mouth causing more pain. Plastic oral screws can be introduced on each side between the teeth to take the strain. A few layers of gauze can be placed over the open mouth.

Reduction procedure Lie the athlete down. Somebody else should hold the athlete's head. Place both thumbs inside the mouth (not on the teeth; preferably between the cheek and the molars), and index and middle fingers of each hand above and below the angle of the jaws, respectively. Cradle the jaw by placing the carpal tunnel region of the base of your hands either side of the angle of the jaw, outside the mouth. Your objective is to disengage the condyle of the jaw allowing the soft tissue to relocate the jaw. There may be so much spasm in a full dislocation that a general anaesthetic may be required before a relocation is possible.

Mandibular fracture

As with other fractures, these fractures of the lower third of the face are generally classified as simple, comminuted or compound. These fractures result from blows to the point of the jaw, from any angle. There may be more than one fracture and there may be other fracture sites in the face and/or skull associated with them. In the case of suspected fracture the jaw should be stabilized, with either a four-tailed bandage or a Barton (barrel) bandage.

Maxillary fracture

These are midface fractures, involving the upper jaw and invariably the face.

Return-to-play criteria after head injury

- After mild grade 1 concussion (see Table 6.1, p. 242) if the athlete has no symptoms at rest or exertion after a short period of observation, he or she may return to play. A second mild concussion means removal from competition for at least 2 weeks. The athletes should only be allowed to return if he or she is asymptomatic during rest and exertion for at least 1 week. It is recommended that three grade 1 concussions terminate a player's season, i.e. the athlete should not be involved in contact sports for at least 3 months.
- Return to competition after a first moderate (grade 2) concussion may be as soon as 1 week after the athlete is asymptomatic at rest and exertion. After a second grade 2 concussion the athlete should stay out for at least 1 month and termination of the season should be considered. Season participation should be terminated after a third grade 2 episode.
- One month has been suggested as the minimum disqualification from participation following grade 3 head injury. Return is only considered after 1 month if the athlete is asymptomatic at rest and exertion. A season is terminated after two grade 3 concussions.

(Adapted from Canto, R.C. and Micheli, L.V. (1991) *ACSM's Guidelines for the Team Physician.*)

SHOULDER AND UPPER EXTREMITY

Anatomy

Bones

The bones of the shoulder and upper extremity are the scapula, clavicle, humerus, radius, ulna and the proximal and distal rows of carpus which from the radial to ulnar side are:

Proximal row – the **scaphoid** has a tubercle anteriorly; its blood supply is from the radial artery into the centre of the dorsum and from the superficial palmar arch into the anterolateral surface distally and the distal pole (tubercle). The **proximal pole** is prone to avascular necrosis with a fracture of the waist or proximal third of the bone. The **lunate** has its blood supply entering into the anterior and posterior poles (in about one-third of the population only one of the two arteries is present). The **triquetrum** articulates with the **pisiform** which is a sesamoid bone in the tendon of the flexor carpi ulnaris (FCU).

Distal row – the **trapezium** has a large groove anteriorly for the tendon of the flexor carpi radialis (FCR). This groove is bounded by a ridge on the radial side. The remaining bones are the **trapezoid**, **capitate** (the largest carpel), and the **hamate**, which has a hook anteromedially.

The remaining bones of the upper extremity are five metacarpals and phalanges with respective interphalangeal joints.

Ossification

Shoulder girdle The scapula forms from cartilaginous tissue in eight or more centres, from the eighth week of intra-uterine life to the 20th year. The clavicle ossifies from two (primary) centres before any other bone in the body, between the fifth and sixth weeks of intra-uterine life. A secondary centre appears and ossifies quickly about the late teens. The humerus first appears in the head at 1 year, greater tuberosity at 3 years, and the lesser tuberosity at 5 years. Three secondary centres fuse together by the seventh year, and fuse with the shaft by the 20th year.

Elbow The first appearance of the distal humerus is in the capitulum at 3 years (epiphysis, contributes to growth in length), the medial epicondyle at 5 years (apophysis, no contribution to the growth in length), the trochlear at 7 years (epiphysis) and the external epicondyle at 11 years (apophysis). The capitulum, medial epicondyle and trochlea fuse together at 14 years, and this fuses with the shaft at 16–17 years; the lateral epicondyle fuses separately with the shaft at about 20 years. The olecranon appears at 11 years (epiphysis) and fuses at 18 or earlier. The radial head appears at 4 years and fuses at 18. The distal radius appears at 2 years of age, the ulnar head at 4 years, the capitate at 1 year, the hamate at 2 years, the triquetrum at 3 years, the lunate at 4 years, the scaphoid at 5 years, the trapezium at 6 years, the trapezoid at 7 years and the pisiform at 10–12 years. The centres follow an orderly progression around the carpals, in a circle.

Hand There is one ossification centre for the heads of the four medial metacarpals, and one for the base of every phalanx and for the first metacarpals (which behave like a phalanx in this respect).

Joints and ligaments

The pectoral girdle and shoulder

The pectoral girdle and shoulder involve a complex of four joints, the scapulothoracic, acromioclavicular, sternoclavicular and scapulohumeral joints. At the scapulothoracic joint the anterior surface of the scapula lies in a bed of muscle and slides on and around the muscle-covered posterolateral wall of the thorax. The articular surfaces of the acromio-clavicular joint consist of the lateral end of the clavicle and the anteromedial part of the acromion. An articular disc is frequently found with this articulation. The ligaments are fairly strong, and are the acromioclavicular ligament which blends with the superior part of the clavicle, and the coracoclavicular ligament, which is made up of two parts: the trapezoid section, from the stem of the coracoid process obliquely upwards and outwards to the anterolateral surface of the clavicle, and the conoid segment, which is short, thick and fan-shaped, and goes from the base of the coracoid straight up to the inferior surface of clavicle (conoid tubercle). The coracoacromial ligament forms an arch over the head of the humerus, and the tendon of the supraspinatus passes under the arch.

The joint movement and plane Due to ligamentous and fibrous capsular structures around the joint there is a limited gliding movement. The flat joint plane has a long axis that runs anteroposterior.

Sternoclavicular (SC) joint
This is without doubt the most important joint in the function of the shoulder girdle. The subtle contribution of this joint is vastly under-estimated. The medial end of the clavicle articulates with the manubrium sterni and the first costal cartilage. Between these surfaces, in the joint, is an intra-articular meniscus or disc. Anterior and posterior ligaments attach to the manubrium, the superior of which is very strong, blending with the superior ligament from the other side, therefore it is also known as the interclavicular ligament. The costoclavicular ligament, which is a strong structure, attaches to the first rib. Behind (posteriorly to) the joint are the sternohyoid and sternothyroid muscles. Behind these muscles are the innominate vein and common carotid artery on the left and the bifurcation of the innominate artery on the right.

Ranges of motion It is important to basically realize that the SC joint follows shoulder motion in normal function, but impedes normal motion in dysfunction. Motion is described as medial head clavicular movement. Elevation of the shoulder – inferior movement; depression of the shoulder – superior movement; protraction – posterior movement; and retraction – anterior motion. The SC joint cannot perform normal combinations of these movements if the starting position is altered; it will run out of movement possibilities.

Scapulohumeral (glenohumeral, GH) joint
The glenoid cavity of the scapula looks upwards and outwards, laterally and 30° forwards. It is very shallow, but is enlarged and deepened by the glenoid labrum, a fibrocartilaginous rim. The humeral head is one-third of a sphere, facing upwards medially and 30° posteriorly; the head/shaft angle is 130°; anatomically the neck separates the head from the shaft, lies

along the border of the articular cartilage, and forms an angle of 40° with the horizontal. Stability of the joint depends on the capsule and ligaments (passive and weak) and the muscles (active). The capsule inserts around the edge of the glenoid labrum and around the superior part of the anatomical neck of the humerus; inferiorly the insertion lies nearer the surgical neck – the proximal humeral metaphysis is intracapsular at this point; the surgical neck lies horizontally at the level of the lesser tuberosity and the proximal growth plate. The coracohumeral ligament is the strongest of the ligaments. The glenohumeral ligaments are three thickened bands in the front of the capsule and consist of the superior (horizontal), middle (oblique) and the inferior (horizontal) forming a 'Z' shape. The muscles of this joint are short and stabilizing, arising from the scapula; their tendons blend with the capsule, forming the rotator cuff muscles. These are: subscapularis (anterior), supraspinatus (superior), infraspinatus (posterosuperior) and teres minor (posteroinferior).

Muscles of the pectoral girdle

Posterior group

Trapezius Origin (O): from the superior nuchal line of the skull, ligamentum nuchae (along the tips of spines of the cervical vertebrae), and all thoracic vertebral spines. Insertion (I): into the lateral third of the clavicle, acromion and spine of scapula above the origin of the deltoid. Nerve supply (N): the spinal accessory nerve, C2, C3, C4. Action (A): elevation of scapula and shoulder, and with serratus anterior it rotates the scapula.

Latissimus dorsi O: from the spines of the seventh to twelfth thoracic vertebrae, spines of all lumbar vertebrae, posterior part of the iliac crest and inferior angle of the scapula. It runs laterally and twists around the inferior border of teres major to form the posterior wall of the axilla, then inserts into the floor of the bicipital groove of the humerus, between the pectoralis major laterally and teres major medially. N: thoracodorsal nerve from posterior cord of brachial plexus C6, C7, C8. A: adduction, internal (medial) rotation and extension of shoulder.

Levator scapulae O: from the transverse processes of the upper four cervical vertebrae. I: to the upper quarter of the medial border of the scapula, above the base of the spine of the scapula. N: special branches from the cervical plexus, C3, C4, C5, and dorsal scapular nerve. A: pulls scapula medially and upwards, squares the shoulders.

Rhomboids O: from the spines of C7 and T1 (minor) and T2 to T5 (major). I: to the lower three-quarters of the medial border of the scapula. N: dorsal scapular nerve, C5. A: similar to levator scapulae.

Anterior group

Pectoralis major O: from medial half of clavicle, sternum and rectus abdominis aponeurosis, runs up and laterally, while tendon twists through 180° as it approaches the humerus, so that the lowest muscle fibres insert the highest, and forms the anterior wall of the axilla. I: into the lateral lip of the bicipital groove, covering the long head of the biceps. N: medial and lateral pectoral nerves, C6, C7, C8. A: adduction, flexion and internal (medial) rotation of the arm.

Pectoralis minor O: from costochondral junction of the third, fourth and fifth ribs. I: runs to medial border of the coracoid process. N: pectoral nerve, C8. A: depression of the shoulder, and with the serratus anterior, it pulls the scapula forwards around the chest.

Serratus anterior O: from upper eight ribs anteriorly by interdigitations. I: to deep aspect of entire medial border of scapula. N: long thoracic nerve, C5, C6, C7. A: pulls the scapula forwards and rotates it (push forwards).

Muscles of the shoulder joint

Subscapularis
O: the entire surface of subscapular fossa of scapula. I: the lesser tuberosity of the humerus. N: upper and lower subscapular nerves, C6, C7. A: internal rotation of the arm. An important point is that a bursa lies beneath this muscle and often communicates with the synovial cavity of the shoulder joint.

Supraspinatus
O: from the supraspinatus fossa of the scapula. I: to the superior facet on the greater tuberosity of the humerus. N: the suprascapular nerve, C5. A: Initiates abduction of the shoulder.

Infraspinatus
O: from infraspinatus fossa. I: to the middle facet of the posterior surface of the greater tuberosity. N: suprascapular nerve, C5. A: external rotation of the arm.

Teres minor
O: from the upper part of the axillary border of the scapula. I: to the lowest facet of the posterior surface of the greater tuberosity. N: axillary nerve, C5. A: external rotation of the arm.

Teres major
O: from the angle of the scapula. I: to the medial lip of the bicipital groove. N: lower scapular nerve, C6, C7. A: internal rotation and

adduction, and with teres minor, prevents upward movement of the humeral head when the shoulder is abducted.

Deltoid
O: this is in three parts, from the lateral third of the clavicle, the acromion, and the spine of the scapula below the insertion of the trapezius. I: all three parts meet to form a common tendon inserting into the deltoid tuberosity on the lateral surface of the humerus. N: axillary nerve, C5. A: this, like the origins, is threefold. The anterior part flexes, the central part abducts the arm, and the posterior part extends the arm. Both the anterior and posterior parts stabilize the humeral head in abduction.

Axillary spaces

These are quadrangular and triangular spaces. Their integrity is clinically vital. They are structured by the teres minor, teres major, the humerus and the long head of the triceps brachii. Narrowing of these spaces is the major causative factor in the presentation of non-conforming myotome and dermatome signs and symptoms. Compression and irritation (chemical or physical) of neurovascular structures to and from the upper extremity can lead to presentations in the upper limb, thorax, neck or head.

The axilla is shaped like a pyramid, having an apex, four walls and a base:

- apex – anteriorly by the clavicle, medially the first rib, and posteriorly the superior border of the scapula;
- anterior wall – two pectoral muscles and the clavipectoral fascia;
- medial wall – upper four or five ribs and serratus anterior;
- posterior wall – superior to inferior: subscapularis, latissimus dorsi twisting beneath teres major, included in the wall is the quadrilateral space of Velpeau, which forms an exit for the axillary nerve and posterior circumflex artery from the axilla and is formed by the subscapularis above, long head of triceps medially, teres major below, and humerus laterally;
- lateral wall – the humerus and coracobrachialis;
- base – the superficial and deep aponeurotic layers.

Contents
The axilla is lined with a tubular downward continuation of the cervical fascia to form the axillary artery and vein, the brachial plexus and the long thoracic nerve. Axillary fat is of particular importance since it gives support to the structures, especially the axillary vein, passing through the region. The loss of this function of the fat is well illustrated by oedema of the arm that sometimes appears after the fat has been removed with the lymphatic glands during the course of radical mastectomy (Cathie, 1974a).

Vascular system of the upper limb

The venous system
The axillary vein lies medial to the artery and brachial plexus, continuing over the first rib as the subclavian vein and continuing as the brachio-cephalic emptying into the superior vena cava. The veins are divided into the superficial veins lying mostly outside the deep fascia, and the deep veins which lie inside the fascial sleeve accompanying the arteries.

- Superficial veins – the fingers drain through the anastomosis on the palmar and dorsal aspect of the hand. Palmar drainage returns through the dorsal veins at the back of the hand, especially into the intercapitular veins. The radial aspect drains through the cephalic veins and the ulnar aspect drains through the basilic vein. This cephalic drainage passes through the clavipectoral fascia ending at the axillary vein, while the basilic vein drains to the axilla continuing as the axillary vein.
- Deep veins – these veins are arranged in pairs, except for the axillary vein, and they drain in pairs following the arteries.

Lymphatic drainage
The lymphatics of the fingers are drained into the palm and then to the dorsal aspect of the hand. Drainage of palmar tissues passes on to the wrist (ulnar border) and the thumb drains to the wrist (radial border). Continuing up the forearm and arm the superficial lymphatics follow the superficial veins. Medial vessels follow the basilic vein continuing along the medial border of the biceps, piercing the deep fascia. Lateral vessels follow the cephalic vein turning medially after the insertion of the deltoid draining into the lateral group of the axillary nodes. The axillary nodes are divided into the lateral group, draining the entire limb, other than those following the cephalic vein; the anterior (pectoral) group drain the areas of the anterior and lateral walls of the thorax, including the level above the umbilicus and central and lateral parts of the mammary gland; the posterior (subscapular) group drain the skin and muscles of the lower part of the back of the neck, those vessels that follow the cephalic vein, the upper and peripheral part of the mammary gland. The nodes drain into the subclavian trunk on the right and the thoracic duct on the left.

Arterial supply
The immediate supply of the upper limb differs on the right and left. The right arterial supply leaves the aortic arch by way of a short, wide vessel known as the brachiocephalic trunk. This trunk then divides into the right common carotid artery and the right subclavian artery. This subclavian artery continues down the upper limb. The left subclavian artery begins directly from the aortic arch. Both left and right subclavian arteries change their names as they pass various landmarks in the upper limb, as follows: the axillary artery on entering the axilla, the brachial artery at the lower border of the teres major muscle, dividing into the radial and ulnar

arteries on passing the cubital fossa, the radial artery continues to the lateral aspect of the wrist, curves around the back of the hand then passes anteriorly through the interosseous space between the first and second metacarpal bones, finally anatomosing with the deep palmar branch of the ulnar artery. The ulnar artery runs from the cubital fossa, on the ulnar side of the forearm, to the flexor retinaculum; here it continues laterally to the pisiform dividing into the superficial palmar arch and a deep palmar branch joining the radial artery to form the deep palmar arch.

The subclavian artery has two branches in the neck: the transverse cervical branch which continues to the deep surface of the trapezius muscle, and through a deeper branch to the levator scapulae, supraspinatous, infraspinatous and subscapular areas; and the subscapular branch which continues anteriorly to the brachial plexus, the suprascapular notch and distributes throughout the supraspinous and infraspinouus fossae supplying branches to the local joints and muscles.

The axillary artery is a continuation of the subclavian artery, entering the apex of the axilla, and leaving at the lower border of the teres major to become the brachial artery. It is divided into three parts by the pectoralis minor and is surrounded by fascia, the axillary sheath, which surrounds the brachial plexus in the axilla. It has three major branches: the superior thoracic artery (from the first part) to pectoral muscles, acromiothoracic and lateral thoracic arteries from the second part and subscapular, anterior and posterior circumflex humeral arteries from the third part.

The brachial artery is the continuation of the arterial system below teres major and has three main branches: the profunda brachii artery, which after stemming from the brachial artery runs down the back of the humerus accompanying the radial nerve, and then divides into two; the radial collateral artery, still following the radial nerve, to the front of the lateral epicondyle and the posterior descending branch passing behind the lateral epicondyle; and the superior ulnar artery, which runs down the back of the medial epicondyle, and the inferior ulnar collateral artery (supracondylar), which supplies branches both in front of and behind the medial epicondyle.

The radial artery branches into the following: the radial recurrent artery, the superficial palmar branch, the palmar carpal branch, dorsal carpal branch, two dorsal digital arteries, princeps pollicis artery and the radialis indicis artery.

Branches of the ulnar artery are the following: ulnar recurrents, common interosseous artery, anterior interosseous artery, posterior interosseous artery, palmar carpal branch and the dorsal palmar branch.

Brachial plexus

This consists of roots, trunks, divisions, cords and branches, which are names given to denote location while the nerves combine and travel down the upper extremity. Always remember it is a three-dimensional structure.

The roots
The roots are the anterior primary rami of C5, C6, C7, C8 and T1 lying deep between the scalenus anterior and medius muscles (which protect them) beneath the floor of the posterior triangle.

The trunks
These are at the lateral border of the scalene muscles. At this point C5 root joins C6 to form the upper trunk, C7 continues as middle trunk, and C8 joins T1 to form lower trunk. The trunks lie in the lower part of the posterior neck triangle.

The divisions
Behind the clavicle each trunk divides into the anterior division to supply the flexor compartments, and the posterior division to supply the extensor compartments.

The cords
These lie in the axilla and are named in relation to their position to the axillary artery: the lateral cord lies lateral to the axillary artery, being formed by the union of the anterior divisions of the upper and middle trunks; the medial cord lies medial to the axillary artery, being formed from the anterior division of the lower trunk; and the posterior cord lies posterior to the axillary artery, being formed from the union of all three posterior divisions. The cords approach the first part of the axillary artery, from the lateral border of the first rib to the upper border of pectoralis major, surround its second part behind pectoralis major, then give off their branches around the third part of the artery, from the lower border of pectoralis minor to the inferior border of teres major.

The branches

1. Branches from roots (3):
   (a) Dorsal scapular nerve (C5) – this goes posteriorly to supply the rhomboids, and a small branch to the levator scapulae.
   (b) Nerve to subclavius (C5, C6) travels downward and forward to supply subclavius muscle.
   (c) Long thoracic nerve (C5, C6, C7) travels posteriorly to serratus anterior.
2. Branches from trunks (1):
   (a) Subscapular nerve (C5, C6) arises from upper trunk, known as Erb's point, and goes posteriorly through the subscapular notch, beneath the fibrous band which bridges the notch. It supplies the supraspinatus and continues on to turn around the lateral end of the scapular spine to the infraspinatus.
3. There are no branches from divisions.
4. Branches from cords (13):
   (a) Lateral cord (3):
       (i) lateral pectoral nerve (C5, C6, C7) travels anteriorly to pectoralis;

(ii) musclotendinous (C5, C6, C7) travels to coracobrachialis, biceps, brachialis and supplies the skin on the lateral aspect of the forearm;

(iii) lateral head of median nerve (C5, C6, C7).

(b) Medial cord (5):

(i) medial pectoral nerve (C8, T1) travels anteriorly to pectoralis minor and pectoralis major;

(ii) medial brachial cutaneous nerve of the forearm (C8, T1);

(iii) medial antebrachial cutaneous nerve of forearm (C8, T1);

(iv) ulnar nerve (C7, C8, T1) supplies flexor carpi ulnaris (C7), the medial half of flexor digitorum profundus (C8) and intrinsics (T1);

(v) medial head of median nerve (C8, T1) – this crosses in front of the third part of the axillary artery to communicate with the lateral head of the median nerve.

(c) Posterior cord (5):

(i) upper subscapular (C6) supplies subscapularis;

(ii) thoracodorsal nerve (C6, C7, C8) supplies latissimus dorsi;

(iii) lower subscapular (C6, C7) supplies teres major and sub-scapularis;

(iv) axillary nerve (C5, C6), looping back through the quadra-lateral space in the posterior axillary wall, continues on laterally then anteriorly around the surgical neck of the humerus supplying teres minor, deltoid and the skin over the deltoid;

(v) radial nerve (C5, C6, C7, C8, T1) – leaving the axilla it passes backwards through the triangular space winding postero-laterally around the humeral shaft. In the axilla the radial nerve supplies a motor branch to the long head of triceps, another to the medial head of triceps (this branch accompanies the ulnar nerve), and the cutaneous branch, the posterior cutaneous nerve of the arm (containing all T1 fibres of radial nerve), eventually supplying all extensor compartment muscles of the arm and forearm.

Nerve root supplies to the upper extremity

- Shoulder: C5 – abduction and external rotation; C6, C7 – adduction and internal rotation.
- Elbow: C6, C7 – flexion; C7, C8 – extension.
- Forearm: C6 – supination; C6 – pronation.
- Wrist: C6, C7 – dorsiflexion; C6, C7 – palmar flexion.
- Fingers: C7, C8 – extension; C7, C8 – flexion.
- Hand intrinsics: T1 (and C8 for thenar muscles).

Function of the upper extremity

As with all parts of the body this extremity functions as an integrated and interlinking unit within itself and with the rest of the body (Fig. 6.8),

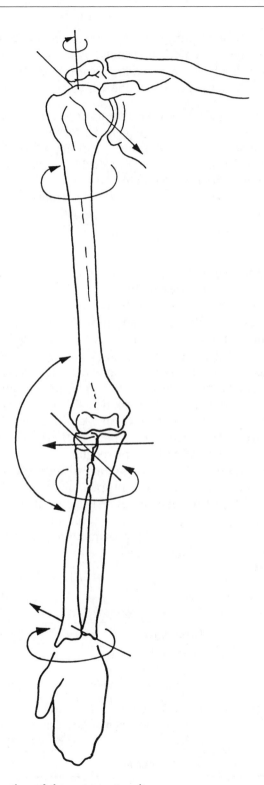

Fig. 6.8 Integration of the upper extremity.

however to communicate information the individual sections of the upper extremity have to be presented separately. Analyses have been carried out in the past, but none, so far as we are aware, have attempted to solve or derive a comprehensive picture of the whole.

> Much of the early work is very contradictory, and nearly all is incomplete, due to lack of an adequate experimental method. For this reason many misconceptions exist, owing to the too ready facility with which investigators have evolved conceptions based on *a priori* reasoning from the inert cadaver.
>
> (Inman *et al.*, 1944)

The shoulder girdle

The shoulder is a girdle of integrated function, and relies heavily on the myofasciotendon system for its stability.

The first action of the shoulder girdle is a fixing and retraction of the scapula to the thoracic wall, before any movement in any direction can take place. Components of the shoulder girdle have been described as **links** (Goldman, 1989) (Table 6.4).

Goldman describes a link as any single part of rigidly linked components that is rigidly attached to a base (frame) and has motion relative to all of the other components. A 'kinematic pair' consists of any two links that remain in contact throughout motion. A 'closed mechanism' exists when the last movement is reconnected back to the frame; conversely, in an 'open mechanism' the last link is not reconnected.

One-third of the humeral head is in contact with the glenoid fossa. The scapula and the humerus must have proper alignment of the surfaces before any true motion can take place, hence the fixing of the scapula before any motion. This is osteopathically important, especially in cases of so-called 'frozen shoulder'. Poor approximation precipitates shoulder dysfunction; this can result from trauma, repetitive minor trauma or poor adaptation (repetitive strain injury).

Table 6.4 Components of the shoulder girdle

Structure	Description
Sternoclavicular joint	The only bony connection of the upper limb to the axial skeleton
Acromioclavicular joint	Consists of articulation between the acromion process of the scapula and the distal end of the clavicle
Suprahumeral articulation	Composed of the coracoid and acromion processes and coracoacromial ligament; serves to prevent upwards dislocation of the humerus and protects from downward blows to the glenohumeral joint and the head

(From Goldman, 1989.)

Motion

The phases of motion described by Goldman (1989) in normal function of the shoulder girdle are a vital basis for the diagnosis of shoulder dysfunction. There are four basic phases.

First phase
The first is considered the 'setting mechanism', when the medial border of the scapula is anchored by action of the rhomboid major, rhomboid minor, serratus anterior, levator scapulae and the lower two sets of the trapezius. The setting mechanism involves relatively little motion of the scapula. During abduction of the upper extremity, phase 1 abducts the arm from 0 to 30°, which allows for maximal contact in the glenohumeral joint. Conversely, during flexion, phase 1 flexes the arm from 0 to 60°, which results in increased incongruity in the glenohumeral joint. In either case, the shoulder is less stable than it is at rest. At the end of this phase, motion ceases because of limitations imposed by the coracoclavicular ligament. This is known as the 'closed link phase', as an imaginary line running through the sternoclavicular joint and through the scapula forms, with the acromioclavicular joint, a triangle. This is linked and moves as one unit.

Second phase
The second phase of motion occurs along a new mechanical link – the clavicular link. This link, which is formed by eliminating motion at the acromioclavicular joint, affords increased stability to the shoulder mechanism. At this point, a rotary axis exists around an imaginary line drawn from the sternoclavicular joint to a point on the proximal scapular spine. Motion occurs during this phase via contraction of the lower fibres of the serratus anterior and ceases at approximately 100° of abduction because of the costoclavicular ligaments.

Third phase
Phase 3 begins with rotation of the clavicle along its long axis. Rotational movement now centres around the acromioclavicular joint. As the serratus anterior continues to pull the scapula inferiorly and laterally, the scapula passively follows the contour of the rib cage and the rotary motion of the clavicle. This process results in a net elevation and rotation of the acromioclavicular joint, which further abducts the upper extremity. In addition, the head of the humerus externally rotates to free itself of the overhanging acromion process. The complicated rotation and abduction of this phase ends at the limits of the trapezial ligaments. This is also known as the 'open link phase'. The triangle in phase 2 is broken and opens up.

Fourth phase
Further elevation of the lateral half of the superior border of the scapula occurs during phase 4 until there is an exhaustion of all motion capacity in the shoulder girdle.

Conclusions

Three conclusions can be made concerning the motion dynamics of the upper extremity.

1. The initial phase of elevation is dependent upon the scapulothoracic articulation and the sternoclavicular joint.
2. Further phases of elevation are dependent upon the glenohumeral and acromioclavicular joints.
3. After the setting phase, every degree of scapular motion corresponds with 2° of humeral motion (that is, for every 15° of upper extremity motion, 10° occur at the glenohumeral joint).

Dysfunction in any component in the system will hinder motion of the upper extremity.

Alterations to this normal function are the result of acute trauma and/or chronic repetitive strain. 'In a large percent of neurologic suffering of the shoulder whether there be swelling or not, I find the outer end of the clavicle pushed too far' (A.T. Still). It has been my experience that not only is the outer end of the clavicle too far back, but the whole shaft is also back and medial. While the position of the clavicle is no doubt the prime consideration in the osteopathic pathology of the painful shoulder there are other considerations (Perrin T. Wilson, DO). Normal shoulder function is impossible without normal myofascial integrated function. The regions that make the walls of the axilla and its spaces are important areas of normal palpatory quality. Irritation of the neurovascular structures passing through the quadrangular and triangular spaces leads to a spectrum of symptoms.

The elbow

This is a complex of three joints: the humero-ulnar, the radio-ulnar, and the proximal radio-ulnar joints. The three joints share one synovial cavity. Normal motion of the elbow relies on even more integrity than the shoulder. The elbow complex has more joints than the shoulder but has more rigid planes of motion, therefore it has much less room for error in functional ability and adaptive compensation than the shoulder. Normal function relies on all the joints remaining healthy. With this in mind, it may be that pain in one area of the elbow could be due to a non-pathological motion dysfunction in another area of the complex.

Upper extremity dysfunction

Impingement syndrome

This term was first used by Dr Charles Neer, to describe a number of pathological presentations that include the subacromial bursa, the rotator cuff, the biceps tendon and occasionally the acromioclavicular joint. As the name suggests, this is an impingement of structures in the space bordered by the acromion process superiorly (particularly the anterior aspect), the corocoid process anteromedially, the acromioclavicular joint superiorly, and the tuberosity of the humeral head inferiorly. Diagnosis is based on ability to name not only the structures involved in a presenting case, but to what level they are inflamed and degenerative. The range of severity with which impingement syndrome can present has been graded from I to III, in which grade I is reversible inflammation and grade III gross degeneration in the cuff and the subacromial space.

Treatment
OMT is directed at decompression of the subacromial region. The use of NSAIDs and ice is indicated in the acute presentation, while heat is sometimes used in the chronic presentation.

Subluxation of the head of the biceps

This is a movement of the long head of the biceps out of the bicepital groove. There will be mild fullness of the anterior aspect of the shoulder. Movement of the arm will still be possible, but will be sore and limited. Generally, this occurs with a history of inflammation in the area with degeneration of the transverse humeral ligament. Any motion that contracts the biceps and reduces the glenohumeral angle anteriorly could precipitate such an event. Active resisted supination will exacerbate symptoms.

Treatment
Ice, NSAIDs and support (sling). OMT should be directed at the original cause of the tendinitis. This usually involves the rotator cuff muscles, cervical spine and upper ribs. Check glenohumeral integrity.

Rupture of the head of the biceps

Sudden sharp, snapping pain and immobility of the arm are the signs. The athlete may experience only a small amount of pain to begin with, which then develops into severe pain. The biceps may show signs of bulging, but this may be hard to see initially. Active resisted supination is impossible due to pain and no muscle attachment. Bruising will appear, with confirmation by palpation that the 'muscle has gone' and moved down to the elbow or up the elbow, depending on the rupture site.

Treatment
This an orthopaedic surgical emergency, depending on the extent of the rupture. Support (sling) and transfer to emergency unit. Ice may be used to control pain. No food or water should be ingested.

Dislocation and/or subluxation of shoulder complex

These can include any of the joints that make up the shoulder complex, i.e. glenohumeral, acromioclavicular and sternoclavicular. Causes of all complex shoulder injuries tend to be similar, e.g. falling on the point of the shoulder or falling with arm outstretched.

Glenohumeral joint

The commonest direction of a dislocation is inferior and slightly anterior. The athlete will not want to move the arm and if standing will tend to bend forward as the humeral head is in the axilla. There will be flattening of the roundness of the injured shoulder, known as a sulcus sign. In the case of subluxation, which is very common, the arm tends not to be able to be elevated above horizontal, there is a poor quality of motion if it can, and there are general aches in the shoulder. Athletes may complain that they can use the arm, but sleeping on the shoulder is a problem. Figure 6.9 shows a lateral view of the glenohumeral joint.

Treatment Check vascular and neurological status first. The glenohumeral dislocation should not be reduced, if it is the first dislocation, at the time of injury. Those athletes who have recurrent dislocations will direct you in the reduction procedure. The commonest reduction procedure involves traction of the upper extremity with the athlete lying on their back, or prone on a bench with the limb hanging over the side and a heavy weight in their hand. Inhalation anaesthesia with nitrous oxide helps to reduce the pain. Subluxations tend to be palpated as a slight humeral head displacement compared with the other shoulder. Anteroposterior shift attempts are resisted by the athlete. A glenohumeral thrust is employed, with the athlete placing the hand of the problem shoulder behind the neck. The osteopath stands behind and grasps the point of the elbow in both hands. Fixing the scapula with chest pressure the osteopath applies a thrust along the length of the humerus to release any restriction to movement.

Acromioclavicular joint

Dislocation is apparent in the presentation of the lateral end of the clavicle pushing up the skin and being more prominent than the other side. The athlete will have pain at the joint. There will be a little swelling due to the stretch/rupture of the ligaments and capsule. Pressure on the distal end of the clavicle relocates the acromioclavicular joint. Subluxations have a similar presentation but not as bad. X-rays will show the extent of the damage. If the ends of the acromion and clavicle still face each other then it is classified as a subluxation; if they are well separated and do not even come close to facing each other then the joint is dislocated. The costoclavicluar ligament will also be affected to some degree.

Treatment Ice, NSAIDs and rest with support. Generally, the dislocation/ subluxation is left alone, even if still displaced. Rehabilitation leading to

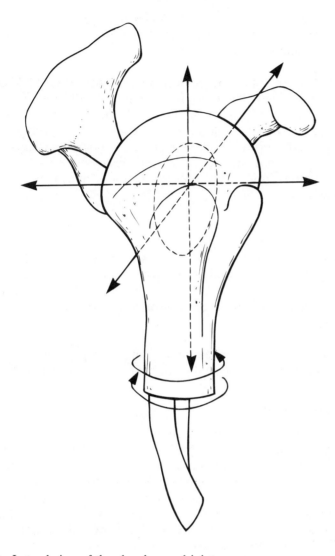

Fig. 6.9 Lateral view of the glenohumeral joint.

pain-free movement and full shoulder function means that the athlete can return to sports within about 6 weeks, or when the return-to-play criteria have been reached.

Sternoclavicular joint
Dislocation is rare. If it does occur it is important to assess the direction in which the clavicle has been shunted. In all cases the clavicle will have moved medially, but it is the additional posterior displacement that is dangerous, as the great vessels and trachea are in the superioanterior mediastinum. The additional anterior displacement may be more visibly distressing, but less potentially dangerous. There will be the usual swelling, immobility of the upper extremity and there may be coughing (if

posterior displacement). The costoclavicular ligament will be affected to some degree. Subluxation of this joint is the most common reason for pain. The displacement is usually minimal.

Treatment Check vascular and neurological status. Ice, NSAIDs and inhalation anaesthesia may be used. Reduction in the dislocation presentation is by retraction of the shoulder by the osteopath but, even in subluxation, may not be possible without anaesthesia. It is best performed with the help of somebody holding the athlete's thorax and other arm. If the displacement is not evident it may be posterior. This is a clinical emergency. Subluxation can be reduced in the same manner with the same treatment.

Epiphyseal plate injury

Injury to any growth areas should be considered in young athletes with shoulder pain. The best method of diagnosis is by X-ray. There may be a displacement but the usual finding is bruising, tenderness (on movement and palpation) and reduced range of motion in the limb.

Treatment
Rest, ice and soluble anti-inflammatory medication. OMT should be directed at reducing the myofacial component by functional techniques.

Shoulder capsule injury

The capsule of the shoulder can be traumatized (stretched or torn) acutely in contact sports or chronically due to activities such as pitching or bowling. Breaking the capsule down into anterior, posterior, inferior and superior compartments allows for a procedural basis for passive testing. The object of testing is to stress components of the capsule that may be inflamed or irritable. In reality, injury presentation has no barriers. Examination is carried out with the athlete lying supine and the arm moved passively. The object is to stress the different aspects of the capsule while trying not to stress the others.

Anterior injury
Pain and discomfort over the anterior aspect of the humeral head. Arm is adducted, externally rotated and extended.

Posterior injury
The elbow is flexed to 90°, the shoulder is flexed to 90°, the shoulder is internally rotated, and the shaft of the humerus is driven, along its long axis, backwards into the posterior aspect of the shoulder.

Inferior injury
Elevation of the shoulder may cause an apprehension response. If it does not, additional stress can be applied by pushing gently in an inferior

direction on the neck of the humerus with the arm elevated more than 90°. Be careful.

Superior injury
This is harder to elicit, but may respond to subacromial discomfort if the arm is placed at the athlete's side (adducted) and then pushed superiorly along the long axis of the upper extremity.

Adhesive capsulitis (frozen shoulder)

This is one of the most misdiagnosed of shoulder presentations. Because an athlete can only raise the arm 45° or just above, this does not qualify the problem as an adhesive capsulitis. An adhesive capsulitis is the end result of gross motion restriction. Case history is important. Shoulder restrictions, infections and vascular disorders can develop into an adhesive capsulitis. Increased motion causes increased shoulder discomfort which leads to reduced motion, increased capsule adhesions, poor joint approximation, more pain on movement etc.

Active shoulder motion is obviously decreased, especially passive motion. Passive motion test is important. The athlete should be relaxed and supine while the shoulder is being examined. The capsule is not an active contracting tissue, but a passive restricting tissue especially when it is forming adhesions.

Treatment
Check vascular and neurological status. Palpation and OMT are directed at finding the original cause for the shoulder restriction and dealing with that first. Check anteroposterior shift of the glenohumeral joint, reduced soft tissue and joint restrictions (thorax, neck, shoulder, elbow etc.). Passive articulation with a 'little and often' approach is useful; NSAIDs can help to control the discomfort that may arise from treatment.

Shoulder contusion (shoulder pointer)

This often involves the deltoid muscle. Examination should eliminate ligamentous and acromioclavicular joint (and other joint) involvement. Bruising may develop after hours or a day due to traumatized soft tissue. Repeated impact to the outside of the shoulder can result in the formation of a lateral humeral periostitis, continuing on to thickening of the periosteum, an **exostosis**. This is often seen in rugby and football, and is called 'tackler's exostosis'. Further chronic irritation may lead to a palpatory lump with the X-ray presentation of a bony spur. This is also known as a 'blocker's spur'. Progression to these stages is generally due to overuse of analgesic and anti-inflammatory medications without proper treatment and rest.

Treatment
The initial contusion should be approached with ice, NSAIDs, support and isometric exercise. There will be bleeding within the muscles during

the active phase of the injury, and no massage of any kind should be used over the injury site when active, due to the risk of bone formation in the soft tissue, i.e. myositis ossificans. Functional techniques of OMT are the best with relocation of any minor joint displacements, in the initial presentation. Later treatments, when the injury is past the active phase, include heat, OMT (including cross-fibre soft tissue) and isotonic exercise.

Thrombosis

Pain resembling effort thrombosis is essentially a deep vein thrombosis involving the subclavian or axillary veins. The history is vital. Overall, there tends to be a deep, aching and occasional pain when the arm is used. This may be accompanied by indiscriminate pins and needles and an ischaemic-like cramping. Check characteristics of pulses (radial and cubital) of both arms after effort. History may include trauma, tight musculature (e.g. scalenes) or infection.

Treatment
Venography is the most reliable method of diagnosis and refer to a physician for treatment.

Fractures

Within the shoulder complex fractures occur in the clavicle, scapula and proximal humerus, or in the humeral mid-shaft. In all cases check vascular and neurological status.

Clavicle
These tend to displace in an anterosuperior direction. They are usually observed and palpated without much problem. Athletes will carry the injured side by holding the elbow. The head and neck will be in a flexed and sidebent attitude towards the side of the injury.

Treatment X-ray will reveal the extent of the damage. Hold shoulder in retraction with figure-of-eight bandage or sling for support. Provide a sling for arm.

Scapula
Trauma to the scapula can lead to what is usually a hairline fracture. There will be pain over the site and the athlete will feel a deep discomfort in the muscle, and will not want to move the arm. Commonly these are stable fractures within the borders of the scapula.

Treatment Rest, ice and NSAIDs. Provide support for the arm. OMT is directed at reducing scapula muscle tension. Keep glenohumeral joint moving and try to keep arm moving as much as possible to prevent wasting.

Proximal humerus
The most common fracture is that of the neck of the humerus. Injury to the axillary nerve may occur. Differention between this kind of fracture and a dislocated shoulder may only be possible by X-ray.

Treatment Stabilization and proper alignment in an unstable fracture is important for the future of the athlete.

Humeral mid-shaft fracture
This is indicated by sudden mid-shaft pain in a traumatic situation, that may or may not result in fracture displacement.

Treatment Check vascular and neurological status. Support. This fracture has to be X-rayed for confirmation if not displaced. It should be plated to avoid problems with a varus or valgus displacement. OMT is directed at the cervical and thoracic regions, especially the upper ribs.

Neural (brachial plexus) injury

This occurs due to overstretch or compression of the neural structures when the angle between the neck and the point of the shoulder is increased or decreased, usually accompanied with a degree of rotation. The stretching results in a combination of symptoms including tingling in the hands, arms and shoulders, and sometimes numbness in these same areas; hence these injuries are called 'burners', 'stingers', 'pinched nerves' or 'hot shots'. The majority of the signs and symptoms are transient, lasting a few seconds with no long-lasting effects. If minor problems occur on a regular basis scarring may occur disrupting nerve function and leading to chronic pain. At worst, sudden violent force will 'tear' the nerves 'out' causing sudden paralysis and numbness. Repetitive minor trauma may interfere with neural function as a result of scarring, leading to a condition of neurapraxia.

Treatment
Check neurological status. Ice, NSAIDs and support of the affected limb side. OMT is directed at reducing pain by a functional technique and improving function of restricted areas of the neck, upper thorax and upper extremity.

Rotator cuff injury

This is a collective term for the structural degeneration, inflammation and/or tearing of the muscles that make up the rotator cuff system. Athletes prone to rotator cuff problems include bowlers, pitchers, quarterbacks, swimmers and tennis players. Diagnosis and pathological findings dictate the treatment protocol.

Elbow dysfunction

As with all other joints, evaluation of total elbow function should be assessed whatever the complaint. Manifestation of pain in the elbow is often due to reduction in function in an area that is asymptomatic within or outside the elbow area. Acute injury and pain should immediately be assessed, and inflammation and pain control instigated.

Capsular strain

This tends to occur as a result of unguarded elbow hyperextension. There is a diffuse type of pain/discomfort that gets worse when the athlete tries to extend the elbow. Active full flexion is also painful towards the end of the movement due to compression of swollen tissue. At its worst it may feel like the elbow is fractured or dislocated.

Treatment
Initially, ice, NSAIDs and support. Isometric exercise is important for maintaining muscle tone. OMT is directed at reducing swelling and improving circulation.

Distal biceps tendon injury

This tendon can be avulsed, torn, ruptured or become inflamed (tendonitis). There will pain and swelling of varying degrees in the anterior aspect of the elbow. Tendon involvement will be diagnosed with a positive sign on active resisted flexion and supination. An avulsion will be seen on X-ray, a tear can be palpated, rupture will additionally be seen as a lump in the arm as the athlete tries to flex the arm, and an inflamed tendon will be sore on use, but not too bad on active resisted movement.

Treatment
In the case of tear or tendonitis, initial administration of ice, NSAIDs and support is necessary to prevent the condition from getting any worse. It is important that the causative factors of tendonitis are found; they include thorax, neck, shoulder, arm and wrist soft tissue and joint problems that may be asymptomatic. Suspicion of a rupture can be narrowed down to signs of pain, initially mild, with immobility of the arm with a bulge, the ruptured bicep, in the anterior aspect of the arm when the athlete even slightly tenses the muscle. This is an orthopaedic emergency and the athlete should be sent to an accident and emergency department immediately, with the arm supported. An avulsion will have similar signs to a rupture and tear except there are no signs of a bulging bicep. X-ray investigation is vital for the final diagnosis.

Olecranon and fossa dysfunction

Poor olecranon engagement when the arm is extended is one of the signs of intra-articular irritation and thickening that may be accompanied with pain. It may also be a sign of dysfunctional progression over time. The result may be a breakdown in compensation elsewhere in the elbow or upper extremity complex. This is sometimes termed olecranon fossitis or hyperextension overload syndrome.

Treatment
Ice, NSAIDs and support are the initial approach. OMT is directed at improving circulation. This is achieved by distraction of the olecranon/fossa joint.

Radial head dysfunction

Dysfunction of the radial head (radial/ulnar/humerus complex) tends to be in an anteroposterior range. Palpation may reveal an anterior or posterior resting humeral head. Symptoms range from 'tennis elbow' to lateral cubital fossa discomfort, especially on gripping.

Olecranon bursitis (student's elbow)

Irritation of the olecranon bursa leads to tenderness and swelling. The appearance at worse is similar to a small sac of fluid over the posterior aspect of the elbow. It can be quite painless.

Treatment
Ice, NSAIDs, compression and padding will help. Aspiration of the swelling may be necessary in severe cases. Swelling tends to occur until the fluid production calms down.

Distal triceps tendon

As with the biceps tendon the triceps tendon can be avulsed, torn, ruptured and inflamed. Signs and symptoms are the similar and so is the treatment approach.

Lateral epicondylitis ('tennis elbow')

This is irritation, swelling and pain over the lateral epicondyle. In the majority of cases it is tender to the touch. It tends to result in a degenerative process of the extensor carpi radialis brevis. It is the end result of dysfunction of the upper extremity in its relation to the body. Referred pain from the thorax (ribs), neck and shoulder can cause pain in the lateral epicondyle, which is also tender to the touch. Poor racquet sport technique, even foot work, is the most frequent causative factor.

Treatment
Immediate approach is ice, NSAIDs and local support. Find the causes (obstructions to potential healing).

Medial epicondylitis ('golfer's elbow')

Irritation of the medial epicondyle from which originate the flexors of the wrist. As with tennis elbow it is a degenerative process, and treatment is the same (look for areas that obstruct healing).

Median nerve compression syndrome

Compression of the median nerve tends to be the result of hypertonic muscle, shortened aponeurosis or fibrotic fascia. The muscles most often involved are the pronator teres and flexor digitorum superficialis with radiations in the anterior aspect of the forearm. The compression by shortened soft tissue causes a neural disturbance with numbness and tingling in areas of median supply. This tends to be of a chronic nature with the hypertonia being associated with a cramping feeling in the forearm.

Treatment
In the chronic presentation NSAIDs tend to be of little help. Increasing the circulation to the area is important as the signs and symptoms seem to mimic ischaemia. OMT is directed at reducing soft tissue tone locally and improving joint function in the upper extremity, and at a local and general level improving the pharmacological effect of the NSAIDs.

Ulnar nerve injury

This ranges from an acute contusion, to subluxation of the nerve, to chronic irritation in an athlete with a valgus deformity. The medial aspect of the elbow over the ulnar groove will be painful on palpation, usually sending 'electric shocks' down the medial aspect of the forearm into the little finger. It shows all the signs of an entrapment neuropathy. Other than contusion, the majority of presentations are usually chronic.

Treatment
In a contusion and subluxation ice can be used, but should not be applied for extended periods as it may cause additional neural damage. NSAIDs will help, as will a compressive bandage. Always examine for fracture and subluxation, and perform basic neurological examination to test integrity of the nerve about 20 minutes after the injury. In chronic presentations check the entire extremity and thorax, neck and shoulder to reduce the active forcing of the elbow into a valgus deformity which will cause symptoms. Examine the entire elbow for restrictions in quality and range of motion.

Osteochondritis dissecans

This may present in young athletes. It is a focal lesion affecting the growth plates in the elbow. The young athlete will present with a painful elbow, usually of a chronic nature with slow onset. Palpatory findings may reveal clicking, grating and lack of a full range of movement due to chronic thickening of local tissue. X-rays will reveal the epiphyseal plate damage.

Treatment
Ice and rest are the baseline treatment. OMT is directed at reducing elbow tenderness and restoring function. Application of a functional technique seems to have the best results.

Fractures, dislocations and subluxations

These usually present as extreme pain, limitation of range of movement and swelling. In the case of dislocation the most common displacement is a superoposterior direction of the ulnar with disruption of the capsule and neurovascular structures. Subluxations are just as painful and may be apparent on palpation rather than on X-ray. Fractures, dislocation and subluxations can occur together. Most of these injuries occur when the athlete falls forward with the hand out or lands on the point of the elbow.

Treatment
All injuries will probably need to be reduced under anaesthesia. In the case of fractures and dislocations immediate transportation to an emergency unit is vital. Subluxations range from the joint being held in a dysfunctional position by muscle spasm after trauma, to the injury mechanism disrupting intra-articular structures. Ice and NSAIDs may suffice, with OMT applied to reduce the muscle spasm and decompress the joint in an attempt to relocate and normalize structures.

Sprains and strains

These respond very well to OMT. They present as limitation of range of motion, swelling, etc. The specific diagnosis depends on examination.

Treatment
Ice, NSAIDs and support. OMT is directed towards reducing swelling and hypertonia and increasing the function of the other joints and soft tissue in the upper extremity.

Wrist injury

Sprains and strains

These tend to occur due to forced extension of the hand. They present with pain on the posterior aspect of the junction between the proximal part of the hand and the distal end of the forearm. This suggests a crushing or compressive mechanism of injury, e.g. putting the hand out when falling to the ground or palming off an opponent. Ligaments on the posterior aspect include the radioulnar, deep radiocarpal and ulnar collateral. Minor displacement or dysfunction of the functional interaction between the distal and proximal row of bones in the hand will maintain a symptomatic picture. Any injury mechanism can include the flexor and extensor apparatus, capsules and palmar ligaments.

Treatment
Ice, NSAIDs and support. OMT is directed at removing dysfunctions in the bones of the hand and distal and proximal radioulnar articulations. After impact with the palmar surface of the hand it would be rational to include the shoulder and upper extremity in your assessment.

Scaphoid injury

The scaphoid in the 'anatomical snuff box' is usually injured when the athlete falls on the outstretched hand, palms off an opponent, or is hit around the base of the thumb. There will be pain in the snuff box, made worse by palpatory pressure. Sprains of the ligament complex between the scaphoid and lunate bones are common. Generally, play on the safe side and treat it as a scaphoid fracture, especially in severe cases, until proven otherwise (Giachino, 1993).

Treatment
Initially, ice, NSAIDs and support. The hand must be X-rayed as soon as possible, and then again in a few weeks, as any fracture may not be apparent initially. The blood supply may be cut in the bone due to the fracture, which will appear as a necrotic lesion on the film.

Colles' fracture (dinner fork deformity)

This is where the distal end of the radius is displaced dorsally. The mechanism of injury is usually excessive force on the palmar aspect of the hand.

Treatment
Check vascular and neurological status. Ice (for not more than 20 min) will help reduce pain while a support is applied. X-rays will reveal the extent and direction of the fracture. Administration of anaesthesia and reduction of the fracture as soon as possible are important. As with all fractures, the quicker you can remove the cast and rehabilitate the better.

Smith's fracture

This is the opposite of the Colles' fracture. This usually occurs when the athlete falls on the back of the flexed wrist. Displacement is in a palmar direction. Treatment is the same as for Colles' fracture.

Epiphyseal plate displacement

In young athletes displacement of the epiphyseal plate may result instead of the usual fracture. The appearances of a Colles' and Smith's deformity in epiphyseal plate displacement will be the same as the fracture. Treatment approach is as for Colles' fracture.

Dislocation

Dislocations of the wrists are quite rare. If they do occur the capsulo-ligamentous apparatus is the major structure disrupted.

Treatment
As for a fracture; the cast should be removed as soon as possible.

Ganglion of the wrist

There seems to be no consistent definition of a 'ganglion'; various structural alterations may present in this fashion. The ganglion tends to occur more on the dorsum of the hand and is a small lump that is defined and mobile. It has also been called a cyst. It results from the degeneration of the scapholunate joint area, damage to the tendon sheaths (e.g. an arterial aneurysm), hernia of the synovial capsule etc. Whatever the reason, the ganglion is asymptomatic and should not unduly worry the athlete.

Treatment
Ice may help to 'shrink' the swelling slightly. OMT can be directed at improving joint mobility and reducing musculotendinous tension, working as high as the forearm/elbow.

Hand injury

Contusion and abrasions

The most common injury is direct trauma to the dorsal aspect of the hand. This presents with swelling and limitation of movement. In contact and collision sports this is usually accompanied by a contusion and abrasions.

Treatment
Initial orthopaedic, vascular and neurological assessment will reveal the extent of the damage. Abrasions should be cleaned and dressed, ice should be applied, support given, NSAIDs prescribed (if not suspicious of fracture), and X-rays taken if deemed necessary.

Carpal tunnel syndrome

Increasing pressure on the palmar aspect of the heel of the hand results in compression of the median nerve. The mechanisms are varied, but the presentations are similar. These include pain, sensitivity and tingling in the heel of the hand; there may be in addition numbness, tingling and pain in the fingers. Symptoms may be felt up the arm. Symptoms are generally worse at night, and when the hand has to be used. Tingling provides a positive Tinel's sign, when gentle tapping of the heel of the hand further irritates the sensitive median nerve, and also Phalen's sign, forced flexion of the palmar surface of the heel of the hand, which is held for over a minute.

Treatment
This involves treating the entire upper extremity. Initially, contrasting cold water and warm water will help with circulation. OMT is directed locally at decompression and increasing fluid drainage. Stretching exercises of the palmar surface of the hand are useful.

Thumb injury

Sprain and dislocation

The most common sports-related injury is damage to the ulnar collateral ligament of the metacarpophalangeal (MCP) joint. In the majority of presentations it is sprained, but occasionally it may be dislocated.

Treatment
Orthopaedic assessment should be carried out. In the case of the sprained thumb ice, NSAIDs and support are useful. When the thumb has 'calmed down' check the functional integrity of the MCP joint. The dislocated presentation can be reduced immediately, i.e. on the sideline, if you have the experience; you only have one chance, because the athlete will not let you do it again. Be aware of any other mid-shaft deformity that may indicate a fracture. Inhalation anaesthesia will help the reduction procedure, then ice, NSAIDs and support.

Injury of the fingers

Mallet finger

The extensor tendon of the distal interphalangeal (DIP) joint may be injured due to an impact at the tip of the finger. This tendon at the tip of the distal phalynx can be ruptured or overstretched, with or without an avulsion of the base of the phalynx.

Treatment
Ice, NSAIDs and support with a splint. X-rays may be indicated in extreme cases. Fingers take around 6 weeks to heal, but may take many months to return to full function, and indeed full function may never be regained. OMT is directed at reducing scar tissue. Care should be taken not to break down the scar tissue too early, which may lead to poor healing and future dysfunction.

Jersey finger

This is an injury to the flexor tendon of the DIP, called jersey finger due to the fact that in rugby and football repeatedly grabbing on to another player's jersey pulls the DIP into extension and the tendon can be torn or degeneratively broken down.

Treatment
As for mallet finger.

Dislocations

Deformity of the phalanx will be obvious. The commonest are flexion and valgus deformities. They tend to stay deformed until reduced.

Treatment
As for thumb dislocations.

Boutonnière deformity

This is a flexion deformity of the finger. It is the end result of hyperextension of the MCP joint, flexion of the proximal intercarpophalangeal (PIP) joint, and hyperextension of the DIP joint.

Rings

Rings should be removed in all activities or at least covered with a plaster. Contact and collision sport participants in particular are at risk from a torniquet effect if the finger swells after injury, and degloving if the ring is pulled along the finger.

Nail infections and injury

Osteopathically there are many reasons for nail infection, while traditional medicine blames infection by organisms. Organisms may be present, but the poor trophic function of nerve supply affects the healthy division of cells in the generation of new tissue, especially the hands and nails. The upper thorax and lower cervical spine areas tend to be pain free accompanied by hypertonus and fibrosis of soft tissue. OMT should be directed at these areas. Infections of nails and fingers are generally overlooked in athletic health care. Many athletes, especially in contact and collision sports, damage nails and fingertips and are repeatedly exposed to minor infections.

Paronychia

This is infection under the cuticle, mainly associated with *Staphylococcus* organisms. There is breakdown of the cuticle, which is sore, swollen and bleeding.

Treatment

Keep the fingers clean, supple and dry. There are many antibacterial preparations on the market.

Subungal haematoma

This is otherwise known as blue black nail and is usually the result of trauma.

Treatment

Putting the finger in iced water for 15 minutes at a time will help to control the inflammation. If the subungal damage is severe enough the nail will eventually be shed and a new nail will form. Protective taping may allow the athlete to continue playing. Check for distal fractures of the phalynx.

Onycholysis

This presents as a structural breakdown of the nail from the nail bed. It is an indication of both local (trauma, tinae unguium) and general (psoriasis, thyroid disease) problems.

Onychogryphosis

This is thickening and curving of the nail. The nail becomes hard to cut and generally will have to be filed down. Repeated minor trauma and infection contribute to this condition. Keeping the nail supple reduces the risk of further injury.

THORAX AND ABDOMEN (INCLUDING UROGENITAL SYSTEM)

Anatomy

Boundaries

The thorax and abdomen are bounded anteriorly by the sternum, ribs and intercostal muscles, laterally by the ribs and intercostal muscles and posteriorly by the thoracic spine, ribs and intercostal muscles.

Superiorly the thorax is bounded by the first thoracic vertebra, the two first ribs with their costal cartilages, the pleural cupola, the upper end of the manubrium sterni and the sternoclavicular joint articulations. This is an area of continuation and interplay, known as the cervico-thoracic junction. This is especially important to remember when looking at the athlete's thoracic outlet region or root of the neck. Therefore, the boundaries of the roof of the thorax must include the investing fascia, scalenus anterior, longus colli, brachial plexus and the brachiocephalic artery which bifurcates, on the right, into the common carotid and subclavian arteries (these are independent on the left), and their branches, the subclavian arteries and veins. Branches of the sympathetic trunks from the middle and inferior cervical ganglia (arterial and cardiac branches), with the phrenic and vagal nerves, supply the trachea and the oesophagus. Osteopathically, one of the most important structures in this region is the thoracic duct of the lymphatic system for drainage of the left half of the body and lower extremities.

The diaphragm is under the control of the phrenic nerve, both voluntarily and involuntarily, from the third to fifth cervical spinal roots. Autonomic nervous control is sympathetically from the first to fourth thoracic segments and parasympathically from the vagus nerves. The outer parameters of the diaphragm receive neural fibres from the intercostal nerves.

Intrathoracic components

Within the thorax the cavities are divided into:

1. the right and left pleural cavities;
2. the mediastinum outside these cavities.

The right and left cavities contain the lungs. The mediastinum should be visualized three-dimensionally, i.e. as sections of the intrathorax that have been portioned into non-anatomical areas in which some structures sit and others pass through. These are the anterior, superior, posterior and middle mediastinum.

The anterior mediastinum is a small zone behind the sternum and the manubrium–sternal angle inferiorly along the sternum to the xiphosternal angle. It is in front of the pericardium and contains fat and lymph nodes. Fluid exchange in and out of this zone relies heavily on thoracic movement.

The superior mediastinum has its base as a horizontal plane lying over the fibrous pericardium at a level running posteriorly from the manubrium – sternal angle to the bodies of the fourth and fifth thoracic vertebrae. It fills the rest of the thorax rising to the cupola over the superior domes of the lungs.

The posterior mediastinum is behind the pericardium. Its upper level is about the level between the fourth and fifth thoracic vertebrae, extending downwards below the pericardium, and tucking further downwards between the posterior dome of the diaphragm and anteriorly to the thoracic vertebrae.

The middle mediastinum holds the contents of the pericardium. Besides the heart it contains the roots of the great vessels passing to and from the heart.

The cardiopulmonary system

The heart has its nerve supply via branches from the cervical sympathetic trunk, the cervicothoracic (stellate ganglion) trunk, and branches from the thoracic trunk. Preganglion supply originates from approximately the first to fifth thoracic spinal cord segments. Parasympathetically, the supply is via the right and left vagus nerves, continuing on to contribute to the cardiac plexus. Arterial supply is via the right and left coronary branches of the aorta. Venous drainage is from the coronary sinus into the right atrium. Lymphatic drainage is mainly through three plexuses:

1. subendocardial, under the endocardium;
2. myocardial, in the muscle;
3. subepicardial, adjacent to the visceral pericardium.

The lungs and pleurae

Lung lymphatic drainage is from superficial and deep plexuses. The superficial plexus is beneath the pulmonary pleura and the deep accompanies branches of the pulmonary venules and the ramifications of the bronchi. Larger bronchi are drained by the deep plexus via two networks: the submucous and the peribronchial outside the walls of the bronchi. Smaller bronchi are drained by a single plexus which extends to the bronchioles but does not reach the alveoli. Superficial efferents of the lymphatic system turn around the borders of the lungs and the margins of their fissures, coming together to end in the bronchopulmonary lymph nodes. The deep efferents drain to the hilus along the pulmonary vessels to the bronchi and end in the bronchopulmonary lymph nodes. At this point it is important to realize that there is no anastomosis between the superficial and deep lymph vessels of the lungs, except in the hilar region.

Particular drainage from the pleura is from the visceral and parietal layers. Visceral pleura drainage is via superficial efferents of the lungs forming a plexus beneath the pulmonary pleura. Parietal pleural drainage is along three routes:

1. The costal pleura, with vessels of the internal intercostal muscles to the parasternal nodes;
2. The diaphragmatic pleura drains along the plexus on the thoracic surface of the diaphragm muscle;
3. The mediastinal pleura drains along the posterior mediastinal lymph nodes.

Oesophagus

Lymphatic drainage of the oesophagus can be broken down into three sections. The cervical region drains to the deep cervical nodes, the thoracic region to the posterior mediastinal nodes and the abdominal part to the left gastric lymph nodes and occasionally directly to the thoracic duct.

The thoracic walls

Lymph drainage is from superficial and deep tissues. Superficial tissues include the subcutaneous structures coming together at the axillary nodes.

Superficial drainage of the trapezius and latissimus dorsi regions runs forwards uniting in 10–12 trunks in the subscapular region (group). Draining vessels of the outer pectoral region (including the skin over the peripheral part of the mammary glands and the subareolar plexus) run backwards; those of the serratus anterior region run upwards to the pectoral nodes. Vessels of the lateral margin of the sternum drain inwards between the rib cartilages to the parasternal nodes. A small number of draining vessels from the upper part of the pectoral region ascend over the clavicle to the inferior deep cervical lymph nodes.

Deep tissue drainage of the thoracic walls collects in vessels from:

1. The muscles attached to the ribs, draining to the axillary nodes.
2. The intercostal vessels that drain the intercostal muscles and pleura, the anterior half of the thoracic wall and the pleura. They end in the parasternal nodes, from the posterior half of the intercostal nodes.
3. Drainage of the diaphragm is via two main routes; first, the thoracic plexus on the thoracic surface of the diaphragm which is sectioned into anterior, middle and posterior regions. The anterior diaphragm drains towards the anterior diaphragmatic nodes; the middle diaphragm drains towards the nodes of the oesophagus and around the termination of the inferior vena cava; the posterior diaphragm drains towards nodes around the aorta. Second, the diaphragm drains along the abdominal surface (plexus). Vessels from the liver, periphery of the diaphragm, with those of the subperitoneal tissue drain into this plexus. Efferents from the right half drain to a group of nodes on the trunk of the inferior phrenic artery and the right lateral aortic nodes. The left half drains into the preaortic and lateral aortic lymph nodes to the nodes on the terminal portion of the oesophagus.

The diaphragm
Essentially, the partition between the thorax and abdomen, the diaphragm is vital for the movement of fluids and for an efficient breathing system. Within the diaphragm there is so much neural tissue (coeliac plexus) that this area is sometimes called the second brain. Changes in tension take place due to physical and particularly emotional stress.

The gastrointestinal tract

Overall, the gastrointestinal tract (digestive and elimination system) from the mouth to the anus traverses many levels of the autonomic nervous system. This system is the most reflective of autonomic nervous function, as it has less higher level conscious intervention than any other system in the body. The digestive system can be broken down into the following:

• oral cavity: buccal cavity, teeth, salivary glands, parotid, submaxillary and sublingual;
• pharynx, oesophagus and stomach;
• small intestine: duodenum, jejunum and ileum;

- large intestine: caecum, appendix, ascending colon, hepatic flexure, transverse colon, splenic flexure, descending colon, sigmoid colon, rectum and anal canal.

Lymphatic drainage
Osteopathically, it important to remember that the lymph nodes, capillaries and vessels are embedded in the deep fascia and membranes that surround the viscera. A network of vessels forms an anastomosis so that when drainage is reduced in one particular region the capillaries alternate their drainage to the nearest vessel. Large areas of lymphatic drainage can be compromised over time by increasing fascial tension or irritation. Chains of nodes along the sides of the aorta (known as the right and left aortic or more significantly the lumbar chains of nodes) receive lymph from the gastrointestinal vessels and continue on to drain into the cisterna chyli, which is on the right side of the aorta, and the right crus of the diaphragm on its right side (Passmore and Robinson, 1976).

Liver

This gland lies under the diaphragm and is partially protected by the lower right section of the rib cage. It consists of two lobes, right and left. The right makes up around 85% of the total liver and is separated from the left section by the falciform ligament.

Intra-abdominal structure location

For ease I have divided the abdomen into four sections. A vertical line travels from the xiphoid process to the pubis symphysis through the umbilicus (following the linae alba). The other travels horizontally from one iliac crest to the other through the umbilicus. These sections can be thought of as four three-dimensional blocks: the upper right, lower right, upper left and lower left. Do not forget that abdominal organs are under the rib cage as well. Some structures overlap into adjacent sections. Vascular, peritoneal and neural structures also travel through these sections.

1. Right upper section: liver, gallbladder, right kidney (and adrenal gland) and ureter, stomach (pylorus), hepatic flexure of large intestine, small intestine, upper half of ascending colon, right half of transverse colon, head of pancreas.
2. Right lower section: appendix, small intestine, caecum, lower half of ascending colon, urinary bladder and right ureter. In the female, the uterus, vagina, right ovary and right Fallopian tube. In the male, the right vas deferens, right testicle, right spermatic cord etc.
3. Left upper section: stomach, abdominal oesophagus, spleen, left kidney (and adrenal gland) and ureter, small intestine, splenic flexure of the large intestine, left half of the transverse colon, upper half of the descending colon, tail of the pancreas.

4. Left lower section: small intestine, descending colon, sigmoid colon, urinary bladder, rectum and left ureter. In the female, the uterus, vagina, left ovary and left Fallopian tube. In the male, the left vas deferens, left testicle, left spermatic cord etc.

Injury presentations

Important: Do not be tempted to manipulate any area that has a history or indications of trauma. Exclude all possibilities first.

Contusions

These are most common over the ribs, sternum, mammary tissue and abdominal wall. Bruising presents in the normal way with localized swelling, tenderness of subcutaneous tissue, muscle and periosteum, and possible abrasion of the skin. Always be aware of possible involvement of deeper tissues, especially when the signs and symptoms are not resolving as quickly as you expect. Check for underlying fractures and displacements. Abdominal muscles should be palpated for contusions with the athlete supine, then asked to raise his or her head and shoulders off the bench. If the muscle and surrounding tissue are severely injured this will be painful; if they are not severely injured it will allow you to palpate the abdominal wall more easily.

Treatment
This is quite straightforward, i.e. rest, ice, NSAIDs and OMT in the early stages. When symptoms begin to subside a rehabilitation programme with warmth before activity, ice after activity and OMT is important.

Costochondral injury

Costochondral injuries involve the rib and the cartilage that attaches to the sternum. The most common presentations result from anterolateral impacts to the chest wall resulting in pain at the costochondral junction. These presentations can range from fractures or sprains to displacement of the cartilage from the rib. Signs and symptoms include pain and tenderness over the area, especially when palpated, discomfort and/or pain on breathing, and there may be palpatory and observational signs of structural displacement. More common in contact and collision sports.

Treatment
A wide long bandage around the thorax should help to ease the discomfort while breathing. In addition, rest, ice, NSAIDs and OMT are helpful.

Chondrosternal injury

These have the same presentations and treatment as costochondral presentations but are closer to the midline.

Tetse syndrome

This is chronic presentation of costosternal irritation. The usual cause is reduction in range of motion at the costovertebral junction, precipitating discomfort on breathing.

Treatment

OMT directed at improving rib motion, especially at the costovertebral joints.

Costovertebral injury

This is a common occurrence in athletes. They complain of pain and/or discomfort in the back just left or right of the spine. Sometimes there may be radiations along the course of the rib or intercostal muscles. More common in contact and collision sports, but also in athletes who use their upper extremities to resist or load as in gymnastics and rowing. A heavy impact to the area may result in a fracture of the rib and/or vertebra, a sprain of the ligamentous structures or a restiction of joint motion with no inflammation.

Treatment

Rest, ice, NSAIDs and OMT; X-ray possibly.

Rib fractures

Fairly common in contact and collision sports, rib fractures should always be suspected with bony point tenderness over the thorax. Remember that the ribs surround vital organs. Rib fractures may be classed generally as displaced or non-displaced. Displaced fractures are particularly worrying due to the risk of infection and are even more dangerous if the displacement is inwards (internal) rather than outwards (external), breaking the skin. Organs and arteries are at risk due to internal displacements. However, non-displaced ribs should not be regarded as any less a threat to vital organs. Force transmission through the body can cause tearing and shearing forces leading to damage of abdominal organs, liver, spleen and kidneys, resulting in internal bleeding. Signs of rib and intercostal muscle trauma include pain and/or discomfort on breathing, general movement, coughing and sneezing. In general, a small amount of movement leading to a great amount of pain indicates an extreme state of injury. Palpation may reveal tenderness, displacement, crepetation on breathing, and contusion (with abrasion) signs. In addition to this always palpate the abdomen, look for displaced trachea (pneumothorax), and ausculate abdomen and thorax. X-rays of the chest may confirm suspicions of rib damage, but do not forget internal organs.

Treatment

Stabilization of thorax movement should be carried out by binding the chest with a heavy duty wide bandage overlain with adhesive elastic tape.

This will control pain, breathing and prevent the development of atelectasis and pneumonia. Resting is important, as is the administration of ice bags to the injury site two or three times a day, and analgesics. OMT to accessory respiratory muscles, diaphragm, neck and breathing exercises all help to improve the athlete's condition.

Sternoclavicular injury

Sternoclavicular joint injury can range from a simple sprain to dislocation. The usual mechanism of injury is as a result of falling on the point of the shoulder with compression of the shoulder and upper thorax and transmission along the shaft of the clavicle and direct compression in a pile-up in contact/collision sports. Dislocation of the sternoclavicular joint can present with displacement of the clavicle, most commonly in the anteromedial or superomedial, and less commonly in the posteromedial direction. Posterior direction displacements are particularly dangerous due to the delicate structures in the root of the neck, major vessels and the airway. The athlete who has fallen will not want to move. If he or she is lying prone, with help, support the upper limb against the trunk, support the head and shoulder, and roll the athlete onto their back, with the uninjured side staying on the ground. An athlete who can walk will tend to support the upper limb on the injured side and will be bending the head towards the injured side. There will be swelling, observable displacement at the joint and apprehension. The swelling has to be reduced. The athlete should be sent to an emergency department to rule out any complications.

Treatment

If you are presented with a slight subluxation on the sideline then the application of an ice bag will act as a local anaesthetic (or use inhalation anaesthesia if available). The reduction of the subluxation is best carried out when the athlete is lying supine. This procedure should be performed in the emergency room with the athlete under sedation. The practitioner should kneel on the ground on the athlete's injured side. A distraction force should be applied to the lateral end of the clavicle and the manubrium with the practitioner's forearms crossed.

Muscle strains and ruptures

Thoracic wall pain of muscular origin is usually due to strains and ruptures of the intercostal muscles. These are generally the result of impact or sudden overstretching, e.g. the fielding cricketer. The second most common presentation is that involving the pectoralis major and/or minor. Sudden resistance to the action of the muscle (pectoralis major), which is adduction, flexion and internal rotation, is the main risk factor in sport. An example of this is grabbing the shirt of a player running past you, or falling forward and putting your hands out as you hit the ground. Signs and symptoms in all cases include sudden pain/discomfort in the damaged area, bruising (later), swelling, tenderness on palpation, and discomfort from breathing. In the case of a rupture of the pectoralis major, for example, there will be a bulging of the area compared with the other side of the chest. There will be extreme weakness in movement of the arm.

Treatment
With minor strains and tears the procedure is consistent with all muscle acute injury, i.e. rest, ice, NSAIDs and OMT. If there are signs of rupture it should be regarded as an orthopaedic emergency. The upper extremity should be stabilized in a sling and the athlete should be sent immediately to an emergency department. On the normal X-ray there is a shadow of, for example, the pectoralis major, which is absent in a rupture.

Breast tissue injury

The mammary glands are susceptible to injury mostly through impact, e.g. with other players' elbows (hockey), knees (rugby) and general running activity. Female athletes with large breast tissue should take particular care and wear proper athletic supports. Many athletes complain of pain a day or two after activity due to strain on the Cooper's ligaments. Additional support can be added by wearing two brassieres or wrapping a large wide bandage around the thorax over one bra.

Treatment
Aching due to stretching or contusion of the Cooper's ligaments can be relieved by mild NSAIDs and wrapping a large cool wet towel around the front of the chest. Do not use just ice; the object is to cool the breast tissue not freeze it. OMT to the thoracic spine and ribs will help control discomfort.

Jogger's nipple

This is irritation of the nipples by the rubbing or friction of the jersey. A combination of sweat and heat is a precipitating factor.

Treatment
Make sure the nipples are clean; there is always a risk of infection. Do not use strong cleaners, just mild soap and cool water. A cool wet towel will control the small amount of swelling that may be present. Do not use a direct ice bag as this can damage the nipple. NSAIDs and OMT will help to control discomfort and swelling. Preventive action includes the use of thick skin lubricant or synthetic skin.

Pneumothorax

This is usually of sudden traumatic or non-traumatic onset. Generally, they are either a simple pneumothorax as a consequence of rupture of the pulmonary tissue integrity, from direct trauma; or a tension pneumothorax due to enlargement of the pneumothorax, as a result of a positive intrapleural pressure. This can be due to poor venous return and a mediastinal shift. In a pneumothorax the athlete will be short of breath, complain of chest pain and be in distress. Blood pressure may reveal hypotension, there will be absent breath sounds on auscultation, and hyperresonance to percussion on the affected side. There is displacement of the trachea and mediastinum away from the side of the collapsed pleura. Looking at the throat, the trachea base moves towards the good side.

Treatment
Monitor the athlete. Needs immediate transfer to accident and emergency department.

Cardiac contusion

Otherwise known as myocardial contusion, this is the result of a blunt impact of high velocity to the chest wall, especially over the sternum. It usually occurs in contact and collision sports. The athlete may complain of discomfort 'somewhere inside', which can mimic deep rib-type pain. Pulse will be rapid and may be erratic. The athlete will be distressed. Dysrhythmias may be apparent on auscultation.

Treatment
Immediate transfer to accident and emergency department.

Vessel trauma

Sudden impact or sudden deceleration can lead to the rupture of vessels within the thorax. The most common area is the aorta, where the root of the great vessels at the isthmus is the commonest site of damage. In sports such as American football, where open field tackling takes place, collisions may be as violent as being hit by a car at 30 miles per hour. Blood pressure will drop and athlete will show signs and symptoms of (hypovolaemic) shock.

Treatment
Immediate transfer to accident and emergency department.

Thrombosis

In the thorax and upper extremity thrombosis tends to present in the subclavian and axillary veins. Precipitation of this condition seems to occur in athletes who undergo hyperabduction and external rotation of the upper extremity, e.g. in football, soccer, baseball, tennis and rowing. Signs and symptoms tend to be those of drainage problems, oedema of the upper extremity, visible and distended superficial veins, pain/discomfort and fullness of the hand on gripping. Diagnostically, venography and non-invasive studies are the best approach.

Treatment

Anticoagulant and thrombolytic medication, and elevation of the limb to aid drainage and reduce usage. OMT is directed at reducing discomfort and improving drainage. Do not use heavy soft tissue techniques over the thrombotic area. Functional and strain–counterstrain techniques are the techniques of choice over the thrombotic area. Improving drainage from the limb is important. Attention must be paid to the thorax (ribs) by using thoracic pump techniques, and to the diaphragm, upper thorax and neck.

Sympathetic outflow irritation

Repeated minor trauma can precipitate sympathetic ganglion irritation. One of the main findings is a reduction in motion of the upper costovertebral joints. This is often due to repeated tackling in rugby and football and also occurs in rowing. It tends to occur whenever there is repeated minor force through a triangle with its apex at the occiput and the base at each scapula. Signs and symptoms vary from coldness in the fingers to altered sensations in the upper extremities, face and lips.

Thoracic outlet syndrome (TOS)

This is characterized by compression of the brachial plexus, subclavian artery or vein or a combination of any of the three. TOS is a collective term for the compression of neurovascular structures within the thoracic outlet, which is an area bordered by the first thoracic rib, the clavicle and the superior border of the scapula. There are various types of TOS, including scalenus anticus syndrome, cervical rib syndrome, costoclavicular syndrome, pectoralis minor syndrome and costocoracoid fasciitis. Scalenus anticus syndrome is where there is a shortening accompanied by fibrotic change of scalenus anterior (anticus). For example, the subclavian artery passes above the first rib and between the scalenus anterior and the scalenus medius muscles, becoming compressed on its route. In cervical rib syndrome the development of a cervical rib, thickened fibrous band or a particularly long C7 transverse process can lead to compression of the brachial plexus, subclavian artery or both. Costoclavicular syndrome is the compression of the brachial plexus or the axillary artery and vein or combination of the three, as they pass between the first rib and clavicle. The pectoralis minor syndrome, also known as the coracoid–pectoralis syndrome or the hyperabduction syndrome, occurs when the axillary artery and brachial plexus are compressed between the pectoralis minor tendon near its insertion point and the head of the humerus. Shortening and chronic inflammation of the costocoracoid facsia lead to neural irritation and vascular compression directly or indirectly reducing musculoskeletal function.

The majority of signs and symptoms are neural, with upper extremity 'pins and needles', discomfort/pain and numbness, in no particular distribution in the majority of cases. Where there is particular distribution, this tends to be ulnar in nature. With vascular involvement use of the limb leads to ishaemic-type signs and symptoms with fatigue, numbness, 'pins and needles', coldness of the fingers (usually small finger) and oedema.

Predisposing factors

After neurovascular assessment, the posture of the patient must be taken into consideration. Postural changes are a major predisposing factor towards the development of a TOS presentation. After a general postural evaluation, more local structural alterations should be considered. Locally, some of the common findings include an elevated first rib, an inferoposterior clavicle at the sternoclavicular joint, an extended cervical spine, a flexed upper thoracic spine, fullness of the supraclavicular fossa, and hypertonicity and thickening of the scalenes. Repeated minor trauma to the shoulder and neck in sports such as rugby and football can precipitate increased resting tone of soft tissue and degenerative changes in the shoulder girdle and cervicothoracic area. Regions distant from the thoracic outlet that could have sympathetic neural connections should not be forgotten. Spinal cord facilitation can lead to increased sympathetic outflow, even if not symptomatic.

Examination

Physical examination should include the following tests (Dobrusin, 1989).

1. The Adson's test is performed with the patient in a seated position. The arm is extended, externally rotated, and adducted while the examiner palpates the radial pulse. The patient is then asked to take a deep breath and rotate the head toward the arm being tested. This manoeuvre raises the first rib and decreases the space in the interscalene triangle. Test results are considered positive when the pulse disappears, the blood pressure drops more than 20 mmHg, the symptoms are reproduced, or a supraclavicular bruit is created. The test often produces positive results in scaleus anticus syndrome. Both arms should be tested for comparison.
2. The costoclavicular manoeuvre is performed with the patient placed in an exaggerated military attention position. The shoulders are lifted and the clavicles are rotated backward. This test compresses the space between the clavicle and the first rib. Test results are often positive in patients with costoclavicular syndrome with clavicular deformities. The criteria for a positive test are the same as for the Adson's test.
3. The hyperabduction test is performed with the patient's arm abducted and externally rotated. The radial pulse is palpated, and the criteria for a positive test are the same as for the Adson's test. A bruit may be auscultated anterior to the pectoralis minor insertion. This test often produces positive results in a pectoralis minor syndrome.
4. The claudication test is performed with both of the patient's arms externally rotated and abducted. The patient is then asked to rapidly open and close his or her hands. Results of the test are considered positive when the symptoms are reproduced or when the symptomatic arm becomes weak or tired. This test can be useful in diagnosis and

treating a TOS when combined with the rest of the information obtained.

Treatment

Treatment is directed to improving function. While the athlete is in pain, ice and NSAIDs are useful in the short term. OMT should be directed generally at the pelvic girdle, spinal passive restrictions, costovertebral junctions, rib motions and soft tissues. Techniques used include strain–counterstrain, muscle energy, cranial and high velocity thrush.

Coeliac plexus injury (winding)

This is one of the most common abdominal injuries. It follows an unguarded impact to areas such as the xiphoid process, abdomen or thoracolumbar spinal region. Brief, high intensity force to these areas results in a stunning of the coeliac (solar) plexus. Commonly, this is a temporary minor paralysis of short duration and is more frightening for the athlete than damaging. They will be doubled forwards, gasping for air and in a distressed and anxious state. Signs and symptoms should settle within a few minutes.

Treatment

Reassurance and rest are the normal approaches. Adult athletes in contact and collision sports tend to be able to rationalize the pain and are aware that they will recover. The diaphragm has been stunned, so help the athlete to breathe by straightening them up and raising their arms and placing them on their heads. Keep them in a kneeling position. Instruct them to perform these actions by themselves to allow you to gauge the extent of the damage. If they are extremely distressed and symptoms do not clear in a few minutes look for signs of intra-abdominal damage. Perform abdominal examination, monitor pulse and blood pressure, and observe for shock.

Abdominal injury

Sporting abdominal injuries can be classified under blunt abdominal trauma or penetrating trauma. Blunt injuries, which are the most common, are usually caused by a combination of direct impact, shear forces, rotatory forces and deceleration. For example, contact and collision events like football and rugby often lead to blunt injury. Shear forces are due to pressure on the abdomen, as in a pile up, and the shearing motion damages vessels within the abdomen. Rotatory forces tend to occur when an athlete falls or is thrown, causing the abdominal contents to feel like they are being centrifuged. Deceleration forces are common in impacts, for example in motor racing, where the body stops moving and the abdominal contents continue on, again tearing vessels.

Signs and symptoms

Generally, all athletes will show to different degrees signs of hypotensive shock and unwellness. The condition may become more dangerous the longer it takes for the athlete to feel the symptoms. On-the-field presentations tend to be acute, sometimes with associated fractures. The best diagnostic techniques are a good history, examination, X-ray and CT scan.

Spleen injury

Rupture of the spleen is not common, but is one of the potentially fatal abdominal injuries in sport. Pain is felt in the upper left section of the abdomen, will refer to the left shoulder and scapula, and it is not uncommon to have associated rib fractures. The most susceptible athletes are those who have a recent history of infectious mononucleosis. Shock, abdominal pain, tenderness and unwellness are the primary signs and symptoms. Transportation to hospital is vital, even if spleen injury is only suspected.

Renal (kidney and ureter) injury

This is probably the second most common injury in sports after coeliac plexus injury. Players in contact and collision sports often 'accidently' contact another player with for example a knee in the other player's back. These injuries can be classified into the following:

- contusions;
- superficial parenchymal lacerations or fractures;
- deep parenchymal lacerations or fractures, often involving renal calacies and infundibula;
- multiple deep parenchymal lacerations (shattering or fragmentation of the kidney);
- renal pedicle injuries (avulsion, intimal tear with thromboses).

Motor vehicle collisions with rapid deceleration may lead to major renal vascular injury (Mills *et al.*, 1985). Darkening of the urine (haematuria) may be evident, but not always, and this should not last longer than the following morning. Flank pain and radiations may be put down to rough play especially if the athlete has stud/cleat marks on his back. Injury does not have to be directly to the back, for example it may occur in an athlete who has fallen heavy on their backside – the force can be transmitted through to the kidneys disrupting the delicate internal structure. Kidney and general abdominal examination will reveal tenderness and rigidity. Transportation to hospital is vital, even if this injury is only suspected.

Liver injury

Blunt impact to the abdomen that affects the liver is potentially fatal. It may result in intrahepatic haemorrhage and/or liver fracture. Again, the athlete will complain of right upper quadrant discomfort and right shoulder and/or scapular discomfort. Signs and symptoms are those of shock and should be approached accordingly. Transportation to hospital is vital even if the injury is only suspected.

Stomach injury

This is quite rare in athletic activity. Acute stomach pain can be due to eating too close to an event or drinking large quantities of very cold water during an event leading to 'cramping'. Overenthusiasm with salt tablets to prevent dehydration can cause gastric irritation. It has been suggested that stress can precipitate gastric mucosa ulceration through the parasympathetic nervous system (Hashiguchi *et al.*, 1993).

Duodenal, intestinal and colonic injury

These are not so common in athletic events. They follow the abdominal signs and symptoms picture. In addition, they are particularly a problem due to the presence of microbes in the gut, which can lead to peritonitis.

Appendicitis

Acute appendicitis is a common abdominal surgical emergency which may occur in any age group. The athlete will first present with pain in the centre or periumbilical region, progressively moving to the right iliac fossa or lower right quadrant within a couple of hours. The athlete will look unwell and be preoccupied with the pain in the abdomen. He or she may be sweating, pallid, feel nauseous and reveal a slight leukocytosis. On examination of the abdomen there will be tenderness and guarding of the right lower quadrant. McBurney's point is usually the most painful point; this is midway between a line drawn from the right superior iliac spine and the pubic tubercle. In chronic appendicitis the athlete will have discomfort in the same region but will tend to show signs of anorexia and weight loss, be pallid, and may have a low grade fever. Immediate transportation to hospital is necessary; if an appendix ruptures there will be a generalized peritonitis which can be an extremely grave situation.

Bladder rupture

Many athletes, especially in contact and collision sports, may forget to urinate before they participate in on-the-field activities. Impact to the abdomen when the bladder is full, especially when the abdominal muscles are off guard, can lead to an intraperitoneal bladder rupture. A general peritonitis will ensue but may delay for several hours if the urine is sterile. Immediate transportation to hospital is essential.

Hernias

The definition of a hernia is the protrusion through a normal abdominal opening of a piece of viscus. Hernias in the abdominal region tend to be inguinal (above the inguinal ligament) or femoral (below the inguinal ligament). Inguinal hernias are generally classified as indirect or direct. Indirect or oblique inguinal hernias occur when the viscus tracks obliquely along the inguinal canal; a direct hernia protrudes straight forward.

Treatment
True hernias need surgical intervention. OMT can be directed at treating the reason for the structural breakdown – check, for example, abdominal, quadriceps, adductor and gluteal muscle tension. A hernia is likely to be the end result of structural adaptational breakdown in thoracic and pelvic/lower extremity interaction.

Ovarian injury and pain

Impact to the lower abdomen in female athletes may cause ovarian contusion. The athlete will have lower abdominal tenderness, usually over one ovary region, with nausea and deep abdominal discomfort. Palpation of the area will be consistent with intra-abdominal trauma and point tenderness. Deep pelvic pain may indicate an ovarian cyst. This may be associated with deep lower thoracic and upper lumbar referred pain.

Treatment
Ice, analgesia, and NSAIDs will reduce pain. Athletes should be referred to a gynaecologist for a check-up. Even when cleared, a viscerosomatic reflex may continue to be present. A manipulative approach is very beneficial in reducing any residual deep pelvic discomfort and the inflammatory condition.

Amenorrhoea

Absence of menstruation in athletes can be primary or secondary. Primary exercise-related amenorrhoea occurs when a young girl is under stress, physical and/or psychological, and fails to begin menstruation by around 16 years of age. Secondary exercise-related amenorrhoea is where athletic activity, stress and poor nutrition prevent menses for a minimum of 3 months. Helping the athlete to change these factors is a delicate process. Try to identify the problem areas, and build a picture of the athlete's circumstances. If the athlete is legally the responsibility of a guardian or parent, this must be discussed with them. Tackling this problem may be equally difficult with an adult patient. See screening, p. 204.

Treatment
Alterations in diet, training and stressor factors will be very helpful. Refer the athlete to the relevant specialists.

Testicular lumps

Every testicular lump should be considered a possible carcinomatous tumour until proven otherwise. There is no age predisposition for testicular cancer. All male athletes should be encourage to palpate their testicles at least once a week. Generally, this is done by being comfortable in the bath, shower or in bed. Each testicle should be felt by checking the continuity of the shape of the testicle, the skin and the groin area for glandular swelling. Any sign of tenderness or inconsistency of shape should be further investigated as soon as possible.

Testicular contusion

It is surprising how few contact sport athletes wear testicular protection. Some wear athletic supports that contain the testicles but do not protect them from the damage of impact. The main reason for this is that hard protectors are cumbersome and can even be dangerous when the athlete hits the ground and the legs get crossed. Hard case protectors are usually worn in cricket. If you have seen a cricket 'box' that has been hit by a ball you will understand why it is an essential piece of equipment. Signs and symptoms of testicular contusion are fairly obvious. The athlete will be in pain and usually lying on the ground doubled over.

Treatment

In mild cases the player will be bent over, standing or lying on his side. The following procedure will give instant relief. With a clenched fist the medial aspect is used like a hammer and the athlete struck sharply and firmly over the sacrum around the S2 level. The impact will shock the reflex cremaster contracture into releasing and should give a sense of relief. In more severe cases athletes should be examined for rupture and excessive swelling where the internal structures become indistinguishable. The athlete should sit in cold water (whirlpool or bath with additional ice if necessary) and should be administered analgesics and NSAIDs. A better athletic support should be worn in the future.

Testicular rupture

This is a medical emergency. There is damage to the tunica albuginea, bleeding within the scrotum, which 'fills up', and pain. Signs are consistent with testicular trauma and the athlete should be sent to hospital immediately.

Testicular torsion

This is characterized by a sudden or advancing onset of pain and discomfort which is felt deep in the abdomen and inguinal region. As with most genital problems there is a feeling of nausea and shock as the symptoms get worse. A torsioned testicle tends to twist away from the midline in the direction in which the cremaster fibres run with twisting of the spermatic cord. The torsioned testicle usually lies higher than the other testicle and may show slight signs of scrotal oedema.

Chronic bowel dysfunction

This is general term which includes dysfunction due to:

- irritable bowel syndrome;
- lactose deficiency;
- drugs (laxatives/cathartics, magnesium-containing antacids);
- diverticular disease of the colon;
- psychiatric disorders [depression (often with weight loss), somatization disorders];
- parasitic infections (*Giardia lamblia, Entamoeba histolytica*);
- inflammatory bowel disease [Crohn's disease, ulcerative colitis (both can be accompanied by fever and/or rectal bleeding)];
- malabsorption (accompanied by weight loss and/or steatorrhoea; chronic pancreatitis, coeliac sprue, postgastrectomy syndrome);
- metabolic disorders [diabetes (with nocturnal diarrhoea); thyrotoxicosis (with weight loss)];
- bacterial infections [salmonella, *Campylobacter jejuni, Yersina enterocolitica, Clostridium difficile* (associated with antibiotics)];
- endocrine-producing tumours (with high volume diarrhoea);
- gastrinoma, carcinoid, vasoactive intestinal polypeptide tumour;
- other neoplasias (villus adenoma, adenocarcinoma of the colon).
  (Harber, 1988)

Irritable bowel syndrome (IBS)
This condition should not be overlooked when treating musculoskeletal (soft tissue) injuries. It retards healing and exacerbates symptoms. In the majority of cases paraspinal soft tissue reflects colon tension by being hard in constipation and soft in diarrhoea, while the skin will be spotty and greasy. Abdominal pain is the consistent symptom, but can vary from athlete to athlete, from a dull ache to extreme severity. The usual location of the pain is in the lower left quadrant, i.e. indicating spasm of the sigmoid colon. Pain tends to be worse in the morning and after eating. A bowel movement usually reduces the pain.

The most important factor in the diagnosis of IBS is a good case history, which should include characteristics about the patient's personality, and stressful life events that tend to be low grade and of a long lasting nature, e.g. relationships, work, parental pressure or event pressure. Symptoms of IBS tend to be the following, in patients who otherwise appear normal and well-nourished.

- Specific: abdominal pain, abdominal distension, pain with bowel movements, hard pellet-like stools, frequent loose stools, mucus in stools, feelings of incomplete evacuation.

- Non-specific: fatigue, depression, anxiety, dyspepsia, excessive bloating, weakness, palpitations (Harber, 1988).

Treatment

An approach to this condition involves initially helping to relieve the athlete of concern about the problem. In this condition the athlete has to work closely with the practitioner. Treatment approaches include dietary changes, OMT, pharmacological intervention, exercise and sometimes psychotherapy.

1. Diet. The diet should be tailored to the athlete's needs. For example, if the athlete is primarily suffering from diarrhoea then you want to reduce foodstuffs that promote colonic motility and bloating, e.g. beans, cabbage, caffeine, nicotine and fatty foods. Those suffering from constipation should be advised to drink plenty of water, i.e. at least 2 litres/day. Bran is useful. Not eating between meals is advisable. Eating small meals often, e.g. four meals a day instead of three, may be helpful.
2. OMT. OMT is directed at the intervertebral joints, the paraspinal soft tissue and the abdomen, to improve venous and lymphatic drainage of the abdomen. This reduces the effect of spinal cord facilitation and the autonomic nervous imbalance which heightens any musculoskeletal injury pain. OMT should ideally be applied at least twice a day.
3. Pharmacological therapy. This is never a desirable step to take, but may be used for symptomatic relief. Anticholinergics can be prescribed to decrease gastric motility and colonic spasm. Side effects of these medications include urinary hesitancy and retention, tachycardia, mydriasis and palpitations. Tranquillizers may be prescribed to control stress and anxiety. They may not be useful for the IBS, but are a short-term symptomatic control measure. Antidepressants and anti-diarrhoeals are also useful.
4. Exercise. Activity should not be stopped if it can be helped. Musculo-skeletal activity helps in a high percentage of IBS sufferers due to a circulatory shift. The type of exercise is dictated by any injured areas, e.g. an upper body training programme should be employed with lower extremity injury.
5. Psychotherapy. This kind of management may be indicated if the practitioner feels the athlete has a basic personality or stress problem. The autonomic nervous system will be involved. The psychotherapy will aim to reduce stress.

Cardiac assessment of children

Heart murmurs are caused by turbulent, non-laminar flow of blood through the heart or great vessels. More than 50% of normal children will have an audible heart murmur at some stage. The presence of dysmorphic features or extracardiac abnormalities should alert the general practitioner to the possibility of structural heart disease. It is essential to exclude cyanosis and clubbing of the fingers and toes.

Observation

1. Palpation of the pulses and the precordium should be normal. In all children, coarctation should be excluded by normal and equal pulses in the upper and lower limbs.
2. Auscultation should be directed firstly at the heart sounds. The second sound is of particular importance in children. To be normal it should split physiologically (that is, it should split on inspiration and be single on expiration). A persistently split second sound is characteristic of an atrial septal defect. A single second sound is abnormal and occurs with tetralogy of Fallot and other causes of severe pulmonary stenosis, pulmonary atresia, common atrial trunk and transposition of the great arteries. A loud pulmonary component to the second sound suggests pulmonary hypertension. Then attention is turned to the presence of any abnormally added sounds such as a fourth sound or ejection clicks. Systolic ejection clicks are caused by semilunar valve stenosis or a dilated great arterial root. An aortic click is best heard at the apex, while a pulmonary click is heard at the upper left sternal border and is loudest or only heard in expiration.

Manoeuvres affecting the intensity of heart murmurs
(↑ increased ↓ decreased)

Respiration

Inspiration:
- ↑ Systemic venous return
- ↑ Right heart murmurs, e.g. pulmonary stenosis, tricuspid regurgitation.

Expiration:
- ↑ Pulmonary venous return
- ↑ Left heart murmurs, e.g. ventricular septal defect, mitral regurgitation, aortic stenosis.

Valsalva manoeuvre

- ↑ Intrathoracic pressure
- ↓ Venous return
- ↓ Intrathoracic volume
- ↓ Flow murmurs
- ↓ Innocent murmurs
- ↑ Subaortic obstruction
- ↑ Mitral regurgitation.

Posture

Supine position:
- ↑ End-diastolic volume
- ↑ Cardiac stroke volume

- ↑ Increase flow murmurs
- ↑ Innocent murmurs
- ↓ Subaortic obstruction
- ↓ Venous hum.

Sitting/standing position:
- ↓ End-diastolic volume
- ↓ Cardiac stroke volume
- ↓ Flow murmurs
- ↓ Innocent murmurs
- ↑ Subaortic obstruction
- ↑ Venous hum.

(Source: Ladusans, 1993.)

SPINE

The spine is the axial skeleton of the body. In addition to this, its osseo-cartilage make-up contains an enormous amount of potential energy. This energy is released when the muscles initiate bending forces. Like the initiation of a fly-wheel, the muscles control the kinetic energy which drives the pelvis and lower extremity. This is added to by the counter rotation of the shoulders to produce the basis of movement, especially in running.

> Locomotion was first achieved by the motion of the spine. Then limbs came after, as an improvement, not as a substitute; and yet, analysis of bipedal gait concentrates almost exclusively on the motion of the limbs. This theory of locomotion requires the central nervous system to control the torque at those intervertebral joints and suggests that a breakdown of the control system would result in tortional failure of the spine.
>
> (Gracovetsky, 1985)

Anatomy

The anatomy and function of the spine are totally integrated, within the spine and with the pelvis and extremities. This integration is not through the axial bony skeleton, but through the autonomic nervous system and the spinal cord.

Bones

The bones consist of five cervical, 12 thoracic, five lumbar, one sacrum, coccyx (and two pelvic bones).

The cervical vertebrae
These consist of two atypical first (C1) and second (C2) vertebrae and five (C3–C7) typical vertebrae. The atlas (C1) is named after the Greek god,

Atlas, who holds up the world. This vertebra has no body, but functionally combines with the odontoid process of the axis (C2). The anterior arch continues with the two lateral masses with a small articular facet on the posterior surface. Both lateral masses have superiorly an articular facet which articulates with the occipital condyles forming the occipitoatlantal joint (OA joint). Movement at this level is primarily flexion and extension due to the concave and horizontal nature of the facet planes. Small articular facets under the lateral masses articulate with the axis inferiorly. These facets allow for rotation. It is important anatomically not to forget the presence of the transverse ligament, running between the lateral masses, behind the anterior arch from tubercles on the medial aspect of the masses. It does not appear on X-ray.

Protruding laterally from the lateral masses are the transverse processes (TPs), which provide muscle attachments. Clinically important is the region where the TPs are palpable anterior to the mastoid process and posterior to the jaw, just under the ear. This I have called the 'C1 TP recess'. It receives the tip of the finger except when oedematous when the TPs seem prominent. The vertebral arteries pass up through the foramen transversarium; the first cervical nerve runs over the posterior arch laterally then behind the lateral masses, under the vertebral artery and then divides into an anterior division running forward and along the lateral border of the lateral mass, medial to the vertebral artery, and the posterior division which enters the suboccipital triangle. The posterior arch of the atlas brings together the lateral masses as they continue backwards. There is a groove on the superior surface of the posterior arch for the vertebral artery and the first cervical nerve. There is no spinous process of C1, but there is a small posterior tubercle.

The axis (C2) has a body that is in fact the odontoid peg rising superiorly to lie posterior to the anterior arch of C1. This odontoid peg ossifies in three centres and fuses with the axis at about 4 years old. The blood supply to the odontoid peg is by the anterior and posterior branch of the vertebral artery, a small branch from the internal carotid continuing along the alar, apical and accessory ligaments. The articular facets are superior and inferior. The superior facets lie posterolaterally to the odontoid peg at the junction between the body and transverse process. They articulate with the inferior facets of the lateral masses of the atlas, which slope down and laterally. The inferior facets lie posteriorly to the TPs, looking downward and forward like the typical cervical inferior facets to articulate with the third cervical vertebra. The TPs of the axis have the foramen transversarium for the vertebral artery passing upwards and outwards continuing through the foramen of the atlas and the nerve root, which passes out behind the artery. The posterior arch marks the uniting of the TPs and pedicles posteriorly; it carries the inferior facet anteriorly at its junction with the pedicle, and the spine of the axis is bifid.

The typical cervical vertebrae (C3–C7) each have a small, oval body which is concave superiorly in a transverse (coronal) plane. The TPs are attached to the posterolateral region of the body and anterolateral area of the pedicle, and are concave superiorly for the nerve root, which runs laterally behind the vertebral artery. It contains the foramen transversarium for the vertebral artery, lying in front of the nerve root, and the vein, which lies in front of the vertebral artery. Pedicles of the cervical vertebra project backwards and laterally and unite the posterior arch, the lamina, with the body. Articular facets sited at the junction of the pedicle and lamina are angled at about 45°. The superior facets look up and back, the inferior facet down and forward. They are flat and oval. The architecture of the cervical vertebra continues backwards to form the lamina, which is thin and quite weak; the spine is bifid and small except C7, which is longer and not bifid, and the vertebral canal forms a large triangular space for the spinal cord.

The thoracic vertebrae

The typical thoracic vertebra has a body which is heart shaped. The bodies become larger as you descend the thoracic column. Due to the attachment of the ribs to the thoracic vertebrae they have two demifacets for the synovial joints of the rib heads on the body. The superior demifacet lies just in front of the pedicle and the inferior demifacet lies in front of the inferior vertebral notch. Pedicles are attached to the posterosuperior angle of the body just behind the rib facet. They unite the body with the lamina, and form the superior border of the inferior vertebral notch. Thoracic spine TPs are thick and strong and arise from the junction of the pedicle and lamina. The TP has a facet on the anterior surface of the tip for the synovial joint with the tubercle of the rib. This is not the case for the 11th and 12th vertebrae. Superior and inferior articular processes are present. The superior articular processes begin from the junction of the lamina and pedicle. They have a flat surface, and the facets look back and slightly up and laterally. The inferior articular facets begin from the junction between pedicle and the lamina, but this time below and just posterior to the plane of the superior facets. These facets look forward, slightly medially and downwards. These inferior facets form the posterior wall of the inferior vertebral notch. The pedicle of the vertebra below forms the inferior margin of the notch, called the intervertebral foramen, through which the nerve roots leave the vertebral canal. Lamina of the thoracic vertebrae are wide and strong, and overlap each other. Their spinous processes are long, narrow, and slope down and back, and have a vertebral canal that is narrow and circular.

The lumbar vertebrae

The typical lumbar spine has large, strong and heavy bodies, increasing in size as they descend. The pedicles are short and thick, project back from the proximal half of body, join the body to the lamina and form the superior border of the inferior intervertebral notch. The TPs begin from the base of the pedicles, increase in length from the first to the third, then decrease again; they are mostly thin except for the fifth, which is a short, thick process. The superior articular processes are from the junction of the pedicle and the lamina superiorly; the facets are concave and look medially and backwards. The inferior articular facets form from the junction of the pedicle and lamina inferiorly; the facet is convex and looks laterally and forwards, locking the superior facet of the vertebra below. The pars inarticularis is the junction of the superior and inferior facets, the pedicle and lamina. Due to its structure it is at this region that there is concentration of stress passing through the lumbar vertebrae. The pars is viewed clearly on an oblique X-ray as a 'Scotty dog', where the head is the transverse process, the eye the pedicle, the ear is the superior articular process, the front leg is the inferior articular process, the body the lamina, and the neck is the pars inarticularis. A 'collar' around the dog's neck is the presentation of a spondylolysis. Lamina and spinous processes of the lumbar vertebra are thick, short and strong. The spinal canal is triangular, larger than the thoracic, but smaller than the cervical canal.

Joints

Occipitoatlantal joint
These are synovial joints, large and oval in the anteroposterior direction, whose action is mainly flexion and extension. A capsule surrounds the joints, with anterior and posterior membranes.

Atlantoaxial joint
The odontoid peg articulates with the anterior arch of the atlas in front and the transverse ligament of the atlas behind by a synovial joint. These synovial joints allow rotation between the axis and atlas, being surrounded by a capsule. The ligaments include the apical ligament, which runs from the tip of the dens to the anterior margin of the foramen magnum; the alar ligaments, one on each side, running from the side of the apex of the dens laterally to the occipital condyles; the accessory ligaments from the lateral mass of the atlas close to the attachment of the transverse ligaments; the cruciate ligament consists of a vertical band from the back of the body axis, upwards to the transverse ligament, a horizontal band, and on to the superior surface of the basiocciput just in front of the foramen magnum; the membrana tectoria is posterior to these ligaments and is a continuation of the posterior longitudinal ligament of the vertebral column from axis to basiocciput; and the ligamentum flavum between the posterior arches.

Intervertebral joints
In the typical cervical spine there are three intervertebral joints. The two apophyseal joints and the intervertebral disc allow limited anteroposterior flexion, extension, lateral flexion and rotation. There are no discs between the occiput, atlas and axis. Apophyseal joints are synovial joints that are surrounded by a capsule. Ligaments around the vertebrae include the longitudinal ligament, which is continuous in front and behind the vertebral bodies, being wider as they run over the intervertebral discs. The ligamentum flavum attaches near the anteroinferior margin of proximal lamina, and runs downward to attach to the superior border of

adjacent lamina below; this tissue allows movement between vertebrae, and protects the spinal cord posteriorly between the laminae. The ligaments are the weak interspinous ligament and the strong supraspinous ligament, the ligamentum nuchae, which travels from the occiput to the spine of C7, and the strong intratransverse ligament.

The thoracic spine has the three joints, two apophyseal and the intervertebral discs. The ligaments are the same as the cervical spine. Lumbar spine joint and ligament make-up is essentially the same as above. In addition the lumbosacral region has very strong ligaments, the iliolumbar (fascial derivative) and lumbosacral ligaments.

Spinal muscles

It is important to remember that spinal muscular function is integrated: although a muscle stops at one point it may still influence another muscle's ability to function properly elsewhere. The neuromyofacsial skeletal system makes up the patient's 'back' and it must be remembered that this is a sensory system.

The suboccipital region has more than 20 muscles attaching to this area. There are eight posterior occipital muscles that control and guard this delicate area of the head–spine junction. An interesting anatomical finding is that they are striated and are considered as only voluntary muscles in action. Due to their position they are under the long-term emotional and physical stress influence of reflex autonomic contracture.

The superficial muscle of the cervical and upper thoracic area which influences spinal joint and shoulder girdle function is the trapezius. Overlapping at the lower thoracic region with the trapezius, the latissimus dorsi is the other long lever muscle of the back. These two muscles are powerful movers and as a consequence are instigated in long-term limitation of range of motion. They act to keep the back within its total limit of motion, to prevent overtaxing the deeper structures. The other main muscle that works with these two as a major flexor is the psoas.

Spinal cord and nerve roots

The spine 'houses' the spinal cord. The cord travels through the canal from the foramen magnum to the lower border of L1. It then continues on as a fibrous cord, the filum terminale, which is in fact a continuation of the pia mater. It descends in the middle of the cauda equina from the tip of the spinal cord, the conus medullaris, ending in the sacral canal. Nerve roots are classified as peripheral and are split into motor nerves, from anterior horn cells, and sensory nerves, which enter the spinal cord at the posterior horn and column.

Osteopathically, particular importance is placed on the superior sympathetic ganglia. It is the largest of the cervical ganglia and is essentially several ganglia in one. Its anatomical relation is anterior to the axis and third cervical vertebral transverse process, near the internal carotid artery. Vasomotor impulses travel up this region from the thoracic spinal cord centres. From the superior cervical ganglion postganglionic impulses continue on superiorly via the carotid plexus, controlling the blood supply to the brain, eyes, ears, thyroid, and possibly also the Gasserian ganglion and the pituitary body. Posteriorly, impulses travel to the articulation of the spinal joints controlling the arterioles of the suboccipital region. Anteriorly, connection is made with the heart, thyroid gland, the phrenic nerve, the vagus and other cranial nerves. Figure 6.10 shows neuroendocrine pathways in the cervical region.

Vascular drainage

Osteopathically, emphasis is always on drainage rather than supply. Cathie (1974b) described the vertebral venous system:

> The veins of the body fall into two general classifications, the caval system and the portal system. From functional and clinical points of view, a third or internal vertebral system should be added. This system is unique in several ways and requires special consideration. It lies within the vertebral canal and is composed of the longitudinal veins and plexuses connected almost at every spinal level with the external venous vertebral plexus. The internal plexuses are located in the extra or epidural space, and in relation to the pia mater. Into these passes the venous blood from the spinal cord. Associated with these veins should be mentioned the sinusoidal arrangement of veins within the vertebral bodies. These veins drain, in large part into the anterior longitudinal meningo-rachidian veins. The internal venous vertebral plexus is deprived of the benefit of actively contracting and relaxing muscles and heavy fascial specialisations that elsewhere assist in the propulsion of venous blood. They depend, to a great degree upon the motion of the spine for this function. They are devoid of valves. Engorgement and dilatation of these veins and their connections are frequently found with the result that chronic passive congestion and increased fluid in the perivascular tissues, or oedema, is an important clinical consideration. The veins are also influenced by changes in intra-abdominal and thoracic pressure as has been pointed out by Baston of the University of Pennsylvanina.

From this we can see the importance of motion in the venous and lymphatic drainage systems. We can also see that the effects of oedema, as the result of injury around the facet joint, would affect the integrity of the intervertebral foramen. Inflammation will always find the point of lowest resistance disturbing local circulation. The longer the increased pressure is present, the greater the risks of further, initially unrelated, tissue becoming involved. The formation of anastamoses is unlikely to solve the problem. There is a surprisingly large volume of venous blood in the vertebral canal, much larger than required to return blood brought to it by the arterial system; indeed, if required, it could carry a volume equal to that carried by the inferior vena cava.

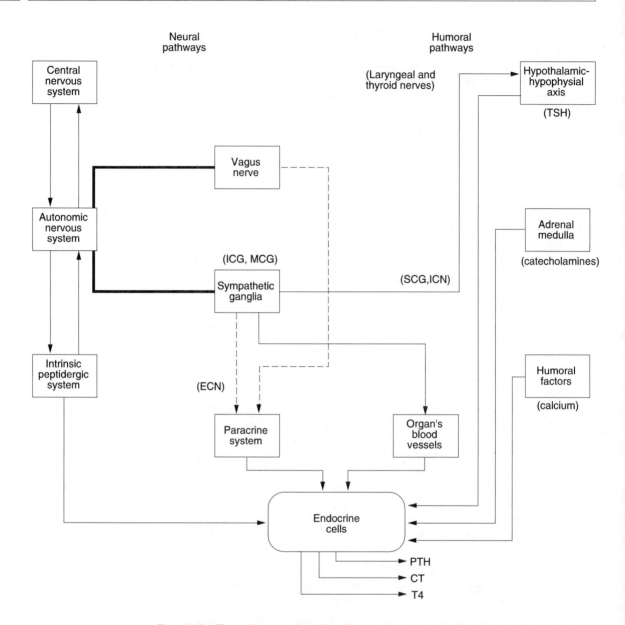

Fig. 6.10 Flow diagram depicting hierarchical and parallel organization of neuro-endocrine pathways in the cervical region. ICN, internal carotid nerve; ECN, external carotid nerve; SCG, MCG, ICG, superior, middle and inferior cervical ganglia; TSH, thyroid stimulating hormone; PTH, parathyroid hormone; CT, calcitonin; T4, thyroxine. (From Cardinali and Romeo, 1990.)

Function

The spinal column is part of a complex of muscles, tendons, fascia and ligaments. It should not be thought of as a weight-bearing column, as it relies on the soft tissues, and vice versa. Soft tissues 'house' the spinal column which in turn contains the spinal cord. Spaces between each vertebra allow exit and entrance points for the central nervous system. Soft tissue absorbs most energy in the back in health, not the discs; soft tissue also exerts the most energy. The spinal column is bound by ligaments that provide potential energy for movement. Here I would like to present extracts from Gracovetsky (1985):

> The demand for torque transmission imposes specific constraints on the intervertebral joints. It is known that the resistance of the facets to a static torsional load approximately equals that of the entire annulus. Unfortunately, the fibre orientation of the annulus has been traditionally viewed and modelled as a system designed to retain a pressurised nucleus, although the resulting calculations indicate that with such representation the joint would fail at about one quarter of its ultimate value. Although it is tempting to visualise the 'X' patterns fulfilling both compressional and torsional function, it must be remembered that the vertebral body will fail in compression long before the annulus. Hence, the available data suggest that the structure of the annulus is primarily determined by the requirements of the torque transmission; further experimental evidence would be necessary to reverse this argument.

Gracovetsky continues with a description of spinal function during walking:

> As the left foot advances and the right leg is in extension, contraction of the lateral flexors forces the spine to flex to the left, as viewed from the back. The left facet engages and the spine flexes in the saggital plane, as it bends to the left. Spinal flexion must not be confused with forward bending. The spine flexes whenever the lordosis is reduced; this effect is evident when the left heel strikes (LHS) and the hip extensors' moment rotates the pelvis backwards. Furthermore, the intervertebral joint is axially loaded and torqued to the left by the combined effect of lateral flexion and the gravitational field acting on the trunk. Under such conditions, an axial torque is generated and the pelvis is forced to rotate clockwise.
>
> While the spine reverses its rotation, it is necessary to correct the lordosis, maintain the axial compression, and reduce shear; that requires a downwards and forwards pull on the convexity of the spine. The right psoas is the only muscle which can perform this task, provided that the facet joints overlap from above, downwards. The coupled motion of the spine is reversible, and the psoas induced and controlled axial counter-clockwise torque, forces the spine to bend to the right; the spine begins to straighten up. The electrical activity of the psoas has been studied and its cyclic nature well documented. With this representation, psoas is a controller of the spine. It is interesting to note that in the rabbit, psoas is attached to the pelvis and not to the femur, which would indicate that the function of psoas is not fundamentally related to

leg motion. The action of the psoas is enhanced by the combined action of the erectores, the right latissimus dorsi and trapezius. The spinal motion is repeated at each step, as the spine resonates in the field of gravity walking requires a relatively low frequency and a small amplitude of oscillation. The low power required for walking can be supplied entirely by muscles of the trunk. Note that this theory requires the spine to transmit the required torque to drive the pelvis, and that enough energy be stored (and released) by the oscillating spine.

The key to restoring spinal and pelvic function as an integrating unit is to first know how an integrating unit functions. Atheletes take this functionability to an extreme.

Physiological movements of the spine

All joint motions may be divided into four types: flexion, extension, rotation and lateral flexion (sidebending). The normal range of each of these types of motion varies considerably in the different joint structures throughout the body. When a spinal joint is in what we might loosely term a 'neutral' position, i.e. when it has a normal range of each of the above physiological movements remaining to it, we say that it is in 'easy normal'. Another way of describing this condition is to say that the joint is in a position in which no bending movement is being applied to it about any axis. All physiological movements of the spine have a specific relationship with one another. The simple example of this is that rotation and lateral flexion always occur together as complementary motions, although in varying degrees in each type in different areas of the spine. Likewise, other physiological types of motion occur under different conditions, and so specifically that two laws of physiological movements of the spine can be stated. The principle of these two laws should could be kept in mind, as they constitute the key to the relationship of posture to health and disease.

1. **First Law**: when any area of the spinal column is in the easy normal position and lateroflexion is introduced, rotation of the vertebral bodies occurs into the convexity of the curve thus produced. The movements occur in the order named, i.e. easy normal, lateroflexion, rotation.
2. **Second Law**: when any area of the spine is in either marked flexion or marked extension, lateral flexion and rotation when introduced occur to the same side and are coexistant and complementary. Rotation occurs into the concavity of the curve and probably precedes lateroflexion to a slight degree, and for this reason it is said that these movements occur in the following order: flexion or extension, rotation, lateroflexion.

From a practical point of view, these two laws of spinal motion have very definite diagnostic palpatory findings, which are listed below. Since in any spinal motion involving lateral flexion we have a convex and a concave side, the findings are given for each side separately.

First law

On the convexity:

- superficial tissue tension and tenderness;
- deep tissue tension and tenderness;
- spinous processes separated and in the convexity;
- transverse processes separated and posterior;
- facet motion restricted.

On the concavity:

- transverse processes approximated;
- facet motion relatively free.

Second law

On the convexity:

- superficial tissue tension and tenderness;
- spinous processes in the convexity, either approximated or separated;
- transverse processes separated;
- facet motion comparatively free.

On the concavity:

- deep tissue tension and tenderness;
- transverse processes approximated and posterior;
- facet motion severely restricted.

(From Nelson, 1948.)

Presentation of injury

History and physical examination

All neck and back injuries should undergo a simple neurological evaluation at presentation. The degree of the signs and symptoms and the history should formulate the extent of the examination procedure.

Acute spinal pain

There are common factors between acute presentations of pain anywhere in the spinal column. All acute spinal presentations can be broadly classified as emotional (psychosomatic), physical, infective and combinations thereof.

Emotionally based presentations vary. Repeated minor emotional trauma is an accumulative contribution to the presentation. Physical discomfort close to past experiences can precipitate an emotional crisis.

Extreme anxiety can leave the athlete with very high resting tone of neck and back muscles, and may be associated with digestive problems. This happens at all ages, for different reasons.

In practically all cases of physical back and neck pain presentations there has been some functional breakdown. The majority of cases result from poorly integrated spinal–spinal, spinal–extremity or extremity–spinal interaction. Like emotional disorders, there is usually a history of repeated minor physical trauma. Athletes will tell you that a particular action, at work for example, cannot be the problem because 'I have always done that'. Due to the focusing of the poor motion at a spinal level you may be presented with a spinal lesion that is tender to the touch and painful to the patient when an attempt is made at moving. There will be hypertonia of the tissues long before the onset of acute pain. Structure has to change to meet changes in functional demand; if this is taken too far a breakdown can occur. Therefore, in the majority of cases you are presented with an acute lesion following on from a chronic lesion. Look for the chronic lesion complex and this will help the acute presentation. This is the basic osteopathic principle of removing obstructions so that the body can correct itself. No drugs, manipulation, physical therapy, machines or surgery can heal the body faster than its own vitality can. All we can do is improve conditions and remove obstructions.

Generally the superficial muscles of the back and neck 'drive' active gross function, while the smaller muscles deal with qualitative motions. The major back and neck muscles are the trapezius, latissimus dorsi, psoas, sternocleidomastoid and scalenes. The majority of acute pains in the back and neck are at the lumbosacral and C5–C6 region. Attachments of these two superficial muscles, latissimus dorsi and trapezius, are at the sacrum and occiput respectively. Common points of attachment include the shoulders and an overlap at the midthorax.

The most common acute presentations of spinal trauma are sprains, strains and combinations thereof. Dramatic presentations of pain are generally due to the fact that the back is the axis of body motion and it is almost impossible to perform any kind of function without involving the back.

Torticollis (wry neck, acute facet lock)

The athlete presents with acute restriction of movement, especially of the head/cervical spine. Usually the patient is holding the neck in a rotated, flexed and sidebent position. The cause may be either psychological (emotional) or physical. The emotional presentation tends to occur more in children, but may also occur in adults who have not 'grown out' of this physical presentation of an emotional crisis. This is a psychosomatic presentation, but joint irritation may occur due to repeated episodes, which then trigger a neck muscular spasm. Where the cause is physical, the majority of 'facet locks' are the result of long-term myofascial contracture and restriction of movement. In practically all cases athletes will have a history of a tight neck and shoulders, and they may remember pain in the area some months or even years before.

Neck sprain/strain

Usually there is a history of trauma, especially in contact and collision sports. The most common regions are the sternocleidomastoid, erecta spinae and trapezius areas. Evaluate as for any normal sprain/strain presentation. Never use a spinal compression test: if there is a disc problem, this will make it worse. Gentle cervical traction in the seated position may give some relief; this is not a sign that it is a disc problem. Pain on traction is due to tissue that may be torn, crushed or in protective spasm due to underlying bony or soft tissue damage being exacerbated by the traction force.

Treatment
The application of ice or cold will immediately control pain. Oedema and bony point tenderness may be present initially and should calm down within a few minutes. Never use high velocity thrust techniques at the injured spinal level on an immediate presentation of an acute neck (sprain/strain). Allow the symptoms to calm, to prevent risk of further damage. Additional anti-inflammatory medication and a supportive collar should be used. All acute neck presentations should be X-rayed if there is suspicion of more serious injury.

Trapped nerve (neuritis)

This is a common diagnosis in the patient who has neck pain, limitation of movement, and deep pain in the upper extremity. There is usually a chronic history with an acute onset, i.e. it comes and goes on a regular basis, until one day it does not go. In the cervical spine C6–C7 is the most common level for the root of the problem. Irritation of the nerve can be due to disc prolapse and joint hypermobility associated with chronic inflammation and possible scarring. There may be alterations in extremity power and sensations. Upper thoracic and upper cervical vertebrae are reduced in active function and when passively examined are reduced in motion. This is the baseline for the focusing of movement at the level of pain leading to nerve irritation.

Treatment
The aim of treatment is remove obstructions to healing and integrate spinal function. Initially traction, sitting or supine, will be painful because you are pulling scarred and fibrosed tissue; traction must be very gentle. A cervical collar can make things worse; see how the athlete responds. NSAIDs may not work initially until treatment has progressed a little. Manipulative treatment should be directed at improving function of the

upper cervical and upper thoracic region. For best results treatments should be short (5–10 minutes) and frequent.

Spinal stenosis and cord neurapraxia

This is a narrowing of the cervical spinal canal that may be congenital, or as a result of continued minor trauma due to cervical axial loading, forced hyperextension or hyperflexion. Narrowing of the spinal canal, resulting in cord stenosis, can be as a consequence of thickening ligament within the canal (ligamentum flavum) and osteophytes. This can lead to cord neurapraxia and transient quadriplegia. The phenomenon of cervical spinal cord neurapraxia occurs in individuals with developmental cervical spinal stenosis, congenital fusions, cervical instability or intervertebral disc protrusions when associated with a decrease in the anteroposterior diameter of the spinal canal. Athletes with diminution of the antero-posterior spinal canal diameter can on forced hyperextension and hyper-flexion compress the spinal cord causing transitory motor and sensory manifestations. A transient neurological episode includes paresis of either both arms, both legs or all four extremities, with burning, numbness, tingling or loss of sensation (Torg, 1990). Spinal stenosis is a descriptive X-ray finding that has to put into the proper clinical arena.

Treatment
Torg (1990) describes how measuring the narrowing percentage of the spinal canal allows the risk factors to be weighed up. This is the ratio between the vertebral body and the spinal canal, i.e. Pavlov's ratio = a/b. Lateral roentgenograms of the cervical spine were taken. The distance from the midpoint of the posterior aspect of the vertebral body to the nearest point on the corresponding spinolaminar line (a) is divided by the anteroposterior width of the vertebral body (b). In the 'normal' control subject this is 1:1 (1.00) while in a stenotic patient it is 1:2 (0.50). In the majority of cases this does not mean that they will have permanent neurological injury. Those who have spinal instability or acute or chronic degenerative changes should be precluded from further participation in contact sports. In clinical presentations this should be assessed by a orthopaedist or neurologist.

Straight spine syndrome

Otherwise known straight back syndrome, this is a skeletal deformity of the thorax resulting in a narrowing of the anteroposterior diameter of the thorax. A non-pathological systolic murmur, somewhat distorted X-ray appearance of the heart, and non-specific electrocardiographic changes may be seen in patients with this syndrome. In addition, mitral valve proplapse has been found in up to 67% of patients with straight spine syndrome. Accurate recognition of this deformity may disclose underlying cardiac abnormalities. Early discovery may identify those patients at risk for developing bacterial endocarditis (Gordon and Cox, 1983).

Sciatica

A general term used to describe any dysfunctional or pathological process that causes irritation along the distribution of the sciatic nerve.

Intervertebral disc prolapse

This is not a common presentation. Discs and apophyseal joints are only put under strain when the soft tissues of the spine are not absorbing or exerting energy properly during function. Deep soft tissue tends to be fibrotic on palpation. Add to this fibrosis of the superficial muscles, e.g. erecta spinae, latissimus dorsi and trapezius, and you have a situation where the potential for a disc prolapse is extremely high. Pressure in the disc increases, sitting becomes uncomfortable, and cervical and lumbar movement is poor and painful. There may be radiations down the extremity, with reductions in reflexes, and motor and sensory function may be disturbed (peripheral nerve compression). Onset may be slow, with degeneration of the annulus fibrosis, or acute due to trauma. At its extreme a prolapse may cause paralysis. Symptoms are exacerbated by coughing, sneezing or anything that increases intra-abdominal pressure. A common misconception is that the athlete who is laterally shifted and cannot put his or her foot to the floor has a prolapsed disc. The most common finding, that is not caused by disc injury, is deep hip soft tissue hypertonia and sciatic nerve irritation.

Treatment
Where this condition is not too severe, it is treated like an instability. This includes rest, NSAIDs, a gentle manipulative approach (e.g. traction), improvement in function of the rest of the spine (manipulatively), and gentle isometric exercises. Where this is severe, on the other hand, it is an orthopaedic emergency. The best way for visualizing the damage is by MRI. Relief can be obtained by lying down and remaining still in low back presentations, and sitting upright in neck presentations.

Ankylosing spondylitis

This is a rheumatological disorder of unknown aetiology that is slow in onset, and presents as aches and pains, and stiffness, especially in the morning (this in itself is far from enough for a diagnosis). Common areas include the thoracic spine and sacroiliac joints. When presented with these symptoms, chronic progressive polyarthritis should also be considered. The majority of patients are male and aged from mid-teens to mid-thirties. X-rays will show a blurring of joint continuity, erosions and narrowing. The term 'bamboo spine' is used to describe the widespread formation of syndesmophytes along the anterior and lateral surfaces of the discs, presenting as bridging between vertebrae.

Treatment

Gentle manipulative approaches are used, with NSAIDs. Exercise helps, as does general movement.

Spondylolysis and spondylolisthesis

Spondylolysis and spondylolisthesis are variations of the same condition. On posterior oblique X-ray, presentation of the 'Scotty dog' with a defect (stress-like injury) in the neck (pars interarticularis) like a 'collar' indicates spondylolysis, the simpler form of the spondylolisthesis. This defect can be unilateral or bilateral. In spondylolisthesis, which is a bilateral spondylolysis, the defect at the 'Scotty dog' neck is a complete break allowing a slip of the upper vertebral body on the lower one. The amount of slippage is described as Grade I (0–25% slippage) to Grade IV, which is a complete anterior displacement. The most common slip is L5, then L4. The greater the axial loading of the lumbar spine the greater the risk of the injury. Common sports where this injury occurs are rowing, football (linesmen) and gymnastics.

Treatment

A conservative approach to treatment of the 'spondylo' conditions is recommended. Stop all activity, improve the mobility of the rest of the spine (HVT, ST manipulation), use anti-inflammatory medication in acute cases, and gentle stretching exercises, until pain subsides, as with a fracture.

Apophyseal joint instability

This is usually a chronic degenerative condition that has an acute presentation. Instability tends to occur on one side of the L4–L5 or L5–S1 levels. A history of hard manual labour that involves, for example, digging holes, may precipitate joint irritation and/or ligament distruction. Stresses or minor injuries from a contact sport like rugby may combine to precipitate acute pain. After resting for a few days the symptom of one-sided back pain will subside and the player will return to the sport and work that will again precipitate the problem. Recurrence of this acute attack will become more and more frequent. In the majority of cases there are no neurological signs. A common description of the pain is that something is 'out', and they will have a protective posture. Age groups affected vary depending on the combination of work intensity and athletic intensity. A retired athlete who has a history of contact sports may present with the condition.

Treatment

As with any unstable joint, rest and anti-inflammatory medication reduces pain and restores mobility, temporarily. However, the joint will still be unstable. The objective is to reduce movement at the joint level and improve ligament stability. The lumbar erecta spinae and thoracolumbar fascia will be hypertonic. Manual restoration and improvement of high vertebral and soft tissue level function is important. Active rehabilitation may exacerbate the symptoms, so this should be monitored. Rest from twisting and flexing is vital, but heavy lifting is not a factor in a healthy back; in reality however it is recommended to cease all such activity. A back support may help to reduce mobility, but it is important for the back soft tissue not to have any stimulation at all. Stationary cycling is a good supportive modality. In all back and pelvic presentations check for intra-compartmental disease.

The acute back pain

All practitioners will encounter acute back pain at some time in their professional lives. We all develop our own approaches to relieving the athlete's suffering, and what I describe here is an approach that I have developed over the years.

It is important to recognize the 'fear factor' in acute back pain. This must be rationalized with the athlete before treatment is begun. Fear is not unfounded: it is based on the athlete's own physical and emotional experiences, and on second hand information from others. The practitioner should explain in simple terms why the pain is so bad and what the injury is doing to them, and that if they calm down they can help you to get rid of the pain.

In the majority of cases the damage is minimal. Let the athlete assume the most comfortable position for them. Neurological examination can be difficult under these conditions: if you do not feel experienced enough to take control of the situation, refer the athlete to hospital.

The following are principles of approach towards the acute low back. The following procedures should only be followed when you are sure that the athlete has no neurological deficit or remarkable findings.

Principle 1

The spine functions as a unit; the spinal cord is the medium through which impulses are passing and also creating more nociceptive input from other areas of the spine. Most walk-in acute presentations have a history of back pain, but have put things off until something has finally 'gone'. In the past they have treated themselves by resting or have been treated by somebody else who has only worked locally. The facilitated spinal cord has become sensitive from aberrant 'silent' information from the entire back over a long period of time.

Principle 2

It will be painful for the athlete to move the affected part. If the acute pain origin, e.g. lumbosacral level, is passively moved or stretched out it will hurt. Your main objective is to reduce the athlete's perception of pain. Treat other areas to reduce the 'total' neural bombardment of the spinal cord. If you want you can even start from the occiput and work downwards with OMT of your choice. Calm the spinal cord down. This will reduce the physical stress on the painful injured level. One of the most common findings is increased tension and immobility at the lower thoracic and upper lumbar region, the root of the diaphragm. HVT applied to this region tends to act as a 'circuit breaker'. Soft tissue manipulation of the spine is necessary with or without the HVT procedure.

Principle 3

Know when to stop. Your overall plan is to get the athlete to return to activity as soon as possible, not to get them better in one visit. They may leave still in pain, but you have begun the process of 'debriefing' the spinal cord and removing obstructions to healing.

Principle 4

Advise the athlete to rest. Explain to the athlete the principles of your approach. You will be able to reach a more accurate diagnosis once the acute situation has calmed down a little.

Principle 5

Only the body can heal itself. The more you attempt to treat the level of injury the more the chances are that you will disturb the healing of disrupted tissue. Your objective with OMT is to remove obstructions to the healing process.

Principle 6

Other modalities. Medication, heat, cold etc. can be used in addition to OMT to alleviate the discomfort.

PELVIS AND LOWER EXTREMITY

The osteopathic approach to problems involving the lower extremity is consistent with general osteopathic principles; these are discussed later (p. 368). Although it is important to know the anatomy and physiology of the areas concerned, this will not improve your treatment success unless you have a principle to work from. One of the major approaches of the osteopath is to investigate the quality and quantity of function of that limb in relation to the body, including nutrition and usage (past and present), and the most important aspect is that of the case history. Listen to your patients! A good case history will give you at least 70% of the diagnosis. The trademark of the osteopathic practitioner is his or her ability to reinforce clinical findings in injury and disease presentations with palpation. This tactile ability is one of the most basic of the osteopathic skill, without which you will be unable to make an accurate diagnosis.

Anatomy

Bones

The bones of the pelvis and lower extremity are the sacrum, innominates, femur, patella, tibia and fibula, talus (astragalus), calcaneus (os calcis), navicular (scaphoid), cuboid, cuneiforms, tarsals and metatarsals.

Greater sciatic foramen (GSF) of the pelvis

This is posterior to the anterior inferior iliac spine (AIIS), under the posterior inferior iliac spine (PIIS), and is divided by the piriformis tendon into an upper and lower part. In a similar fashion to the spaces of the shoulder girdle, the superior gluteal nerve and vessels travel through the upper part and the inferior gluteal nerve and vessels, internal pudendal nerve and vessels, sciatic nerve, and the nerves of the obturator internus and quadratus femoris, pass through the lower part of the GSF.

Lesser sciatic foramen (LSF) of the pelvis

This is below the ischial spine, which separates the GSF and LSF. The sacrospinous ligament connects the ischial spine with the sacrum and separates the GSF (above) from the LSF (below). The obturator internus travels through this foramen.

Hip joint

The acetabulum of the innominate forms a socket to receive the ball of the head of the femur. It is formed from the three pelvic bones, the ilium, ischium and pubis. This socket is directed 45° (from the coronal plane) laterally and downward (from the vertical plane). This socket is shaped like half a sphere and is deepened by fibrocartilage. The centre is filled with fat and vessels. The ligamentous apparatus of the femoral head (round ligament, ligamentum teres) has its origin from the transverse acetabular ligament, crossing the fat pad and inserts into the notch on the inferomedial part of the femoral head.

The capsule and synovium are attached proximally to the acetabular rim and transverse the acetabular ligament. They also attach distally to the middle of the femoral neck posteriorly and intertrochanteric line anteriorly. The majority of the femoral neck is intracapsular – this is an important factor when considering the spread of infection of the femoral neck into the hip. The synovium is reflected along the femoral neck to the rim of the head and has an extension beneath the transverse acetabular ligament to cover the round ligament.

The iliofemoral ligament, which is Y-shaped and known as the ligament of Bertin or Biglow, travels between the anterior superior iliac spine

(ASIS), with a strong lateral part to the upper part of the intertrochanteric line and a weaker medial part travelling downwards to the inferior part of the intertrochanteric line. The ischiofemoral ligament, which is posterior to the hip joint between the ischium, travels horizontally to the capsule/iliofemoral ligament. Finally, the pubofemoral ligament, which is the weakest of the ligaments, travels between the obturator crest and obturator membrane.

The knee

The most important structures of the knee are extra-articular, comprising the myotendinous fascial complex above, below and behind.

The capsule
This is attached to the femoral condyles and superior border of the intercondylar notch posteriorly (femur), the anterior margins of the patella and the patellar tendon inferiorly, the periphery of the menisci and the upper margins of the tibial condyles (meniscotibial portions called the coronary ligaments).

The synovium
The synovium lines the capsule and retropatellar fat pad. It covers the cruciates and supplies them with blood vessels, and forms the suprapatellar bursa lying between the quadriceps tendon and the distal femur, allowing the tendon to glide on the femur during flexion and extension of the knee.

Anterior aspect of the knee
Over the anterior aspect of the knee there is the capsule. Over this is the patellar tendon, the quadriceps expansion from the vastus lateralis and medialis, which forms the retinacula to the sides of the patella and patellar tendon, with expansions to the tibial condyles anteriorly, medially and laterally, reinforcing the capsule in these areas.

Medial aspect of the knee
The tibial (medial) collateral ligament is a strong, flat band which originates from the medial epicondyle and condyle of the femur. It has deep fibres (also called the medial capsular ligament) which inset into the medial meniscus and the edge of the medial tibial condyle. The superficial fibres travel down and forwards to the tibial shaft about 10 cm distal to the condyle, beneath the tendons of the pes anserinus (sartorius, gracilis and semitendinosus) and separated from these by bursae. The ligament glides backwards and forwards over the femoral condyle in flexion and extension; it stabilizes the knee against valgus stress (superficial part) and rotation (deep part).

The posterior oblique ligament is a thickening in the posteromedial capsule, blending with the deep part of the tibial collateral ligament in front and with the oblique popliteal ligament behind. It is said to resist rotatory stress of the knee.

The pes anserinus comprises the tendons of sartorius (in front) and gracilis and semitendinosus (behind), which insert into the medial side of proximal tibial shaft protecting the knee against rotatory and valgus stress.

Posterior aspect of the knee

Semimembranosus ramifications insert directly into the posteromedial corner of the medial tibial condyle. They insert indirectly through four expansions, all originating from the direct insertion:

1. The popliteal ligament upwards and laterally to lateral femoral condyle near the origin of the lateral head of the gastrocnemius, reinforces posterior capsule centrally.
2. The expansion into the posterior horn of the medial meniscus and adjacent capsule.
3. The long expansion forwards, in the groove along the margin of medial tibial plateau just below the articular surface and inserts into the tibia beneath the tibial collateral ligament.
4. The distal expansion to the posteromedial part of the proximal tibial metaphysis, and to the fascia covering popliteus.

The semimembranous muscle internally rotates the tibia and shortens the capsule posteriorly and posteromedially, thus helping stabilize the knee against rotatory stress. It also pulls the posterior rim of the medial meniscus backwards during flexion.

The posterior oblique ligament blends with the oblique popliteal ligament and reinforces the posteromedial capsule.

The arcuate complex consists of the posterior capsule, lateral part of the oblique popliteal ligament, the short fibular collateral ligament and expansions from the politeus muscle origin and biceps femoris tendon. It reinforces the posterolateral capsule and stabilizes the knee against rotary and varus stress.

Meniscofemoral ligaments: O: posterior horn of the lateral meniscus; two small ligaments pass upward and medially, and lie anterior (Humphery) and posterior (Wrisberg) to the posterior cruciate ligament. I: into the medial femoral condyle just anterior and posterior to insertion of posterior cruciate. The ligaments help to provide feedback to stabilize the knee through meniscal attachment to the capsule and arcuate complex.

Lateral aspect of the knee

The fibular (lateral) collateral ligament is a round ligament from the lateral epicondyle of the femur that travels down and back to the head of the fibula anterior to the syloid, beneath biceps tendon. It has no capsular attachments and is separated from the lateral meniscus by the popliteus tendon. It provides stability against varus stress, especially with the knee extended.

The short fibular collateral ligament lies posteromedial and parallel with the fibular collateral ligament, may contain a sesamoid bone (fabellar), and reinforces the posterolateral corner of the capsule.

Iliotibial tract: O: a longitudinal thickening in fascia lata. I: the lateral femoral epicondyle, passing between the lateral border of the patella and the biceps tendon to the lateral tibial tubercle (Gerdy's tubercle). A: stabilizes the knee against varus stress. It moves back and forth over the femoral condyle in flexion and extension.

Intra-articular structures of the knee

Menisci Fibrocartilaginous in make-up, triangular in cross-section with the base on the periphery of the tibial rim. Superior surface is concave. Medial meniscus is shaped like a large, open C, the lateral is a small closed C. Vascularity is important in meniscal damage diagnosis, as the outside is vascular while the inside of the C is avascular.

Cruciates Both of the cruciates are intracapsular but extrasynovial. The anterior cruciate originates from the medial part of the anterior inter-condylar fossa of the tibia, upward, backward and laterally to the posterior part of the medial surface of the lateral femoral condyle, in the intercondylar notch. The small anteromedial portion is tight in all knee positions, while the large posterolateral part is taut only in extension. The posterior cruciate originates from the posterior part of the posterior intercondylar area of the tibia, upward and medially to the posterior part of the lateral surface of the medial femoral condyle, crossing the anterior cruciate. The bulk (anterior portion) is tight in flexion, loose in extension. The smaller posterior part is loose in flexion, tight in extension. The cruciates are involved in reduction anteroposterior (sagittal) displacement of the tibia on the femur (maximum normal displacement is about 5 mm). They wind around each other and tighten in internal rotation of the tibia on the femur, therefore limiting internal rotation; they unwind in external rotation, thus permitting greater anteroposterior displacement and external rotation in this position.

Tibiofibular joints

The superior tibiofibular joint, a posterior synovial joint between the head of the fibula and the undersurface of the lateral tibial condyle, is supported by a capsule and anterior and posterior ligaments. The interosseous membrane, deficient above (anterior tibial artery passes forwards into the anterior compartment), and below (perforating peroneal artery), fibres are directed down and outwards. The inferior tibiofibular joint has a strong interosseous ligament 3 cm wide just above the ankle, essential for stability of the ankle, and it has anterior and posterior inferior tibiofibular ligaments (the latter come below distal tibia posteriorly to deepen the socket for the talus).

Ankle joint

This consists of a mortice-type arrangement constructed from three surfaces. The distal tibial articular surface forms the roof (takes five-sixths of standing weight), the medial malleolus, with comma-shaped articular surface, is the medial wall, and the lateral malleolus (fibula) is the lateral wall. The tip of the lateral malleolus is 1½ cm more distal and posterior to the medial malleolus, and slopes obliquely laterally (takes one-sixth of standing weight).

The body of the talus fits into the mortice of the ankle and an important point to remember is that the superior surface of the body of the talus is dome-shaped, broader anteriorly than posteriorly, i.e. lateral stability is greater in dorsiflexion than plantar flexion. The medial articular facet is comma-shaped, matching that on the medial malleolus, and the lateral articular facet is triangular for the lateral malleolus. This bone is vitally important in restoration of full ankle function after a sprain/strain injury.

The subtalar joint consists two joints, the anterior and posterior talocalcaneals, separated by sinus tarsi (a tunnel containing fat, interosseous ligament and an artery). As with the talus, good function of the subtalar joint is important for recovery from injury. Premature isometric and isotonic rehabilitation can impact the joint, slowing recovery.

Capsule and ligaments
The capsule is thin and attached around the margins of the articulating surfaces. The ligaments are the medial collateral (deltoid) ligament and the lateral collateral ligament. General ranges of movements are dorsiflexion (extension) 20° and plantar flexion (flexion) 50°; in plantar flexion some abduction and adduction are possible.

Muscles

The anterior iliac region
Psoas O: from discs and adjacent areas of the vertebral bodies between T12 and L5. Descends in front of iliacus (in iliac fossa), blends with this muscle, travels beneath inguinal ligament, over pelvic brim and forms part of the floor of the femoral triangle, crosses anterior to the hip joint capsule and turns posteriorly to insert into the lesser trochanter. There is a bursa between the tendon and the femur. A: flexion of the spine and a little rotation. The lumbar plexus lies within the muscle and a thick sheath covers the muscle, which limits the psoas abcess of vertebral tuberculosis (Pott's disease). Nerve root supply is from L2, L3 from lumbar plexus.

Iliacus O: from the medial surface of the ilium (iliac fossa), it blends with the psoas and shares the insertion and has a similar action. Nerve root supply is L2, L3 from the femoral nerve.

Short external rotators of the thigh
These are posterior from above downwards and are the following.

Piriformis O: from the front of the bodies of S2, S3, S4, horizontally through the greater sciatic notch, dividing the notch into upper and lower parts. I: into tip of greater trochanter. Nerve root supply is S2, but can vary between S1 and S3.

Obturator internus O: from inside of the obturator membrane and around the obturator foramen. Travels through the lesser sciatic notch, then bends forwards at right angles to insert into the upper part of the medial surface of the greater trochanter, below the priformis. Nerve root supply is L5, S1 and S2.

Gemelli O: from the upper and lower borders of the lesser sciatic notch. The superior gemelli travels along the upper border of the obturator internus, the inferior gemelli travels along the lower border of the obturator internus. I: into the greater trochanter above and below the insertion of the obturator internus. Nerve root supply, for gemellus superior is L5, S1 and S2, for gemellus inferior L4, L5 and S2 from nerve to quadratus femoris.

Obturator externus O: from the outer surface of the obturator membrane and surrounding bone. I: into digital fossa at the base of the medial surface of the greater trochanter. Nerve root supply is L2, L3, L4, the posterior division of the obturator nerve.

Quadratus femoris O: from lateral border of ischial tuberosity, a flat wide muscle that travels laterally below and parallel with the obturator externus. Nerve root supply is L4, L5 and S1.

The glutei and tensor fascia lata (TFL)
Gluteus maximus O: from lateral mass of sacrum, posterosuperior area of the ilium (above the gluteal line) and the back of the sacrotuberus ligament. I: this is in two parts, i.e. into (1) two-thirds of the fascia lata and iliotibial band and (2) one-third into the gluteal ridge (upper lateral margin of the linea aspera of the femur). A: mainly hip extension, but also lateral hip rotation. Nerve root supply is the inferior gluteal nerve, L5, S1 and S2.

Gluteus medius O: from the outer surface of the ilium between middle and inferior gluteal lines, lying beneath gluteus maximus. I: into front of the greater trochanter. A: abduction and medial rotation of the thigh. Nerve root supply is the superior gluteal nerve, L4, L5 and S1.

Gluteus minimus O: from outer surface of the ilium between the middle and inferior gluteal lines, lying beneath the gluteus medius. I: into the front of the greater trochanter. A: abduction and medial rotation of the thigh. Nerve root supply is the superior gluteal nerve, L4, L5 and S1.

Tensor fascia lata O: from the outer surface of the ilium below the anterior third of the crest. I: into the iliotibial tract, and through into the tubercle of Gerdy on the anterolateral margin of the lateral tibial condyle, with a slip to the lateral femoral epicondyle. A: abduction, flexion and internal rotation of the thigh. Assists in extension of the knee. The TFL is important in the accessory movements in functional restoration after injury. It affects the compressive factor of the lateral aspect. Premature rehabilitation of the TFL can compound knee symptoms. Nerve root supply is superior gluteal nerve, L4, L5 and S1.

Hamstrings
O: from the ischial tuberosity (except short head of biceps femoris). A: extend the hip and flex the knee.

Semimembranosus O: from upper, lateral area of the back of the ischial tuberosity. I: into the posteromedial corner of the medial tibial condyle. It has a number of important indirect insertions; these include:

1. into the oblique popliteal ligament, over the posterior capsule centrally;
2. into the posterior horn of the medial meniscus and capsule;
3. into the groove along the margin of the medial tibial plateau, below the articular surface, inserting into the tibia underneath the tibial collateral ligament;
4. into the posteromedial aspect of the proximal tibial metaphysis and the fascial compartment around the popliteus.

A: internal rotation of the tibia, shortens the capsule posteriorly, posteromedially, and moves the rim of the medial meniscus backwards in flexion.

Semitendinosus O: from the inferomedial area of the ischial tuberosity with the long head of the biceps. It is superficial to the semimembranosus and inserts into the medial aspect of the proximal tibial shaft, behind the insertion of sartorius, and behind and below the insertion of gracilis.

Anterior muscles of the thigh
These muscles are concerned with extension of the knee and they have an involvement with the muscle pump action for venous and lymphatic drainage.

Rectus femoris O: anterior inferior iliac spine and superior acetabular ridge by two heads. I: superior pole of patella as the trilaminar quadriceps tendon.

Vastus lateralis O: proximal half of the lateral ridge of linae aspera by an aponeurosis. I: to the quadriceps tendon, retinacular fibres to lateral side of patella (and patellar tendon), and to the anterior aspect of the lateral tibial condyle.

Vastus medialis O: from the spiral line, medial ridge of linae aspera, and supracondylar ridge. I: medial aspect of quadriceps tendon (important) fibres merge with those of vastus lateralis, medial side of patella, and an expansion to the medial tibial epicondyle.

Vastus intermedius The most important muscle in the majority of knee symptoms. O: upper two-thirds of anterolateral surface of femur, I: posterior edge of proximal patella as part of the quadriceps tendon. Nerve supply of the quadriceps muscles is via the femoral nerve, primarily root L4, but may include L2 and L3.

Sartorius O: anterior superior iliac spine. I: into the medial side of the proximal tibial shaft. Nerve supply is from the femoral nerve (L2, L3).

Adductors
Adductor magnus O: inferior pubic, ischial rami and ischial tuberosity. I: linae aspera, medial supracondylar ridge, and middle of proximal border of medial femoral condyle. Nerve supply posterior division of obturator nerve (L2 and L3) and sciatic nerve (L4 and L5).

Adductor brevis O: outer surface of inferior pubic ramus, above and medial to adductor magnus. I: into upper part of linae aspera. Nerve supply is from both divisions of the obturator nerve (L2, L3, L4).

Adductor longus O: from front of body of pubis. I: whole length of linae aspera. Nerve supply is the anterior division of the obturator nerve (L2, L3, L4).

Pectineus O: front of the body of the pubis above the adductor longus. I: femoral shaft below lesser trochanter and anterior to the adductor brevis. Nerve supply is from the femoral nerve (L2 and L3).

Gracilis O: pubis and inferior pubic ramus. I: into proximal and medial surface of the tibia. Nerve supply is from the anterior division of the obturator nerve (L2, L3, L4).

Muscles of the leg
The muscles of the leg are surrounded by a strong fascia which is attached to the anterior tibial border and then sweeps laterally, posteriorly and medially to surround all the muscle groups. It then reattaches to the medial tibial border. The fascia is considered osteopathically as one of the most important structures of the lower limb.

The muscles of the leg can be divided into three groups: anterior, lateral and posterior.

Anterior group Nerve root supply is mainly by the deep peroneal nerve, L5. The anterior group consists of the tibialis anterior, extensor hallucis longus, extensor digitorum longus and extensor retinacula. Relations of tendons are, in front of the ankle in the order in which the structures cross the ankle joint, from medial to lateral side:

- tibialis anterior
- extensor hallucis longus
- vena comitans (one of two companion veins of the artery)
- anterior tibial artery
- vena comitans
- deep peroneal nerve
- extensor digitorum longus.

Lateral group Nerve root supply is mainly by superficial peroneal nerve, L5, S1. The lateral group contains the peroneus longus, peroneus brevis and peroneal retinacula and sheaths.

Posterior group These are all supplied by the tibial nerve, mainly S1. The muscles are the gastrocnemius, soleus, plantaris, popliteus, tibialis posterior, flexor digitorum longus and flexor hallucis longus. Relations of the tendons, behind the ankle in the order in which structures cross the ankle joint, from the medial to the lateral side are:

- tibialis posterior
- flexor digitorum longus
- vena comitans
- posterior tibial artery
- vena comitans
- tibial nerve
- flexor hallucis longus.

Muscles of the foot
The extrinsic muscles of the foot are tendinous; the intrinsic muscles have their origins and insertions within the foot.

Dorsum The dorsum of the foot has only one intrinsic muscle, the extensor digitorum brevis (EDB), supplied by the deep peroneal nerve, L5, S1.

Sole The sole of the foot has extrinsic tendons and intrinsic muscles in four layers.

- First layer: this is the most superficial layer and contains three muscles, the abductor hallucis (medial plantar, S2, S3), the flexor digitorum brevis (medial plantar, S2, S3) and the abductor digiti minimi, and the plantar aponeurosis.
- Second layer: the lumbricals, which originate from the flexor digitorum longus, insert into the extensor hoods of the four lateral toes; the nerve supply to the medial lumbrical is the medial plantar, to the other three it is the lateral plantar nerve, S2, S3. A: metacarpophalangeal flexion, proximal and distal interphalangeal extension. Included in this second layer is the quadratus plantae (flexor accessorius).

- Third layer: this layer includes the flexor hallusis brevis (medial plantar, S2, S3), the adductor hallucis (lateral plantar, S2, S3) and flexor digiti quiniti minimi.
- Fourth layer: this layer consists of the interossei, three plantar and four dorsal.

Arteries

The arterial supply through the lower extremity originates from two arteries. One is a continuation of the external iliac artery giving way to the femoral artery. This travels anterior to the hip joint, in the upper third of the thigh, lying in the femoral triangle between the femoral vein (medially) and the femoral nerve (laterally). The second arterial supply to the lower extremity is from the largest branch of the internal iliac artery to form the superior gluteal artery and the minor branch forming the inferior gluteal artery and the obturator artery. The popliteal artery, a continuation of the femoral artery, ends at the lower border of popliteus muscle (in the popliteal space) where it divides into two terminal branches, the anterior and posterior tibial arteries. In the foot the anterior tibial artery gives way to the dorsal pedis artery; this follows the lateral border of the tendon of the extensor hallucis longus, then passes into the sole between bases of the medial two metatarsals and interossei to anastomose with the lateral plantar.

Nerves

The nerve supply to the pelvis and lower extremity, from a sensory and motor aspect, begins mainly within the organization of the lumbar plexus. This plexus is formed from the anterior primary of T12 to L4 giving off the following branches: psoas, L2 and L3; iliohypogastric, L1, communicating with the skin of the lower abdomen and buttock; ilioinguinal, L1, communicating with the skin of the upper thigh and genitalia; genitofemoral, L1, L2, communicating with the genitalia and front of the upper thigh; and the lateral cutaneous nerve, L2, L3, which passes over the inguinal ligament communicating with the skin over the lateral aspect of the thigh. Below this you have the lumbar plexus. The femoral nerve, L2–L4 (posterior, dorsal division of the anterior primary rami) supplies the pectineus, sartorius and the quadriceps muscles. The obturator nerve, L2–L4 (anterior division of the anterior primary rami) supplies anterior branches to the gracilis, adductor longus and brevis and the hip joint. It also supplies posterior branches to the obturator externus, adductor magnus, and branches innervate the femoral and popliteal arteries of the knee joint.

The sacral plexus in the piriformis comes together from the anterior rami of L4, L5, the lumbosacral trunk, and S1–S3. It supplies the piriformis, obturator internus, gemellus superior and inferior, and quadratus femoris. It also goes on to form the superior and inferior gluteal nerves, the posterior cutaneous nerve of the thigh, the perforating cutaneous nerve, and the sciatic nerve from a combination of the lateral (common peroneal) division and the medial (posterior tibial) division of the anterior primary rami. The sciatic nerve enters the popliteal space splitting into the common peroneal (lateral popliteal nerve) and tibial nerve (medial popliteal nerve). The common peroneal nerve comes into contact with the lateral side of the neck of the fibula where it divides into its two terminal branches: the deep peroneal nerve, which divides at the ankle into the medial branch, which accompanies the dorsalis pedis and supplies the skin of the first web space, and the lateral branch, to extensor digitorum brevis; and the superficial peroneal nerve, which supplies the skin of the front of the leg and dorsum of the foot and toes except the lateral border and the first web space. The tibial nerve makes a straight course through the limb, from buttock to ankle, where it ends, deep to the flexor retinaculum, by dividing into the medial and lateral plantar nerve.

The medial plantar nerve lies on the lateral side of the medial plantar artery, and accompanies it to the forefoot. Its distribution corresponds to the median nerve in the hand, i.e. it supplies abductor hallucis, flexor digitorum brevis, flexor hallucis brevis, first lumbrical and medial two-thirds of the skin of the sole and the medial 3½ toes. The lateral plantar nerve arises halfway between the heel and the medial malleolus; it lies on the medial side of the lateral artery, and accompanies this across the sole. Its distribution corresponds to the ulnar nerve, i.e. it supplies all the intrinsic muscles of the sole (except abductor hallucis, flexor digitorum brevis, flexor hallucis brevis and the first lumbrical) and supplies the skin of the lateral side of the sole.

Other nerves include the sural nerve, which is a branch of the tibial nerve with fibres from the peroneal via the sural communicating. It accompanies the short (small) saphenous vein forward and beneath the medial malleolus to the lateral border of the foot and little toe. The saphenous nerve is a branch from the femoral nerve and travels with the long (great) saphenous vein, forward beneath the medial malleolus, to the medial side of the leg and foot (not toes).

Nerve root values of movements of the lower limb:

- hip
  - flexion, L2, L3
  - extension, L4, L5
- knee
  - extension, L3, L4
  - flexion, L5, S1
- ankle
  - dorsiflexion, L4, L5
  - plantar flexion, S1, S2
- subtalar
  - inversion, L4
  - eversion, L5, S1
- each joint innervated by four segments except subtalar
- the more distal the joint, the more distal the segment.

Function

Integration of the lower extremity with the rest of the body is important for function. The function of the lower limb relies heavily on the soft tissues and ranges of motion of the pelvis and spine. Internal and external rotation, heel strike point and power are influenced by pelvic and spinal integration. Viewing the body as a unit, particularly during motion it can be seen that function of the lower extremity relies on its point of contact with the ground. The 'heel strike' and 'toe off' phases provide information which reflects functioning above the leg, foot and ankle. Forces of rotation and compression and stride length are some of the main factors influencing function. Soft tissues are the main absorbers of energy in the body, and this includes the lower extremity. Poor energy absorption capacity is the result of fibrotic change and high resting tone of contractile tissue (e.g. muscle and fascia). If forces are not transmitted and dissipated throughout the body, then they will 'focus'.

Focusing is a three-dimensional phenomenon. As a general principle, structures that have the greatest capacity to alter in ranges of movement absorb energy, but still maintain pain and/or discomfort-free function. Shoulders and hips will 'burden' other less capable structures (feet, ankles, wrists). Both chronic and acute presentations are influenced by this higher dysfunction. This is why it is important not just to look at the joints and tissues as a factor of range of movement, but also the quality of that movement. This is where the clinical skill of palpation comes into its own. This will also present as an 'irritable focus', probably located in the posterior horn and created by an abnormal stream of impulses from certain pathophysiological viscera or serous membranes (Denslow and Hassett, 1944).

As mentioned above, lower extremity function relies on factors like rotation and compression. To these we can add joint range of motion, palpable soft tissue quality and, most important, integration to achieve asymptomatic qualitative function.

The interrelationship between muscles and joints, altering the information integrated by the spinal cord, in the spectrum of good function to poor function, is mediated by the somatosomatic reflex system. As mentioned earlier, this term suggests that this reflex model involves a stimulus applied to a somatic structure of the body. Somatic is used here in its broadest sense, including head, trunk, walls of the body cavity, and the appendages, with the response in another somatic structure of the body. Do not forget the somatovisceral reflex system, which is also a two-way communication system. Figure 6.11 shows the lower extremity rotatory integrative function.

> The whole economy of the body is built up of a system of organs whose activities depend on reflexes. A flood of stimuli is continually being poured into the system through the skin and special senses, and each stimulus produces a definite reflex on some part of the body.
>
> (Mackenzie, 1921)

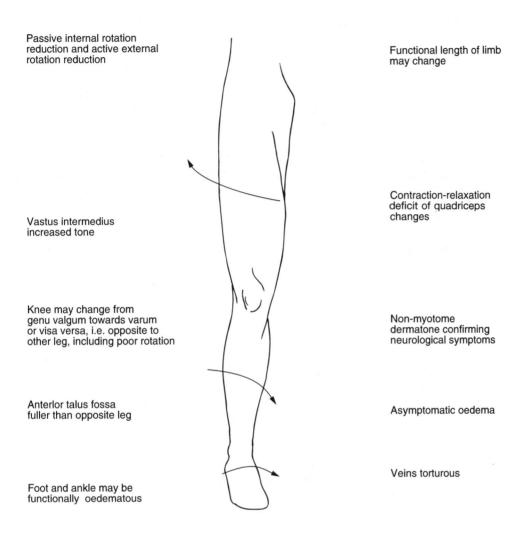

Passive internal rotation
reduction and active external
rotation reduction

Functional length of limb
may change

Vastus intermedius
increased tone

Contraction-relaxation
deficit of quadriceps
changes

Knee may change from
genu valgum towards varum
or visa versa, i.e. opposite to
other leg, including poor rotation

Non-myotome
dermatone confirming
neurological symptoms

Anterior talus fossa
fuller than opposite leg

Asymptomatic oedema

Foot and ankle may be
functionally oedematous

Veins torturous

Fig. 6.11 Signs and symptoms of adaptation.

The somatic reflex is a basic mechanism that is essential to the control of normal physiological activities and that also may be involved in abnormal reactions. It is considered to be the most primitive reflex model mechanism in humans, and may follow either a monosynaptic or (more often) multisynaptic pool pathway.

Thus the concept of the somatosomatic reflex system is not new to the osteopathic profession, but a basic physiological fact. It brings home one of the major principles of osteopathic medicine, i.e. the body is a unit. It does not matter whether the presentation is acute or chronic; there are factors that will both speed and hinder recovery distant from the point of complaint.

Presentation of injury

Bursitis

The bursae include the greater trochanteric, iliopsoas and the ischial bursae. The greater trochanteric bursa is located just posterior to the greater trochanter, and the iliopsoas over the lesser trochanter are palpable over the medial aspect of the groin. Locations of discomfort are palpable and symptoms tend to be chronic in nature. Bursal problems are the result of poor mechanics or breakdowns in adaptive processes following overloading in short, high intensity exercise or prolonged, low intensity exercise.

Treatment
Rest, ice (if active and warm) or heat (if inactive and cold) and NSAIDs (particularly in the active presentation). Postural examinations, dynamic and static, are important as an indication to an interlink functional breakdown.

Psoas abscess

This is can present as an acute condition especially in young athletes and adolesents. Pain may be in the back, hip and/or the groin. There tends to be a history of trauma, even minor, followed hours or days later by sweating at night and loss of appetite. A psoas abcsess usually tracks into the femoral triangle lateral to the femoral artery. Abdominal palpation continuing into the iliac fossa generally detects the abscess.

Treatment
Rest and antibiotic therapy are indicated initially. Scarring from the abscess is a residue of the infection. OMT is directed at reducing this scarring as soon as possible. In the early stages a functional technique approach will help to relieve pain and discomfort; later more direct techniques can be used.

Psoas bursitis

A psoas bursitis presents in the femoral triangle as a tight swelling. The athlete commonly adopts a position of flexion, abduction and external rotation as this gives relief.

Treatment
As for bursitis above.

Iliac crest/hip contusion

Also known as the 'hip pointer' this usually presents as an abrasion of the skin accompanied with hip soft tissue damage. It usually results from direct blows to the edge of the iliac crest and/or to the soft tissue between the head of the femoral trochanter and the iliac crest. Common mechanisms of injury are sliding on the ground, e.g. in baseball or soccer, direct impact, usually without skin abrasion, from an opponents' knee, e.g. in rugby or martial arts, or due to internal forces resulting from activity where the athlete functionally overuses the area. Iliac crest injury involves not only the hip muscle, but can also involve the abdominal muscles that insert along the subcutaneous edge of the crest. Where the abdominal muscles attach to this crest there is the risk of tearing and/or avulsion along the insertion line. A common mechanism for this is forced lateral flexion to the opposite side of the injury under a state of high muscular tone on the resulting injured side. The athlete will guard the area and have problems placing weight on the foot of the injured side. All these can result in deep soft tissue damage and bruising may appear on the surface. Structures associated with this injury include the trochanteric and associated bursae, tensor fascia latae and musculotendinous units. Like all soft tissue damage there may be combinations of hot and cold temperature presentations.

Treatment
Initial limitation of movement, bandaging, improvement of any circulatory disturbance (hot/cold application), reduction of resultant hypertonia (traction, functional technique in hot injury cases) and NSAIDs.

Piriformis syndrome

Here, the piriformis muscle shortens causing irritation of the sciatic nerve. This is usually an acute presentation with a chronic history. The piriformis muscle is not 'pinching' the sciatic nerve, but producing chemicals resulting from a metabolic disturbance that trigger neural mechanisms in the sciatic nerve conduction and/or function. This can be part of sacroiliac/soft tissue complex dysfunction. As with acute spinal pain, the athlete may show signs of postural compensation, in the form of weight bearing on the good side. Pain may present in the low back or posterior hip with or without sciatic nerve referred pain. In chronic cases the pain may be easier with slight exercise, initially. Causes include postural change, performing sit-ups on a hard surface with knees bent and feet on the floor, direct trauma, foot pronation/supination and poor quadriceps.

Treatment
Postural examination is vital. It is very limiting to just 'dig' into the soft tissue to 'work it out'. Analgesia, muscle relaxants and NSAIDs are recommended if immediate manipulative intervention is not immediately successful. OMT is directed at reducing irritation by gentle hip traction, compression over the piriformis, and functional techniques to the area.

The sacrum

This may present with anything from stress fractures and periostitis to tumours.

Sacroiliac joint dysfunction

Like the piriformis syndrome, the athlete will have pain and discomfort over the buttock region with or without referred sciatic pain. This joint should always be examined in lower extremity or back presentations. Hypo- and hypermobility in movement of the joint should be considered as well as its functional positional range. Innominate function and direct or indirect active and passive testing will localize pain over the area. Passive prone athlete examination is useful as the sacrum can be made to move in many directions while searching for areas of hypo- or hyper-mobility or combinations.

Sacroiliac strain

Pain over the sacroiliac joint is, in the majority of cases, indicative of sacroiliac joint strain. This is usually of slow onset and there may be a history of similar discomfort on the same side and/or other side. Both sides of the pelvis work together as a unit and with the rest of the body. Palpation may reveal tenderness and oedema on the symptomatic side. It may also reveal hypertonia, fibrosis and limited function on the asympto-matic side. Increasing deep muscular activity around the painful joint (i.e. 'putting weight through it') by standing on the limb on the bad side makes things worse. Pain may radiate down the limb with a sciatic distribution. Internal rotation of the symptomatic side tends to be poor. Acute traumatic presentations tend to be combined with soft tissue bruising as a consequence of direct impact in the buttock by a knee or other object, or indirect trauma when 'missing a step' while running.

Treatment
In acute presentations with oedema due to recent trauma, ice, NSAIDs, isometric activity, soft tissue techniques and analysis of spinal, pelvic and lower extremity function are important. Cases of a chronic history with acute presentation should be treated as acute presentations with addi-tional investigation and treatment emphasis placed on the opposite side of the pelvis. All acute presentations benefit from 'little and often' treat-ment. Chronic non-acute presentations need further assessment.

Sacroilitis

This is an inflammation of the sacroiliac joint.

Treatment
Vascular drainage is the most important procedure to perform. Applica-tion of heat and/or ice, with medication, will help to control pain and inflammation.

Sprains

Simple sprains are the most common injuries to this area, especially the low back.

Pubis symphasis dysfunction

One of the least considered areas of pelvic dysfunction. Poor function can result in symptoms presented in areas such as the sacroiliac joints, low back, medial knee, and even fallen arches. When localized symptoms are presented, you must examine all tissues that can cause dysfunction as well as the local presentation. X-rays may be useful where there is a periostitis in the area. There may even be an exostosis related to the adductor or rectus abdominus attachments.

Osteitis pubis

Inflammation of the public symphysis. This is usually a consequence of motion dysfunction of the pelvis, as a result of myofacsial dysfunction.

Treatment
Initially rest and NSAIDs. Functional gait analysis, integrating limb and pelvic and spinal function should be carried out. If poor function of the sacroiliac joints and associative soft tissues is evident, treatment provides symptomatic relief.

Bursitis

Commonly presents over the iliopsoas, ischium and greater trochanter. In all cases increased action of the muscle increases symptoms. Palpatory findings will rule out muscle tears (heat), but may reveal chronic but tender area over bursa (cool), except over iliopsoas. Iliopsoas bursitis tends to present over the lesser trochanter, with groin pain medially, and is commonly exacerbated by flexion, abduction and external rotation when actively resisted. Ischial bursitis can be indicated by the athlete who puts his or her hand over the hamstring origin. This can be made worse by active resistance of hamstring contraction and direct palpation. Just posterior to the greater trochanter is the point of tenderness for the greater trochanter bursitis. This can be made more tender by active resistance of the hip abductors and direct palpation.

Treatment
Acute presentations tend to be due to repetitive actions such as long-distance or cross country running. If there is heat, ice and NSAIDs are the initial treatment of choice. Reduction or cessation of activity is helpful. Appropriate manipulative and passive stretching, accompanied by wet heat later when the inflammation calms down and becomes cooler, are useful.

Sacrococcygeal dysfunction

This can be one of the most depressing conditions. It usually results in combinations of torsion and/or flexion of the coccyx which may or may not include the sacrococcygeal junction. It is often the result of direct trauma as in falling backwards and sitting down or being kicked (especially in children playing), and can be caused by soft tissue contraction dragging the coccyx into a position of discomfort. It is rare to fall directly on the coccyx, as the body tends to fall to the dominant side.

Treatment
Posterior hip soft tissue techniques. Per rectal procedure is indicated in difficult cases where joint dysfunction does not respond to soft tissue techniques. This will be primarily due to the length of time that the athlete has had the condition, which has led to shortening of the surrounding ligaments and connective tissue.

Hip joint dysfunction

As with all joints, this should be considered from a positional sense. The ability of myofascial tissue to exert and absorb energy is a vital component in the integration of the hip and the structures above and below this level. Hypertonia of hip soft tissue does not have to be symptomatic in its own right to cause or contribute to dysfunction of the entire lower limb. As with the shoulder, resting positional analysis is important. A joint with such a large range of motion will have an infinite range of accessory resting positions.

Hip dislocation

Fortunately this is rare. This occurs following a large amount of force, usually along the shaft of the femur. The most common position of injury is a combination of flexion, adduction and internal rotation at the hip, with the dislocation in a posterior direction. This may or may not be accompanied by fracture of the rim of the acetabulum. An injury of this magnitude completely disables the athlete's entire body. The ensuing muscular spasm and neurohormonal response is so great as to prohibit reduction without medication. Palpation around the pelvis should reveal a misplaced greater trochanter compared with the other side. Shock can make a detrimental contribution, although I have seen an athlete control his pain by controlled breathing until he was removed to hospital. Complications may arise through blood vessel damage and neural stretch.

Groin strain

This is the most common strain around the hip area. The location of this strain is usually in the region of the hip adductors, flexors and the abdominal insertion. Like any other muscular strains these vary in severity, and damage can be so bad as to warrant surgical intervention.

Hypertonic and shortened extensors and external rotators of the hip are the most common finding. Deep inhibition of these muscles can cause pain awareness over the site of complaint (somatosomatic reflex). If this is the case then some spinal facilitation is present. The slow shortening of extensors and external rotators is the commonest cause with overactivity of the flexors, adductors and rectus abdomini to maintain normal function. This is a common injury presentation in many sports, especially soccer where poor all round athletic development emphasizes the lower half of the body. Environmental conditions can precipitate this condition, e.g. heavy muddy ground in field sports. An intrapelvic haematoma may occur leading to symptoms in the region of the groin.

Treatment
Reduction of tone in hip extensors and external rotators primarily. However, even internal tibial rotation at the knee may precipitate groin symptoms on the same side. Manipulation of the insertion points as well as the belly of rectus abdominus can bring on symptoms. Strapping (hip spiker) is useful with the usual strain treatment modalities. The basic approach is rest and NSAIDs. Be aware of herniation and referred ovarian symptoms.

Other sprains around the hip should be treated in the normal way with hip spiker strapping for support.

Sprains

Damage to the ligamentous and synovial structures around the hip are uncommon in adults, but are more common in children, and often of a minor, repetitive nature. This can lead to the undesirable state of an avascular necrosis around the joint. Watch for the 'limping child'; they can adapt very quickly so that the injury becomes part of their functional make-up and they can still run around.

Fractures and avulsions

Fractures around the pelvis, hip, sacrum and proximal end of the femur are rare but should always be considered in cases of pain, especially when it is not very acute. Epiphyseal damage and avulsion in children and adolesents will present as pain in the hip, back or thigh and should be considered as part of the differential diagnosis. A slipped epiphyseal plate at the head of the femur will represent a similar picture to the subluxed hip.

Legg–Calvé–Perthes disease (osteochondritis juvenilis)

Due to circulatory disruption, the head of the femur passes into a stage of aseptic necrosis and the head collapses. This is a slow process. The head of the femur on X-ray shows a characteristic mushroom shape. The athlete does not show signs or symptoms of fever, night sweats or pain in the hip.

Routine examination for some other condition may reveal reduced hip movement especially in abduction and internal rotation. The young athlete may begin to limp for no apparent reason and there is no memory of trauma. Trendelenburg's sign is negative. It is more common in boys than in girls, and X-ray is vital for diagnosis.

Treatment
Any treatment is based on the X-ray finding. Techniques of choice include gentle rhythmic hip traction, a functional approach, and soft tissue relaxation.

Snapping (clicking) hip syndrome

Usual explanations for this include a thickening of the iliopsoas bursa, a trochanteric bursitis and flicking tendons 'catching' the edge of the joint etc. Chronic alteration in soft tissue tone (becoming fibrotic) and the resultant change in functional joint position can eventually cause structures to 'click' on certain movements, especially flexion.

Treatment
Palpate the region and find the 'clicking', using a stethoscope if necessary. Fibrotic tissue, which may be a little way from the audible noise, may be the cause. Deep stretch of these tissues eventually aids in reducing the snap and any discomfort caused by it. Success is based on the extent of the fibrosis and chronicity.

Contusions (gluteal, quadriceps, TFL and hamstring)

This area is particularly vulnerable to direct blows, especially in contact sports. Crushing of soft tissue may occur through contact with an opponent's knee, the ground, or other hard object. The skin may show signs of abrasion, especially if there is contact with a rough surface. Sliding on the hip on a grass field will present with a combination of abrasion (grass burn) and contusion which may reach as far up as the iliac crest (hip pointer). Impact to the lateral aspect of the thigh, especially with a knee, may lead to a 'dead leg' with temporary paralysis due to crushing of neural tissue. There may be deep bleeding, pain and numbness with an inability to weight bear. A similar picture will be seen on the anterior aspect of the thigh (Charley horse), where running into players or pile-ups are a more common cause. Hamstring contusions are less common. There will be increased temperature over the impact site while active; later there will be bruising and then coolness around the impact site, when becoming inactive.

Treatment
NSAIDs and analgesic medication, ice and compression over injury site when hot; warmth above the injury site when cool. Restriction of thigh muscular action is desirable until acute signs and symptoms begin to

resolve. Gentle isometric exercises should be introduced within a few days with the objective of improving circulation.

Do not manipulate soft tissue acute (active) muscular injuries.

Myositis ossificans

This is a process of metaplasia, where bone forms in the muscle tissue. It usually occurs in the belly of the quadriceps muscle after a direct blow or contusion and results from irritation of the muscle injury site while it is healing, especially from massage or ultrasound.

Treatment
While active, treat with NSAIDs, ice, lower extremity traction and a degree of immobilization (bandage). Once the injury site is starting to show signs and symptoms of healing, a gentle isotonic protocol can be introduced, with ice and NSAIDs still being administered. Eventually, depending on the extent of the original injury, the injury site will become inactive, cool and begin to scar. At this point moist heat is applied with a flexibility and stretching programme.

Iliotibial band syndrome

This is caused by increased resting tone of the tensor fascia lata (TFL) resulting in numerous signs, symptoms and sequelae. This increased functional tone can present as or lead to a trochanteric bursitis, hip ache, burning down the lateral aspect of the thigh, lateral knee pain and knee instability. Hypertonia of TFL, referral down the lateral aspect of the thigh to the knee on deep pressure of the TFL, tenderness posterior to the greater trochanter (possibly a bursitis), and weakness on active resistance of the TFL are common findings.

Treatment
Postural analysis, soft tissue to tensor fascia and tensor fascia lata. Examine for poor accessory motion of the hips, knee and ankles/feet.

Knee dysfunction

The knee, like the elbow, relies heavily on its accessory movements for good healthy function. Accessory movements should therefore always be examined qualitatively for interference with function. These movements include compression, distraction, medial and lateral tibial shift, internal and external tibial rotation, as well as the normal flexion, extension and anteroposterior shift. It is especially relevant to look for these movements in knee injuries that are chronic and do not clear up when internal derangements have been ruled out. The main control factors for the knee are outside the knee, i.e. the quadriceps, hamstrings, anterior compartment and triceps surae. Another main factor in knee dysfunction, therefore, is the quadriceps. Too many athletes have quadriceps that are hypertonic, especially vastus intermedius, which acts more as a postural muscle. Deep manual stretch of this muscle can improve knee function, reduce oedema and reduce patella femoral discomfort in a very short period of time, even minutes. One word of warning, when treating vastus intermedius: it is a postural muscle, and if the treatment is too long and heavy the patient may fall over when he or she weight bears. A feeling of lightness on weight bearing is desirable.

Knee dysfunction, especially when walking or running, can also be due to hip dysfunction. The heel strike shown on a pair of training shoes will confirm an over-externally rotating hip, which should be treated. While the knee pain may be resolved by insoles in the training shoe, the hip problem will remain.

Bursitis

Bursitis in the knee is mostly caused by increased muscle tone. There are about 13 bursae around the knee, four anteriorly, four laterally and five medially. Other than being irritated by tight structures, direct trauma is the other usual cause. The most common presentations are suprapatella, prepatella and infrapatella bursitis. The anserine bursa is the other common presentation; this is situated between the pes anserine tendon insertion and the medial collateral ligament.

Sprain (superior tibia/fibula and knee)

It is important to consider the superior tibia fibula ligamentous apparatus as a functioning part of the knee complex, with additional consideration of the inferior aspect of the fibula. The athlete may have a history of repetitive ankle sprains and strains. Functional hip connections with the outside of the knee should also always be considered.

Strain

Musculotendinous units around the knee joint that are overstretched generally follow the same course as other strains. However, unlike other strains, the effect of even the slightest, asymptomatic strain can upset the accessory movements leading to non-specific discomfort within or around the knee. Full blown strains will naturally be painful at the site of injury, but asymptomatic increased resting tone will perpetuate the symptoms at the knee. A good test to see how much the quadriceps muscles are contributing to the knee pain picture is the contraction–relaxation deficit. This is the time difference between the active contraction/relaxation of one quadriceps muscle and the other. With the athlete standing up and looking straight ahead, tell him or her to contract both quadriceps muscles for at least a count of 3 and then to relax both muscles. The knee complaint side will relax after the non-complaint side. This is not a diagnostic aid, but an indicator of the musculotendinous unit contribution to the symptom picture.

Fat pad contusion

This is a soft tissue contusion and should be approached in the same manner as other such injuries.

Fractures

Fractures around the knee commonly include the superior fibula, tibial plateau, patella and inferior femur.

Popliteal (Baker's) cyst

This name is generally used to describe the distension of the gastrocnemius–semimembranosus bursa but can also be applied to any inflammation and herniation of the synovial membrane in the popliteal region. The usual presentation is a large, soft, painless mass in the popliteal space. The exact cause is not known, however it can result from internal derangement, chronic knee trauma and chronic fluid retention.

Treatment
Postural examination, passive lower extremity examination and particularly qualitative passive knee examination will lead to the finding of qualitative tissue changes and joint problems. These are usually chronic presentations and should be approached with all the precautions of any chronic problem.

Neuromas

These can occur as a result of repeated minor trauma and may be due to previous surgical intervention. The most common nerve involved is portions of the saphenous nerve. Clinical presentation is with altered sensation, e.g. numbness, burning etc.

Treatment
Manipulative release and fascial stretch. The application of warmth usually helps to calm symptoms in chronic cases. In more acute cases the use of anti-inflammatory medication and cooling (not icing) the area with running water is helpful.

Peroneal nerve contusion

Injuries affecting the peroneal nerve as it courses around the neck of the proximal end of the fibula area occur on a regular basis. Causes include direct trauma, compression through bandaging, taping or casting, and indirect trauma such as inversion ankle strains and sprains.

Treatment

Cooling the area (not too cold), NSAIDs and OMT. OMT is directed at decompressing the area to allow better motion and drainage.

Dislocations and subluxations (knee and patella)

Dislocations and subluxations of the knees are rare in sport. They are easy to recognize. On the other hand, dislocations and subluxations of the patella are more common. The patella tends to dislocate (displace) laterally from the femoral trochlea and reduces itself when the knee is extended. This occurs commonly due to a valgus and/or twisting mechanism when the quadriceps are contracting, or if they already have a high resting tone. Other factors include an increased Q-angle, patella alta, vastus lateralis hypertrophy and poor qualitative hip function. The athlete will talk about the knee cap 'popping out', usually on numerous occasions prior to the presenting episode. In cases of subluxation there is usually a partial displacement with spontaneous reduction.

Treatment

This is directed at the establishment of the patella (essentially the quadriceps tracking) by searching for the reason why poor interlink function has led to this presentation. The most common finding is poor control of knee function due to hypertonia of soft tissue and joint range restriction at the hip and the muscles that insert and/or originate from the knee region. OMT is directed at improving soft tissue tone and joint ranges. In the short term steps should be taken to stabilize the knee with a brace, rest and the administration of anti-inflammatory protocols.

Epiphyseal plate injury (proximal tibia, distal femur)

In young athletes it is important that this condition is considered in differential diagnosis. If in doubt X-rays should be taken.

Meniscal tears

These are more common on the medial side than the lateral, and result in a tearing of the semilunar cartilage. The history leading up to their presentation can be varied, and may include slow repetitive injury, sudden onset or a combination of both. Tears can be longitudinal, bucket handle etc. They can also be avascular or vascular depending on the site of the tear. An avascular longitudinal tear that is not attended to surgically can cause more problems to the the healthy knee by damaging the cruciate ligament apparatus, which is vascular. This is caused by pressure on a vascular structure by an avascular structure. Since the menisci are continuous with the collateral ligaments there is always the possibility that the ligamentous structures will also be involved, especially in acute cases. Sudden onset of symptoms can be brought about by twisting while weight bearing, especially on a surface that grips the sole of the footwear such as synthetic turf, or the entire foot in cases of muddy fields, or inadequate footwear. Locking of the knee and an inability to extend the knee fully are classic predisposing factors. A clinical condition named 'pseudo-locking' is due to the loose material interfering with the movement mechanism of the knee. Another important and reliable finding is palpable swelling along the joint line. Symptoms may resolve on activity, and walking may give very little discomfort. X-rays are not useful unless there is long-term meniscal involvement which may present as spurring. MRI and arthroscopy may be helpful.

Treatment
Meniscectomy can be performed to remove or reduce the tear. With good aftercare an athlete can be participating in full competition within about 14 days. Manipulative intervention, as opposed to surgical intervention, can be of symptomatic relief. It can displace the obstruction interfering with the flexion–extension mechanism for a time, but it cannot heal the torn meniscus. Manipulation is indicated in symptomatic relief and especially after surgery to reduce any upsets in accessory joint motion and soft tissue function. Ice or heat and anti-inflammatories are indicated. It is important that the knee is used as soon as possible, but not over-subjected to extension machines as they can retard recovery.

Synovial plica injury

The synovial plica is the embryological remnant of the walls that divide the knee into medial, lateral and suprapatellar portions. It tends to be connected to the underside of the quadriceps tendon (suprapatella plica). The medial plica is a free edge along the medial patellofemoral joint, and injury can present a symptom picture very similar to that of medial meniscal locking. The plica is irritated as a consequence of overuse, direct trauma etc. The athlete will complain of pain over the anterior, supra-patella or medial infrapatella region of the knee.

Treatment
Decompression of the irritated area is the objective of OMT. This is achieved by a combination of soft tissue techniques and qualitative joint palpatory analysis. Initially, NSAIDs and ice are used to control any inflammatory response with any knee support deemed necessary.

Osteochondritis dessicans

Here, there is a reduction in blood supply to the bone, secondary to trauma, leading to a rarefication of bone material. There is localized tenderness usually over the medial aspect of the femoral condyle. It occurs mainly in adolescents. There is usually pain and effusion on palpation and a lateral view X-ray shows an area of reduced bone density.

Treatment

Treatment includes reduced weight bearing, OMT to hip and foot and surgery to improve blood supply.

Chondromalacia patella

This is basically degeneration of the cartilaginous articular surface of the patella. Factors that contribute to this condition are usually past by the time the pain in the knee presents. These include past events such as direct trauma to the knee or quadriceps mechanism, an increased Q-angle, and the result of increased work load within the femoral groove. Gently compressing the patella in the femoral groove and then pushing it distally may reveal crepatus and a positive apprehension sign. Tenderness and/or pain on the articular surface of the patella does not always result in degenerative changes, especially in acute presentations that are the result of direct trauma to the patella.

Treatment

OMT objective is to decompress the patella from the patellofemoral articulation by decreasing the tone of the quadriceps. Initially, the use of NSAIDs and ice is indicated. An X-ray taken from a sunrise or skyline view will show clouding or thickening of the articular surface of the patella.

Osgood–Schlatter's disease

This presents as a chronic discomfort and/or pain over the region of the tibial tuberosity. It tends to be more apparent just after activity initially, then during activity, and then at most times of the day. It presents almost exclusively in children and adolesents. It is possible to have symptoms in both knees with enlargement of the tibial tuberosity. Remember when comparing both sides that both tibial tuberosities could be enlarged but only one may be symptomatic. X-rays will reveal an enlarged tibial tuberosity with a tractioning of the tibial tuberosity apophyseal plate. Locally, it can be caused by excessive mechanical demand. It is often put down to 'growing pains', but postural and functional stresses become focused, especially during activity.

Treatment

Rest, ice and NSAIDs initially. OMT is directed at reducing the tractioning of the tendon attachment to the bone. This is achieved by reducing the resting hypertonia of soft tissue through the response of the central nervous system input.

Neurovascular compression

Sharp direct trauma, e.g. a kick, to the anterior subcutaneous surface of the patella, or any bone, can lead to tenderness and extreme sensitivity on palpation. Palpation often reveals a ridge of (neurovascular) tissue that has been crushed by the impact and is sensitive.

Treatment
Desensitization is the treatment objective and can be achieved with a combination of hot and/or cold (depending on findings) and quadriceps cross-fibre work. OMT is directed at reducing the sensitivity of the athlete to the condition. Soft tissue manipulation of the quadriceps, glutei and hamstrings is useful. Initially, rest, NSAIDs and ice will control the local discomfort. X-ray may be indicated to eliminate a hairline fracture.

Patella tendonitis

The athlete complains of discomfort inferior to, under or on the inferior border aspect of the patella. Initially it will ache after exercise and then calm down until the next activity, but it will linger longer each time until it aches when not active. It usually presents as pain and/or discomfort beginning at the inferior aspect of the patella, travelling distally along the patella tendon. There is an exacerbation of symptoms if digital pressure is applied to this inferior part of the patella while it is being held steady by the other hand. Usually the athlete has a history of stepping up training, jumping etc. When there is no apparent reason, it may be that there is reduced function elsewhere and this area is becoming overworked.

Treatment
Look for reduced lower extremity postural function. Reduce activity and apply ice (three times per day) and anti-inflammatory medication. Strapping may help. Do not apply strapping around the tendon area which can irritate the tendonitis. Apply elastic strapping to the superior part of the patella to push the patella down a little, reducing traction on the tendon.

Patella tendon rupture

This is not common. There is extreme pain and the athlete may show signs of shock. There will be a massive effusion around the area after a few seconds to a minute or so. If you can identify the patella it will be higher than normal in a complete rupture, as opposed to the tearing of a large number of fibres. The usual cause is excessive sudden loading of the extensor mechanism, especially in older athletes.

Treatment
Immobilization as in a severely broken leg. This is an orthopaedic emergency.

Compartment syndrome

This occurs due to an increase in tissue pressure within one or more of the fascial compartments of the leg. A poor arteriovenous gradient develops leading to poor venous and lymphatic drainage. Symptoms include pain, discomfort, tightness, fatigue and numbness, usually over the anterior aspect of the leg. The onset of symptoms may be slow, but eventually they occur whenever the athlete is active. In dark-skinned athletes there may be signs of trophic skin changes over the anterior muscular bulk, and a shiny, tight appearance. The expanding or hypertrophic tissue is actually cutting off its own drainage system. There is usually a history of increased activity in a short space of time, changes in weight (usually an increase) or just unaccustomed activity. An athlete who has no apparent reason for the onset of symptoms is more likely to show signs of postural and/or reduced function elsewhere in the lower extremity. Poor metabolic clearance leads to irritation and tissue damage.

Treatment
Restriction or cessation of activity, local fascial stretch, postural analysis, and lower extremity, back, pelvis and hip treatment. Warmth may help to aid drainage in the short term. If symptoms are too advanced, decompression of the compartment may be necessary, but causative factors must be dealt with. Scarring after decompression is superficial, but is improved with OMT; this is especially important for female athletes and dancers. Differential diagnosis should include shin splints, carcinoma and stress fracture.

Shin splints

Also known as medial tibial stress syndrome, this appears as a periosteal inflammation or avulsion of the posteromedial distal tibia. In the acute form there may be a myositis of the posterior tibialis, anterior tibialis or the peroneal muscles. Athletes complain of discomfort over the medial distal aspect of the shin. An acute presentation will usually be due to preseason enthusiasm, new shoes and/or new training techniques. Symptoms may be exacerbated on activity, especially in the toe-off phase of running, and may occur in both legs. The symptoms decrease when activity stops. The shin may ache in the morning on rising due to local metabolic disturbance. On palpation there are ridges of tissue on the medial distal edge of the bone; these are where fatty fibrous tissue has filled in the inflamed or avulsed areas. The athlete will confirm pain or discomfort in this area. There may be signs of calcaneal inversion; this is not the cause but the result of posterior compartment tissue shortening, and is why the toe-off phase increases pain.

Treatment
Treatment for posture, lower extremity, back, hip etc. If inflamed then ice massage/bag will help. NSAIDs, posterior compartment soft tissue treatment and general and local stretching are useful. Search for adaptive lower extremity, spinal and pelvic joint restrictions. Differential diagnosis should include compartment syndrome, stress factures and carcinoma.

Fractures

Fractures to the tibia and fibula usually occur due to direct impact, especially in contact sports. Injury mechanisms include shin-to-shin contact, planting the foot hard to change direction while running (severe rotation), a low tackle against the leg while the foot is firmly planted on the ground, a glancing kick (foul in soccer), falling on the back of the leg in a pile-up and binding failing to release in skiing. Minor fractures of the tibia tend to cause more pain and discomfort on walking than those of the fibula, due to the fact that the fibula is not a major weight-bearing bone. Nevertheless, the fibula is an important bone in lower extremity function. It is usually fractured by impact on the lateral aspect of the calf or falls when running. Crepitus with swelling may be more apparent in a fractured fibula than in a tibial fracture. Crepitus is suspected when the athlete notices that the leg is clicking, especially when it is days after the injury. To examine for crepitus hold the whole leg just above or below the fracture site and squeeze lightly and repeatedly. A stethoscope may help.

Treatment

On suspicion of a tibia and/or fibula fracture, reassure the athlete. Make sure the fracture is not open; even the smallest break in the skin is important. Check the distal pulses and sensorimotor status. If there is no obvious deformity, swelling or crepitus, palpate gently with graded finger or thumb pressure to locate fracture zone. Traction leg gently holding on to the bone below the fracture site, not the foot unless the fracture is low. If an open splint is used (wood and bandages) a bag of ice and water at the fracture site will ease the pain. When a closed splint is used (pneumatic splint) a bag of ice and water can be applied to the low back on the side of the injury. Transport to hospital.

Non-union fractures

Even after months of casting a tibia/fibula may appear to not have united. The athlete will still be on crutches and will be unable to put the foot to the floor. There may still be metabolic activity at the fracture site, which is a good sign, and is indicated by heat at the fracture site. It is important that the athlete puts weight on the foot or the fracture will not unite, but this cannot happen until the sensation of further pain and 'stress' at the site is reduced. Examine the joints and soft tissue above and below the fracture site. You will find that they are reduced in movement and the muscles are hypertonic and maybe fibrotic. There will be postural compensations as far as the occiput. When the athlete attempts to put the foot to the floor there is no energy absorption in the other structures so the energy is focused at the fracture site. Reduce the hypertonia and improve joint function in the entire lower extremity, hip, pelvis, low back, all the way to the upper ribs and occiput. The athlete should be able to weight bear, with less reliance on crutches, with one to two treatments (or in 3–5 days). Continue treatments into the athlete's retraining phase.

X-rays

X-rays (4–6 weeks old) should be obtained as soon as possible with a non-united fracture, and again after treatment has improved the condition, usually 6–8 weeks later.

If you have an athlete with a non-united fracture that has not been X-rayed in the last 4–6 weeks, you should obtain a new set as soon as possible. When the athlete's condition has improved after treatment have them X-rayed again usually 6–8 weeks later.

Achilles tendonitis

This occurs at the distal end of the calf and posterior part of the heel. Under the skin is a subcutaneous bursa and between the posterior part of the heel and the Achilles tendon is the retrocalcaneal bursa. The Achilles tendon has a mesotendon or 'pseudo-sheath' which contains the main vascular component of the tendon–sheath complex. Achilles tendonitis can occur in three places:

1. at the site of the tendon itself; this ranges from irritation with mucinoid degeneration to actual extensive micro-tearing;
2. the mesotendon or so-called 'sheath' becomes swollen and thickened;
3. irritation of the retrocalcaneal bursa associated with changes in the adjacent tendon and mesotendon.

If the diagnosis is of retrocalcaneal bursitis on its own then it is not Achilles tendonitis. This condition frequently presents in middle- to long-distance runners, basketball players and ballet dancers. It is usually of slow onset, and initially gets easier with activity but then returns after activity about an hour or so later. Sometimes in the early stages it may not give problems until the following day.

The best way to examine the athlete is to have them lying prone with feet over the end of the couch. Comparing the posterior distal end of both legs, look for swelling, stretched skin, discoloration or slight fullness in the area. If the swelling is along the length of the tendon then it is likely to be the mesotendon that is the main problem; if the swelling is localized the tendon itself is more likely involved; if the swelling is more over the heel, then retrocalcaneal bursitis is making some contribution to the picture. Subcutaneous bursitis should be more easily palpable than observed.

Palpation will reveal heat at the site of the discomfort in inflamed conditions. If it is cooler in the swollen area then you have a chronic condition. Feel for integrity of the tendon; it may be ruptured. At the point of greatest discomfort take the tendon between your index finger and thumb. Gently pinch the tendon to confirm the slight discomfort; you should also be able to feel a thickening of tissue at that level. Pinching either side of the tendon at its most distal end with a positive response will help confirm the involvement of the retrocalcaneal bursa.

Causative factors include rotation imbalance at the hips and sciatic nerve irritation.

Treatment

Reduced activity, or controlled but stopping if symptoms worse. Ice or heat application, taping and medication. Surgical intervention may be necessary. This involves making an incision in the medial aspect of the tendon to avoid the sural nerve; the skin and subcutaneous tissue are taken in one layer to expose the tendon. An incision of the mesotendon is made longitudinally to expose the area of mucinoid degeneration. This region may present as glistening tissue due to mucinoid presence; sometimes a small cavity is present, or a clumping of vascular tissue. Recovery from such intervention requires a minimum of 3–4 weeks. Permanent casting of the leg was common in the past, but should be avoided. If any casting is needed it should be with a removable cast so that icing and rehabilitation can take place daily. A lateral X-ray should show a deposition of calcium salts in the tendon, but their absence on the film does not mean that they are not present.

Achilles tendon rupture

This is an actual tearing of the fibres of the tendon that occurs to varying degrees, from a simple strain to a full separation of the tendon. Here, I will describe the full tear.

The athlete cannot weight bear on the injured leg. The athlete may describe the injury as the back of the ankle 'feels strange' or it feels like 'someone has hit me hard'. Although the majority of athletes will be in severe pain and not able to move the foot, a minority will not feel any significant pain immediately; it is not until they realize something major has happened that they may go into a state of shock and pain grips them. There may be 'bunching' of the calf muscles above the injury site. Definition of the area will be lost; this may be obvious only after a few minutes. If you can palpate the area you will feel 'nothing' by placing your index finger at right angles on the distal end of the Achilles tendon. Squeezing the calf will elicit some plantar flexion of the foot if the tendon is intact (Simmonds' test).

Treatment

This is an orthopaedic surgical emergency and should be handled like a fracture. Immersing the leg in a bucket of iced water will help to control pain and swelling before transportation to hospital.

Ankle injuries

Ankle sprain/strain

This is probably the most common injury of the lower leg/foot. Contrary to popular belief, the most common ankle injuries in sport are not inversion injuries, but are injuries due to a combination of inversion and plantar flexion. Like other injuries the surrounding soft tissue cannot heal quickly unless there is good bone-to-bone approximation. Pain on the medial, lateral, anterior and posterior areas of the ankle in the majority of cases indicates movement of the talus within the mortice of the complex. After the injury, oedema, pain and supportive contracture will maintain discomfort for weeks if not months, meaning a slow return to competition. Possible adaptations elsewhere also contribute to the slow progress of the injury and slow oedema drainage.

Treatment
All sprains/strains should be iced, NSAIDs administered, taped and properly assessed once the structures have calmed down enough to be passively moved without causing major discomfort. This examination should reveal restricted areas that need OMT. In the case of chronic presentations the entire posture has to be assessed, and the interlinking of the lower limb with the pelvis, spine etc.

Ankle dislocation and subluxation

There is a disengagement of the subtalar region. In many cases the athlete does not realize they have actually dislocated the ankle; distracting them may delay shock and distress by a few minutes. Dislocation is obvious, but subluxation may not be so obvious.

Treatment
These are orthopaedic emergencies. Check neurovascular status, stabilize as for a broken leg and transport to hospital. Administration of inhalation anaesthesia or ice to the ankle or low back will help control pain.

Venous drainage of the foot

Osteopathically, the drainage (lymphatic and venous) is of paramount importance. Below is a quotation from Gardner and Fox (1989).

> The deep veins of the foot were not even mentioned in a recent anatomical atlas of the foot and ankle or in Grant's Atlas of Anatomy, although the Atlas does depict the dorsal vein of the clitoris. The main reason for this neglect seems to be that in normal anatomical preparations, the deep veins of the foot are collapsed and during dissection are excised as amorphous tissue, better to expose the arteries to which they are the *venae comites*; indeed it was in only one of a series of five foot dissections that we performed that the venous footpump – anatomically the *venae comites* of the lateral plantar artery – was sufficiently filled with blood to be easily identifiable. Perhaps unlike the majority, this patient died in the sitting position. Ideal subjects in the past would have been those from the gallows!
>
> The foot is routinely ignored by pathologists, and an eminent radiologist has stated that 'in contrast to the situation in the rest of

the leg, veins of the foot have no real haemodynamic importance'. A venous footpump was first postulated by Le Dentu in 1867. He, like more recent authors, concluded that the plantar venous pump is emptied up into the superficial veins of the foot by the direct pressure of weight bearing and by contraction of the plantar muscles. As we shall see, neither contention is true. Muscular action is not necessary for footpump function. Indeed repeated observations have shown that weight bearing on a paralyzed limb with the knee braced excites a strong Doppler signal in the femoral vein of the groin. To understand fully the method of emptying of the plantar venous pump, we must first consider the mechanics of the foot.

The way in which the foot adapts to its mechanical function during normal locomotion is extremely complex; it is able to act in turn either as an arch, a truss or a level. During walking, the foot is in contact with the ground for 60% of the time and remains off the ground for 40% (swing time). In the mid-segment of the foot, a transverse arch is present which is high medially and low, or non-existant, laterally, so that weight bearing takes place almost entirely on the ball of the toes, the heel and the lateral aspect of the plantar surface of the foot. There is little if any direct pressure on the medial aspect of the sole of the foot. It is this medial aspect of the arch of the sole of the foot that the plantar veins cross and therefore avoid significant direct pressure, except in individuals with flat feet. The muscles of the sole of the foot are in a relaxed state during plantigrade weight bearing. They contract on heel strike-off, thus opposing forced dorsiflexion of the toes. Much of the body weight is now supported on the toes, the foot acting as a lever. During the stance phase, rotary movements of the tibia serve to control the rigidity of the mid-tarsal joint. The ankle and sub-talar joints act as a universal joint to convert the rotation along the axis of the tibia into rotation about the long axis of the foot, internal rotation of the tibia being converted into supination of the foot.

When the foot is pronated, flexion and extension are possible at the mid-tarsal joint, but when the foot is supinated, this joint is effectively locked. At heel strike, the tibia is undergoing internal rotation, thus pronating the foot so that the tarsal arch may extend; the foot is now acting as a truss. As weight bearing is transferred to the forefoot, the foot supinates, the arch becomes rigid, the plantar muscles contract and the foot becomes a lever to enable weight bearing to occur on the toes. Thus we see that on plantigrade weight bearing, the tarsal arch extends, causing the foot to flatten. Most of the apparent flattening at the medial aspect of the arch of the foot is accused by extension of the first tarso-metatarsal joint. The first metatarsal has been regarded as too large for skeletal function; it seems possible that its large size is related to a role in venous return.

What then is the normal mechanism of footpump emptying? Function could be explained as follows. The plantar veins are slung rather like a bow-string from between the base of the fourth metatarsal in front and the medial malleolus behind, so that when weight is borne and the tarso-metatarsal joints are extended and the tarsal arch flattened, they are stretched causing them to 'neck down' forcibly and eject their content of blood. Video phlebography has shown that this indeed is precisely what happens. If the subject bears weight on transverse bars with pressure only on the ball of the toes in front and the heel behind, with no direct pressure whatsoever on the sole of the foot, the whole length of the plantar venous pump is seen to empty up into the calf. This concept fits with the normal distribution of weight bearing on the sole of the foot. Weight bearing on a transverse ridge under the mid-foot usually empties locally.

The deep veins of the foot do not empty into the superficial veins of the foot on weight bearing as previously thought; but since there are no valves in the perforating veins of the foot to stop this happening, how is it prevented? It is probable that on weight bearing, tension in the plantar aponeurosis closes the perforating veins passing through it. We believe that weight bearing on the forefoot occludes the anterior transverse section of the pump and that the interosseous muscles may also compress the large interosseous vein between the first and second metatarsal heads, thus preventing retrograde emptying of the plantar veins.

Pes planus (flat foot)

Flat feet are blamed for many lower limb conditions, and one suspects that the practitioner uses this diagnosis when he or she can find no other. Flat feet can be static and/or dynamic. The static flat foot is where the athlete has no arch when standing still. This is more common in negroid athletes. Dynamic flat feet occur when during running there is no arch formation, as a source of energy absorption and propulsion. Fitting hard insoles and arch supports into running shoes forces the arch into an unnatural position and reduces natural foot flexibility. Pain in the arch and other foot structures is due to restriction of movement and/or overcompensation of the capsuloligamentous joint apparatus. A hard insole reduces the movement that causes discomfort and, therefore, removes the pain, but does not deal with the problem.

Treatment

The muscles of the leg that maintain both the foot and the arch should be treated. Examination of the entire posture and lower extremity is important to make sure the foot dynamically functional. There is nothing wrong with a static flat foot, unless it does not move or is hypermobile. Piriformis irritation of the sciatic nerve is one of the common causes of a unilateral flat foot in the static presentation. OMT is directed at reducing foot and lower extremity restrictions, and removing restrictions elsewhere that may cause overcompensation at joints in the foot.

Pes cavus (high arch)

As with the flat foot, this may not cause problems. Do not be distracted by the formation of the foot. Pain and discomfort due to what appears to be a high arch may be caused by asymptomatic tissue elsewhere.

Treatment
Postural examination. Check entire lower limb and pelvis.

Plantar fasciitits

This is due to shortening of the plantar fascia around the medial tubercle of the calcaneum. This is tender to palpate (point tenderness) as well as when running, walking long distances, or when putting the foot to the floor on rising in the morning. It may lead to the formation of a calcaneal spur. Expansion of the triceps surae tendon over the calcaneum leads to traction irritation of the plantar fascia. Other structures that can cause plantar fasciitis include shortening of the abductor hallucis and flexor digitorum brevis.

Treatment
This tends to be a chronic presentation so it is important to find the cause of the problem. Locally, a warm foot bath, NSAIDs and triceps surae stretching are used. OMT is directed at improving function of the foot and entire lower extremity. Check the other lower extremity. Shock-absorbing insoles tend to be used, but can make the long-term situation worse. Many athletes do not strike the ground with the heel when they run. The contraction of loading the triceps surae irritates the condition. Surgical fascial release is the last resort, even at the expense of not using cortisone.

Arch pain

This usually presents as a sudden sharp pain in the arch of the foot, so intense that the athlete cannot put the foot to the ground. The most common cause is a reduction in movement of the talonavicular or navicular–medial cuneiform articulations. Other causes of pain include shortening of the abductor hallucis, flexor hallucis brevis, tendon of flexor hallucis longus and stress fracture.

Treatment
This depends on the diagnosis. Common findings include a restricted range of motion at the talonavicular and naviculocuneiform articulations.

Stress fractures of the foot

These result from poor soft tissue energy absorption and dissipation in the lower limb; they have very little to do with being 'unfit'. Over-training will increase resting contractable soft tissue tone. Resting does not significantly reduce this tone, but it will allow the fracture time to heal.

Treatment

OMT is directed at restoring the energy absorbing characteristics of soft tissue, and good joint motion of the entire body. Rest in the mean time is important.

Athlete's foot

Otherwise known as tinea pedis, this fungal infection is common in sport due to the combination of sweat, heat and damp feet after showering. There is itching and a whitening of the skin between the toes. It feels worse when the feet get warm. To prevent this condition it is important to keep the feet dry and aired especially after a shower or bath.

Treatment

There are many preparations on the market. It is advisable to clean with dilute hydrogen peroxide initially and then add the antifungal preparation. After this keep feet clean and dry following the instructions of the preparation or your osteopath/physician.

Turf toe

This is a sprain or damage of the flexor tendon in hyperextension of the metatarsophalangeal (MTP) joint at the base of the great toe. It occurs commonly in soccer players, football linesmen and tennis players. There is tenderness, swelling and pain at the MTP joint on the plantar surface which if continued to be irritated will stiffen, i.e. halux rigidus. Further long-term irritation and weight bearing can lead to degenerative changes. Generally, the mechanism of injury is any situation where the athlete is required to weight bear, push and twist on the base of the great toes. The playing surface and footwear may be contributing factors in the aetiology of the injury; the coaching and playing technique of the athlete must also be considered.

Treatment

Ice (cold foot bath), NSAIDs and support (taping). OMT is directed at all joints in the foot and ankle complex. Find the reason for the focal loading of this joint: it may be a consequence of a poor energy-absorbing hip or quadriceps, for example.

Corns or callus formation

This is thickening of the outer layer of the skin due to excessive pressure on the 'pad' areas of the feet. This is adaptation to pressure loading and activity, but it has to be controlled. Athletes should file or shave down these areas of hard skin, but not all the way to very soft skin otherwise blister formation may occur. There are various foot care preparations on the market. Corns are an indication of incorrect loading, and postural analysis may find areas of lower limb/pelvis etc. with hypertonic tissue or joint restrictions that are affecting energy absorption capacity.

Bunion (hallucis valgus)

Poor weight distribution and/or dissipation through the lower limb can lead to rotation (pronation) of the foot and the development of a valgus deformity at the base of the great toe. A postural examination is vital.

Treatment
In the short term, this can be helped by a wedge of foam or similar material between the great toe and the next toe to straighten the toe. As a long-term measure, improve the quality of the tissues of the pelvis and lower limb.

Nail infection and injury

Poor nail care includes lack of attention and over-enthusiastic care. Poorly cleaned nails and generally poor foot hygiene are precursors to infection. Further problems are subungal haemorrhage (from trauma) and ingrown toenails. Besides lack of general hygiene, causative factors for ingrown toenail include cutting the nails too far back, especially at the corners; pressure from tight-fitting shoes; and too much work load in too short a time, e.g. ballet dancers én-point. Onychogryphosis or thickening of the nail is usually due to trophic changes and/or trauma.

Treatment
General foot hygiene is of primary importance. For an ingrown toenail, bathing the foot in warm water, adding a small amount of mild disinfectant to the water, and drying properly are the basics. Topical antibiotics will help to control any infection. Systemic antibiotics may need to be prescribed if the condition gets worse. There are many over-the-counter preparations on the market that will help. As the corners of the ingrown toe nail begin to grow, let them 'grow out', only cutting the nail across the tip. In the case of subungal haemorrhage cool the area down with ice or a cold footbath. NSAIDs can be administered if the injury is particularly painful. In both cases OMT should be directed at the MTP and mid-foot joints to keep the foot freely functioning. This is important for blood supply and blood and lymphatic drainage.

Blisters

Blisters are extremely frustrating to athletes. Usually they occur on the feet, especially the base of the toe, and less often on the hands. The athlete will usually be fit and healthy, but may be unable to run or in some cases walk properly. Blisters are caused by shear forces that move the outer layer of the skin (epidermis) apart from the next layer (dermis). Due to the friction fluid accumulates between these two layers from the blood vessels. If the pressure continues, then fine blood vessels become damaged and the space is filled with blood. Some of the causes include badly fitting footwear, slow walking over a long period of time, or any unaccustomed activity that brings the body in contact with equipment or the ground.

Treatment
Initially, cool the area. Submerse the foot in cold water or apply an ice bag to the area, for not more than 20 min. This will immediately help to control the pain and discomfort. Check for signs of infection. The blister may need to be aspirated: clean the area first; perforate the blister at its lowest point with a sterile scalpel blade, then gently push the contents of the blister out using a piece of gauze. The application of synthetic skin covered by a ring of foam (doughnut pad) will help keep the pressure off the injury. Do not remove the outer layer of skin unless it is dead. Remove dressing at least once a day, ice and then re-dress.

Treadmill analysis

Most athletes have problems while running. Running is a series of pushes. You cannot push on a treadmill as you do on the ground. Lower limb and body muscles used in running mostly switch off when running on a treadmill, this is why it is awkward to stand up when you get off the treadmill. Treadmills are a very poor (if not useless) tool in motion analysis. They should be used only for cardiorespiratory analysis in a laboratory.

General approach towards manipulative procedures of the lower extremity

Never forget that the objective of treatment (in any form) is to improve function, reduce pain and then take preventive measures (by exercise, nutritional changes, further treatment etc.) against recurrence. This means that, although the pain may be in the lower extremity, this is not necessarily where all the treatment should be concentrated.

Osteopathic manipulative procedures are based on the ability to palpate. The techniques are based on the ability to relax reflex muscle tension. Movement of the joint towards the position that relieves pain and muscle tension will produce reflex voluntary muscle relaxation. Osteopathic manipulative procedures should only be performed as and when the presenting dysfunction demands. The intensity, power, number of treatments, etc. are determined by palpatory findings, history etc., and should not be a procedural approach. No two injuries are the same, so no two treatments or diagnoses are the same. There are only trends in injuries and treatments.

> Traditional medical treatment of the sprained ankle is directed primarily toward reduction of swelling and protection of the ankle, usually through immobilization, until the patient is able to walk without major discomfort. Follow-up treatment with attention to residual difficulties associated with ankle sprains tends to be overlooked. The osteopathic approach to treatment includes traditional medical techniques but extends beyond them and uses systematic, sequential manipulative therapy to eliminate residual as well as immediate physiologic disabilities. This approach includes treatment of anatomic areas that influence the lower extremities, with particular attention to the vertebrae of the upper thoracic and lumbar regions, ribs, and pelvis. Subluxations should be treated, with special attention to the fibula and tibiotalar joints. Somatic dysfunctions of the foot and hip joint should be identified and treated, and isokinetic and isotonic exercises directed to strengthening the muscles involved in supination, pronation, plantar flexion, and dorsiflexion.
>
> (Blood, 1980)

Treadmill analysis

Diagnosis and rehabilitation of the athlete's injury and treatment often involve the treadmill. Sometimes the step machine may also be employed. However both these machines are of limited or no use in the care of the athlete – they give false readings and a false sense of achievement; the muscles of forward motion and anti-gravity are poorly used. Use of the treadmill is similar to running on a moving walkway the wrong way and staying in the same spot – the muscles of forward movement are the last to be employed, hence the shaky start when the athlete stands on normal ground and tries to walk forward. The step machine is similar to walking up an escalator the wrong way; again the athlete stays in the same position. Both these machines should be avoided if possible except, because of their design, for physiological testing.

REFERENCES

Blood, S. (1980) Treatment of the sprained ankle. *Journal of the American Osteopathic Association*, **79**(11), 680/61–692/73.

Cardinali, D.P. and Romeo, H.E. (1990) Peripheral neuroendocrine interrelationships in the cervical region. *News in Physiological Sciences*, **5**, 100–4.

Cathie, A.G. (1974a) Application of anatomy to the regions of the neck, shoulder and upper arm, in *American Academy of Osteopathy 1974 Year Book*. pp. 146–9. American Academy of Osteopathy, CO.

Cathie, A.G. (1974b) The veins of the spine and craniospinal junction – the vertebral system of veins, in *American Academy of Osteopathy 1974 Year Book*. pp. 94–5. American Academy of Osteopathy, CO.

Denslow, J.S. and Hassett, C.C. (1944) The central excitatory state associated with postural abnormalities. *Journal of Neurophysiology*, **5**, 393–402.

Dobrusin, R. (1989) An osteopathic approach to conservative management of thoracic syndromes. *Journal of the American Osteopathic Association*, **89**(8), 1046–57.

Dutia, M.B. (1989) Mechanisms of head stabilisation. *News in Physiological Sciences*, **4**, 101–104.

Friedman, W.A. (1983) Clinical Symposia, *Head Injuries*. CIBA Pharmaceutical Company, **35**(4).

Gardner, A.M.N. and Fox, R.H. (1989) The return of blood to the heart, in *Venous Pumps in Health and Disease*, John Libbey, London.

Giachino, A.A. (1993) Injury to the scapholunate ligaments. *The Physician and Sports Medicine*, **21**(5), 51–8.

Glover, E.D., Flannery, D. Albritton, D.L. and Scott, L.G. (1990) Smokeless tobacco: questions and answers. *Athletic Training*, **25**(1), 10–14.

Goldman, S. (1989) Biomechanical osteopathic approach to shoulder pain. *Journal of the American Osteopathic Association*, **89**(1), 53–7.

Gordon, C.J. and Cox, J.P. (1983) Straight spine syndrome. *Journal of the American Osteopathic Association*, **83**, 4, 99–102.

Gracovetsky, S. (1985) An hypothesis for the role of the spine in human locomotion: a challenge to current thinking. *Journal of Biomedicine and Engineering*, **7**, 205–16.

Hallgren, R.C., Greenman, P.E. and Rechtien, J.J. (1994) Atrophy of suboccipital muscles in patients with chronic pain: a pilot study. *Journal of the American Osteopathic Association*, **94**(12), 1032–8.

Harber, C.J. (1988) Current concepts in the irritable bowel syndrome. Clinical rounds. *Journal of Osteopathic Medicine*, **2**(9), 22–35.

Hashiguchi, J., Ito, M. and Sekine, I. (1993) The effect of the autonomic nervous system on cell proliferation of the gastric mucosa in stress ulcer formation. *Journal of the Autonomic Nervous System*, **43**, 179–88.

Inman, V., Saunders, M. and Abbott L.C. (1944) Observations on the function of the shoulder joint. *Journal of Bone and Joint Surgery*, **XXVI**(1), 1–30.

Kawato, M. and Gomi, H. (1992) The cerebellum and VOR/OKR learning models. *Trends in Neurological Science*, **15**(11), 445–53.

Ladusans, E.J. (1993) Assessment of children with a heart murmur. *Update*, 1st July, 33–42.

Lisberger, S.G. (1988) The neural basis for learning of simple motor skills. *Science*, **242**(4), 728–35.

Mackenzie, J. (1921) The theory of disturbed reflexes in the production of symptoms of disease. *British Medical Journal*, **29**, 147–53.

Mills, J., Ho, M. T., Salber, P.R. and Trunkey, D.D. (eds) (1985) *Current Emergency Diagnosis and Treatment*, 2nd edn, Lange Medical Publications.

Morrow, R.M. and Bonci, T. (1989) A survey of oral injuries in female college and university athletes. *Athletic Training*, **24**(3), 236–7.

Nelson, C.R. (1948) Postural analysis and its relation to systemic disease. Clinical and theoretical significance of posture and imbalance.

Passmore, R. and Robinson, J.S. (eds) (1976) *Anatomy, Biochemistry, Physiology and Related Subjects, Volume 1, A Companion to Medical Studies*, Blackwell Scientific, Oxford.

Peterson, B.W. and Richmond, F.J. (1988) *Control of Head Movement*, Oxford University Press, Oxford.

Prichard, J.J., Scott, J.H. and Girgis, F.G. (1956) The structure and development of the cranial and facial sutures. *Journal of Anatomy*. **90**. 73–87.

Sharr, M. (1984: Mechanics of raised intracranial pressure. *Surgery*, **1**(8), 187–90.

Stein, J.F. and Glickstein, M. (1992) Role of the cerebellum in visual guidance of movement. *Physiological Reviews*, **72**(4), 967–1017.

Torg, M.D.J. (1990) Cervical spine stenosis with cord neurapraxia and transient quadriplegia. *Athletic Training*, **25**(2), 138–46.

FURTHER READING

Burns, L. (1947) Certain cardiac complications and vertebral lesions. *Journal of the American Osteopathic Association*, **47**(4), 199–200.

Goldman, M.D., Loh, L. and Sear, T.A. (1985) The respiratory activity of human levator costae muscles and its modification by posture. *Journal of Physiology*, **362**, 189–203.

McCully, K.K., Boden, B.P., Tuchler, M., Fountain, M.R. and Chance, B. (1989) Wrist flexor muscles of elite rowers measured with magnetic resonance spectroscopy. *Journal of Physiology*, **67**(3), 926–39.

Orani, G.P. and Decandia, M. (1990) Group I afferent fibers: effects on cardiorespiratory system. *Journal of Physiology*, **68**(3) 932–7.

Raphael, K.G., Dohrenwend, B.P. and Marbach, J.J. (1990) Illness and injury among children of temporomandibular pain and dysfunction syndrome (TMPDS) patients. *Pain*, **40**, 61–4.

Spitzer, I.E. (1980) Acute abdominal pain in children: important considerations in diagnosis. *Journal of the American Osteopathic Association*, **80**(3), 195/81–198/84.

Whitelaw, W.A., Ford, G.T., Rimmer, K.P. and De Troyer, A. (1992) Intercostal muscles are used during rotation of the thorax in humans. *Journal of Physiology*, **72**(5), 1940–4.

Principles of rehabilitation 7

Physical medicine is considered as 'that science which deals with the management of diseases by means of physical agents such as light, heat, cold, water, electricity, and mechanical agents,' while osteopathy deals with the structural integrity of the organism and the consequences, in terms of health and disease, of impairments of that integrity.

(Denslow, 1947)

EXERCISE

Exercise in physical therapy is the scientific application of bodily movement designed specifically to maintain or restore normal function to diseased or injured tissues. It is important that careful consideration is given to the type of exercise ordered on the results of physical therapy in a large number of patients. Each condition, as well as each individual, calls for a specific exercise programme. It is vital that a working diagnosis and the rehabilitation protocol are tailor-made for the athlete. A structured protocol does not mean a non-dynamic approach. As the athlete's sign and symptom picture changes so should the therapy applied. An intelligent approach is needed, not a procedural approach. It is also important to remember that in the majority athletes being prescribed exercise have tight hypertonic soft tissues. Active exercise on top of this condition is self-defeating. **Always** give a stretch programme **before** an active exercise programme in those who have tight tissues.

All pre-rehabilitation protocols are only of value after history taking, observation and palpation have been performed and flexibility, strength and function have been assessed. There should then be a controlled programme of rehabilitation with the following basic principles.

1. To maintain the fitness of the athlete.
2. The use of ice and/or heat to control pain, circulation etc.
3. Introduction of isometric exercises to reduce joint motion but involve muscular contraction. These are usually split into sets, with a number of repetitions (reps) per set. The number of sets and reps depends on the ability of the athlete. It is useful to begin with 10 reps in 1 set at a reduced capacity. This can be built upon later.

4. Passive and gentle resistance isotonic exercises.
5. Resistive exercises with weights as the range of motion increases. This is best with the athlete trying to move the weight between no less than 8 and no more than 12 reps. Then try 50% of the weight for the first set, 75% of the weight for the second set and 100% for the third set. All must be through a full range of motion.
6. The only problem with weights is that you do not get resistance through the full range of motion. This is better achieved through the use of isokinetic machines. Linear actions are unnatural, possibly leading to further problems, so they should be monitored carefully.

Types of exercise

Passive exercise

This prevents contractures and adhesion formation. It is used to start motion after fractures and to stretch tight areas. Joint manipulation is also placed in this general category of exercise i.e. tight shoulders, low backs, neck and any other body joint where loss of motion or adhesions is a problem.

Active exercise

This is used for correction of muscular and circulatory disturbances and to hasten restoration of function following trauma. Variations of the above six basic principles would include active assistance and active resistive exercise.

Specific corrective exercises

- William's flexion exercises: positional exercise for the back.
- Exercise for scoliosis, kyphosis and lordosis.
- Breathing exercise, for asthma, bronchitis and emphysema.
- Burger–Allen exercise, for peripheral vascular disease.
- Frenkel exercise, for slight to moderate central nervous system pathology such as cerebrovascular accident, multiple sclerosis and cerebral palsy.
- Codman exercise, for frozen shoulder or shoulder joint pathology.

The following is an example of a programme of low back rehabilitation.

In rehabilitating the low back, the primary concern is stretching of the low back, hamstring and quadriceps, before strengthening. The first exercises used are William's flexion exercises. These are performed when the athlete has acute pain (with minimal tissue damage) or as warm-up exercises. If pain persists or if pain shoots down the hips or lower legs, these exercises should be stopped immediately.

William's flexion exercises

1. One knee to chest, lie supine, right hip and knee flexed. Grasp right knee with both hands and pull toward chest. Hold for 6 seconds.

Release knee gently and let the leg back down. Perform 15 times on each leg alternately. If this is too easy add additional stretch taking right knee to left shoulder, hold for 6 seconds, and the same with left leg. Perform 15 times on each side.

2. Both knees to chest. Same as first exercise, but pull both knees to chest, hold for 10 seconds. Repeat 10 times.

3. Abdominal curls with knees bent. Lie supine, hips and knees flexed with feet lifted and head and shoulders raised 10 inches off the floor. This exercise should be repeated 10 times for the first 5 days, then up to three sets of five (five straight up, five rotating to the right, and five rotating to the left). Increase to 20 each side.

Pelvic tilt
Lie supine, hips and knees flexed, hands on abdomen. The pelvis is rotated backward by tightening the lower abdominal muscles. Feel the pressure of the low back on the floor. This is a postural exercise. Practice the wall test using pelvic tilt. Maintain tension in abdominal wall when standing and walking.

Hamstring stretch
Sit on the floor with the legs straight. Reach forward and grasp the ankles or soles of feet. Pull chest towards knees and hold for 10 seconds. Do not bounce. Repeat 10 times.

Hyperextension
Lie prone with a pillow under the stomach. Raise head, shoulders and arms keeping head in line with the shoulders. Place hands on the floor in a push position but do not lift hips off the floor. Stretch gently for a count of six then release gently going back to lying flat on the floor. Repeat 15 times. Increase number of repetitions to equal the number of repetitions of abdominal curls. **Warning**: this is the most misused exercise of any pre-scribed for back pain, and is also potentially the most dangerous. You must make sure the athlete has no joint inflammation, degenerative change, disc or ligament damage or possible foraminal encroachment. Misuse of this exercise has been responsible for ending many athletes' careers.

Intensive low back strenthening programme
The integrity and strength of the low back is a reflection of the integrity and strength of the whole back.

1. Gluteal setting – pinch buttocks together 10 times every hour.
2. Alternating straight leg hyperextension prone.
3. Double straight leg hyperextension prone.
4. Chest lift – prone, hands clasped on buttocks, pinch shoulder blades together and lift chest off floor.
5. Rocking chair – combine chest lift with double straight leg hyperexten-sion.

6. Alternating arm and leg raise prone – with arms over head, hyper-extend left arm and right leg then right arm and left leg.
7. Over the table back extension – lie face down, edge of table at hips, partner holds legs. Bend at the hips until arms and head touch floor. Then lift upper body until past level of table top.

Do three sets of 20 repetitions of each exercise every day; increase each exercise by five repetitions every week. You should also include abdominal exercises with this programme.

BASIC ORTHOTRON–ISOKINETIC REHABILITATION

Isokinetic or speed-controlled exercise allows for preselected speeds to meet specific rehabilitation goals. Isokinetics also provides more work per repetition and higher intensity levels than any other form of exercise. Isokinetic devices also allow high speed exercise at functional speeds to build both muscular power and endurance. The Orthotron/Cybex system provides resistance in both directions of joint movement. Force levels are measured in psi (pound force per square inch) output on the pump mechanism.

Actuator

This is the resistance mechanism. The Cybex is an electromechanical device, while the Orthotron is hydraulic. Force applied to the actuator arm pumps hydraulic fluid from one side of the cylinder to the other; force applied in the opposite direction pumps the fluid back.

Tare load

The tare load (TL) is the force required to get the device moving. The Orthotron II has a TL of less than 4 ftlbs, while the Cybex has a TL of less than 1 ftlbs. However, the old Orthotron had a TL of 10+ ftlbs. The athlete should be able to easily lift 5+ lbs before working on an isokinetic device.

Gauges

The gauges are accurate (at the time of writing) to ±5%. The visual error may be greater, however. The gauges register the psi of hydraulic pressure that the torque of the shaft pumps through the cylinder. Torque measurements are independent of lever arm length, because the length of the input arm is cancelled out by the equal length of the limb segment.

Testing capability

While the Orthotron is primarily a rehabilitation machine, it can have some limited testing capacity. The absolute accuracy of the Orthotron is effected by the tare load, ballistic momentum of the gauges and the limitations of hydraulic fluid (viscosity and contamination). If absolute accuracy is needed, use the Cybex for testing.

Guidelines

Positioning and stabilization of the affected limb can minimize unwanted movements which produce undesired substitutive force input. Select appropriate speeds of exercise to meet the functional demands of the body part. Some types of pathologies or injuries will respond best to higher exercise speeds. These higher speeds allow lower joint contact forces and tension levels without sacrificing desirable muscular work rates.

ULTRASOUND

Ultrasound is mechanical vibration produced by passing electric current over a quartz crystal. Ultrasound provide a powerful micromassage for cellular tissues. These mechanical vibrations supposedly increase blood supply, influence the sympathetic and parasympathetic nervous systems, stimulate metabolism and produce an analgesic effect. Research indicates that the effect of ultrasound is mainly on prostaglandin production.

Indications

- Bursitis
- Neuritis
- Sciatica
- Haematoma
- Sprains
- Myositis
- Neuromas
- Soft tissue inflammation
- Plexus neuralgia
- Most athletic injuries
- Torticollis
- Back problems
- Indolent ulcers.

Contraindications

- Malignant tumours
- Pregnancy
- Orbit of the eye
- Developing bones in children
- The gonads
- Infectious processes

- Over plexus areas
- Over heart, spinal cord, brain or accessory nasal sinuses.

WHIRLPOOL

Hydrotherapy is one of the oldest therapeutic measures used by humans for the alleviation of pain and spasm. Hot and cold water were used for therapeutic purposes in the days of Hippocrates. With modern whirlpools, we not only get the effect of application of hot water, but also the sedative effect of mild massage from the small bubbles passing the tissue. Ideal temperature of the water varies with the condition. If there is frank mass swelling, the temperature should stay below 2°C; if there is just soreness, the temperature can be as high as 43°C, but no higher.

Indications

- Arthritis
- Adherent scars
- Abscesses or infections
- Impaired circulation
- Post care of fractures
- Sprains, strains and contusions
- Sprained or strained feet
- Superficial burns
- Tender and sensitive feet.

Contraindications

Cold (0–2°C):
- Spastic paralysis and cerebral palsy
- Very young or very old
- Hypertension
- Raynaud's syndrome
- Persons sensitive to cold.

Hot (36–43°C):
- Respiratory involvements
- Pulmonary tuberculosis
- Osteomyelitis
- Persons with fear of water.
- Persons sensitive to heat.

Treatment time is from 15 to 40 min depending on the condition. If you are treating the back and the athlete is sitting in the water, the time should be reduced as the whole body temperature will be elevated and the patient may become overheated.

INJURY PREVENTION AND TRAINING PRINCIPLES

It is quite surprising the large number of amateurs that take part in regular activity only to become injured and then wonder why. It is even more surprising the number of Olympic and professional athletes who have very little knowledge of the principles of injury and illness prevention. On a regular basis I see amateur athletes who have a far better understanding of these principles than their professional counterparts. Understanding these principles is important enough for the athletes, but it is just as important for the osteopath who has to explain what went wrong, the possible reasons for what went wrong, and what can be done to help to correct the situation. Never assume that athletes know what they are doing – make them describe what they actually do or, even better, make them show you.

The use of training techniques is not only useful as pre-event conditioning, but also for a return to activity while the athlete is being treated. Understanding the principles of training allows the osteopath to help the athlete, both from a physical point of view and psychologically.

In this section I will discuss the basic principles of:

1. warm-ups and cool downs;
2. stretching and flexibility;
3. weight training and lifting;
4. speed, power and reaction time;
5. plyometrics;
6. overload principle;
7. training sessions (pre-season, in-season and post-season);
8. training as rehabilitation;
9. jogging.

All of 1–6 are relevant in training for a particular event or events on a regular basis. Practice is the repeated simulation and breakdown of the event so as to improve technique and/or team coordination. Our concept of sports training and practice is formed during our school years, and therefore correct training at this stage is vital. The majority of people who train and coach children are to be commended for their commitment; however the majority of these coaches have no or very little understanding of child psychology and physiology.

Warm-ups and cool downs

Many athletes do not appreciate the importance of these stages of the training procedure. The purpose of warming up is to increase metabolic and neuroendocrine activity in preparation for increased performance. This does not mean dashing around for 10 minutes until you break out into sweat, but should be an ordered procedure. Warm-up is usually performed just before increased physical performance. It can be performed individually or as group calisthenics. Warm-ups have to be performed regularly to be of benefit, not only just before activity as this could predispose to injury. There are different kinds of warming up: some athletes swear by hot baths, hot rubs, or a massage before an event. All these have different merits, but are superficial from a physiological point of view. Hot baths will stimulate skin receptors, increasing heart rate and causing sweating, hot rubs irritate the skin generally causing an erythematous response, and the effect of massage is negligible in warming up the individual. However, the psychological component of these activities may be important for the athlete. Proper warm-up that improves physiological activity affects the ability of myofascial tissue (especially deep structures) to respond to the demands of the event. This response is a physiological total, i.e. the myofascial skeletal system is a sensory system, and the better the sensory input the better the response via the neuroendocrine system. Changes due to warm-up include those of the cardiorespiratory mechanism and improved drainage of metabolites. Organs also have to 'warm-up'. Physiological changes to the heart, due to a sudden increased work rate, can lead to latent coronary flow with periods of ischaemia. There is an increase in heart rate, stroke volume, arterial flow and venous drainage. Warm-ups should precede all other activity, allowing the body to generate heat and stimulate support organs (viscera), slowly bringing 'on-line' communication systems within the body. Hot baths etc. do not perform this physiological function. An increase in metabolic chemical activity raises muscular temperature facilitating a better contraction–relaxation range of muscular tissue, improving metabolic clearance rate, and improving plasticity of the tissue. An improvement in plasticity allows for better force generation, absorption and dissipation. Poor or inadequate temperature increase is activity time and intensity related. The extent of the warm-up must reflect the maximum needs of the performance demands: Snooker and pool players do not need to warm up as much as track and field athletes. If there is not sufficient warm-up then there will be a poor reaction time, speed and energy factors. This increases the risk of injury and illness. The timing of the warm-up is important: it is no good warming up a few hours before the event.

Cool-downs prevent venous pooling and reduce post-exercise muscle soreness. Keep walking around after activity for at least 15 minutes.

Stretching and flexibility

After warming up stretching and flexibility should be considered. Again, many athletes do not perform effective stretching and flexibility exercises.

Flexibility is the range of joint motion. Flexibility exercises can be either passive or active: passive is when the athlete relaxes and is helped to stretch, and active flexibility exercises are when the athlete performs the stretching. Finally there is dynamic flexibility, which is the active speed and range in which the athlete can perform flexion and extension at a joint. These are specific rather than general factors for each joint; therefore any flexibility test, e.g. toe touch or arm curl, only indicates the degree of flexibility in the joint involved.

Any exercise that involves moderate, steady stretching of the joint will improve flexibility. These exercises can be performed passively or actively. Active stretching is the safest form. Here, the athlete stretches the muscle or group of muscles as far as they can functionally be stretched, and the chances of over straining them are low. Passive stretching is very useful as part of a rehabilitation programme after injury. The key to stretching is concentration, and especially concentrating on tight areas. The athlete should stretch the muscles to the point of tightness (and often slight discomfort) and hold for 10 seconds. This can be increased to 30 seconds. It is important that athletes learn how to stretch correctly. The athlete should concentrate on 'think', 'relax' and 'stretch'.

There are various types of stretching and flexibility exercises. The objective is to have longer and more relaxed tissue before beginning activity. Regular stretching increases myofibrillar elements, increases sarcomere length (Aten and Knight, 1978; Cooper and Fair, 1978; Corbin and Knoble, 1980; Glick, 1980; Klafs and Arnheim, 1981; Shelton, 1977), and increases lymphatic and venous drainage by 'necking down' of veins. One of the most common methods of stretching is proprioceptive neuromuscular facilitation (PNF), which is similar to the muscle energy technique (MET). Unlike MET, PNF is said to work on the antagonist/ agonist principle, which may be a little simplistic. The overload of sensory stimulus increases the gamma gain causing a reflex reduction in myofascial-tendon unit tone. Since the spinal cord works longitudinally there should be a functional approach to stretching not a muscle isolation approach.

An athlete may ask 'why is it that even though I stretch I still get stiffness in a muscle?' One of the reasons is that poor sensory input to the spinal cord on resistance leads to poor relaxation of muscle. This can result from microscarring from small haemorrhages due to eccentric contraction in sporting activity. Muscle will increase in overall resting length, but with an area or areas of maintained shortened tissue. It is these regions that suffer from poor neurovascular function, setting the stage for injury.

Weight training and lifting

This is a common form of training in athletes, and has potential to cause problems due to lack of understanding of the basic principles. There is often a lack of understanding of the difference between weight training and weight lifting. Weight training is the use of weights at a submaximal level with the objective of conditioning and toning. This is used by athletes as part of a much wider training programme. In weight lifting the object is to train to lift the heaviest weight possible. Types of weight lifting include power lifting, clean and jerk and dead lift.

The priority for any team osteopath is the teaching of safety protocols in the gymnasium. Overzealous behaviour and bad conduct in the weights room are the commonest reasons for injury, from both accidents and poor training methods. Safety is the primary concern. Before the weight room is used check the equipment. Notices should be put up to keep the weight room clean and tidy. No bags or food should be allowed in the gym. Drinks in closed containers can be permitted. A general warm-up is important before beginning weight training. This includes both increasing body metabolic activity and stretching.

Weight training by children

Weight training by children needs to be considered carefully. First, we should make a distinction between adolescent and preadolescent children, preadolescence being before the onset of secondary sexual characteristics and adolescence after this. Young athletes can benefit from supervised submaximal weight training sessions. Weight training in children, even prepubescent children, under good coaching is safe and will contribute to general health. However, weight training should not be the only activity but should be part of a wider programme of athletic activities. Weight lifting in young children should be avoided, due to skeletal immaturity and the lack of circulating testosterone, a major risk is the disruption of epiphyseal plates (growth centres).

The following are basic guidelines for weight training by children.

1. Check that the equipment is safe. Make sure there are no loose nuts and bolts, worn cables etc.
2. Always begin with a warm-up and flexibility session.
3. Warm-up with the exercises and weights to be used, i.e. taking the joints through their complete range of motion with very low resistance weights. Every weight to be used should be taken through this process.
4. All movements should be controlled and smooth. There should be no snatching or ballistic-type movements.
5. Once the young athlete has used all the weights once, they should stretch again before increasing the weight on the next round.
6. On the next round the amount of weight should be increased. They should be able to comfortably do 15–20 repetitions with the weight.
7. Once they have been round again with this higher weight they should stretch again.

- No pain in a child should be dismissed as malingering.
- All joints should be taken through their full ranges.
- Weight training should only be used as part of a wider sporting programme.
- Begin and finish a weight training session on time.
- Explain what is being taught and why.

Overuse injuries are becoming increasingly common in children with the pressure to compete from parents, clubs and self-pressure of seeing team mates achieve higher goals. The most regular presentation is tendonitis and irritation at the tendon attachment to the bone. The majority of these injuries are due to reduced movement at other joints. Pain and irritation at a particular site is often the expression of poor function elsewhere, poor coaching and possibly not enough rest.

Setting up a strength training and rehabilitation programme

Weight training can be used to increase body size and bulk, dynamic strength and muscular endurance. Size and dynamic strength weight training programmes should be followed during the off season and not during the 6 weeks prior to the season. During the 6–8 weeks prior to the first day of practice, the athlete should switch to an endurance, power or circuit programme to maintain strength without tightening up the body as in the bulk and dynamic strength programmes.

Before starting on these programmes certain rules should be understood by the athletes.

1. You must work out a minimum of every other day, three days a week, averaging 50 min per workout, and with enthusiasm. To work out half-heartedly will be a waste of time, it will not accomplish anything and will only lead to disappointment.
2. You will be working with very heavy weights. If not using a weight machine you will need spotters as a safety factor. Spotters will give you confidence in lifting heavier weights, knowing that they will be there to aid you.
3. You must maintain proper form to gain full benefit of the exercises.
4. You must maintain muscular control of the weight being lifted throughout each exercise.
5. You must believe that you can succeed with each goal.
6. You must balance and complement your weight training programme with agility games and running. This will maintain flexibility of the body.

The following is an example of how to set up a strength training and rehabilitation programme.

1. Find the maximum weight with which the athlete can perform one repetition of the required exercise. Concentrate on proper form rather than on the weight lifted. The maximum weight lifted, one repetition, is referred to as the **single lift capacity** (SLC).
   Example: 200 lbs × 1 rep., bench press
   60 lbs × 1 rep., knee extension, one leg.
2. Select the type of programme needed for the individual:
   (a) Bulk programme for increasing body size and static strength.
   (b) Strength programme for the development of dynamic strength.
   (c) Endurance programme for the development of muscular endurance and repetitive motion.
   (d) Power programme for the development of explosive strength and speed of movement.
   (e) Circuit training programme for the combined purpose of the development of strength and cardiovascular–respiratory endurance.

    (f) Progressive resistance exercise programme for the development and rehabilitation of atrophied muscles following surgery or casting.

3. Use the following formulae for the development of the number of repetitions and sets of the exercise and the amount of weight that should be lifted.

    (a) Bulk programme (3–5 sets with no more than 3 repetitions in any set)

        Example: bench press 200 lbs SLC
        Set 1: 3 reps at SLC 20 lbs* (e.g 180 lbs)
        Set 2: 2 reps at SLC 10 lbs* (e.g. 190 lbs)
        Set 3: 1 rep at SLC   (e.g. 200 lbs)

    (b) Strength programme (3 sets with between 4 and 10 repetitions in each set)

        Example: bench press 200 lbs SLC
        Set 1: 8 reps at 80% of SLC   (160 lbs. Example)
        Set 2: 6 reps at 80% of SLC + 10 lbs* (170 lbs. Example)
        Set 3: 4 reps at 80% of SLC + 20 lbs* (180 lbs. Example)

    (c) Endurance programme (3 sets with about 10–15 repetitions and not more than 25 repetitions in each set)

        Example: bench press 200 lbs SLC
        Set 1: 15 reps at 60% of SLC   (120 lbs. Example)
        Set 2: 12 reps at 60% of SLC + 10 lbs* (130 lbs. Example)
        Set 3: 10 reps at 60% of SLC + 20 lbs* (140 lbs. Example)

    (d) Power programme (1–3 sets with approximately 10 repetitions at a very rapid thrust movement)

        Example: bench press 200 lbs SLC
        One set: 10 reps at 75% SLC (150 lbs. Example)

If performing 3 sets, keep weight in all three sets at 75% of SLC.

    (e) Circuit programme

        Example: bench press 200 lbs SLC
        One set: 10 reps at 60% SLC + 20 lbs* (140 lbs. Example)

This programme is performed in an effort to reduce the amount of time that it takes to complete this exercise.

    (f) Progressive resistance exercise programme

        Example: knee extension, one leg, 60 lbs SLC
        Set 1: 10 reps at 50% of SLC (30 lbs. Example)
        Set 2: 10 reps at 75% of SLC (45 lbs. Example)
        Set 3: 1–10 reps at SLC   (60 lbs. Example)
        Set 4: 20 reps at 25% of SLC (15 lbs. Example)

    *If weights being lifted are less than 100 lbs, then substitute 10 lbs for 20 lbs and 5 lbs for 10 lbs; if weights being lifted are more than 300 lbs, then substitute 40 lbs for 20 lbs and 20 lbs for 10 lbs.

4. The weight lifted should be increased whenever the athlete can perform the number of repetitions required in the last set very easily and in proper form.

5. In the case of progressive resistance exercises, the weight should be increased when the athlete can perform 10 repetitions of the third set

very easily and in the proper form. The increase in weight should be 5 lbs for the exercises in which weight being lifted is less than 100 lbs, 10 lbs for exercises in which the weight being lifted is between 100 and 300 lbs, and 20 lbs for exercises in which the weight being lifted is more than 300 lbs.

Remember: these are guidelines only.

Speed, power and reaction time

These are essential elements in the majority of sporting activity. Speed in the runner is a combination of stride length, stride frequency and anaerobic capability. The technique of holding the head still, pumping the arms, leaning forward, and driving the knees high are additionally important elements. Power can be developed in the same way with more resistance to starting and acceleration, hence sprinting up hills. Reaction time is a combination of experience, training and more importantly initial muscular relaxation.

Plyometrics

The principle of plyometrics is that you perform a movement that allows your muscles to store the energy from the effect of gravity and then you perform an opposite action. This forms a kinetic energy system. An example of this is jumping off a box, bending your knees when you hit the ground with your feet and immediately pushing yourself up into the air.

Examples of drills:

1. Bounding: with feet together the athletes jump forwards repeatedly until they get to the other end. Make sure they use their arms for balance and they bend their knees (not fully flexed). Repeat at least four times.
2. Single leg hops: hop on one foot to the other end. Repeat at least twice on each foot.
3. Cone jumping: cones can be used for the athlete to jump over with feet together for the 40 yards.
4. Bounding strides: this is an exaggerated running drill where the athlete takes the biggest strides possible while controlling height with the arms.

Overload principle

It is important in adult training to progressively increase the work load to a level that can be maintained with comfort. This will impose a physiological response in areas of strength, endurance and speed. Basically, hypertrophy, endurance and strength of muscular tissue will increase only when the muscle performs for a given time period at its maximum strength and endurance capacity. This means that the work loads have to be higher than those normally encountered in normal activity. One of the most renowned experiments demonstrating the overload principle was carried out by Hellebrant and Houtz (1956).

Training sessions

Training sessions are broadly split into pre-season, in-season and post-season sessions. Each has its merits and goals.

Training as rehabilitation

When athletes are returning to fitness they often have residual aches and pains and it is important not to ignore these. All aches and pains need to be examined, assessed and treated continuously. Training while not being treated only slows the recovery and is a naive and poor way of combining rehabilitation and training protocols, i.e. running off an injury.

Jogging

Many patients may ask you about jogging as rehabilitation after an injury or attempt to get fit. There is no correct way to jog. Here are some basic guidelines.

1. A medical history and clinical examination (e.g. blood pressure) should be carried out to make sure there are no health problems.
2. If the patient has not jogged before or for some years a postural examination (dynamic and static) is vital as a precaution to prevent problems. Passive examination is performed with the patient standing still, while they follow a range of movements in an active examination; watching them jog is a dynamic postural examination. For example, it should be checked that when running the head is kept up and not over the feet or knees.
3. Arms should be held slightly away from the body and should be slightly bent at the elbows so that the elbows and hands are approximately the same distance from the ground. Joggers should keep arms relaxed. Do not clench the fists. It helps to periodically shake the arms while working out.
4. It is vitally important for the feet to strike the ground properly. The best technique is to land first on the heel of the foot, then rock forward and take off from the ball of the foot on the next step. Many joggers find it comfortable to land on the entire bottom of the foot, putting most of their weight on the ball of the foot. Landing on the ball of the foot alone should be avoided.
5. Keep steps or strides short while jogging. Let the foot strike the ground beneath the knee instead of stretching it out. If you wish to lengthen the stride, then you may stretch it out. The slower the rate of running the shorter the stride should be.

6. Breathe deeply and in a controlled way while jogging. Develop a rhythm which is comfortable for you. Breathing should be relaxed; do not hold your breath.
7. If you become uncomfortable while jogging, take it easy, slow down or walk.
8. Train, don't strain. Gradually build up, start with short distances and walk for part of it if necessary. You may wish to set a goal. Running too far, too long, too soon has discouraged many joggers. Build up gradually.

REFERENCES

Aten, D.W. and Knight, K.L. (1978) Therapeutic exercise in athletic training. *Athletic Training*, **13**, 123–6.

Barnard, R.J. (1976) The heart needs warm-up time. *The Physician and Sports Medicine*, **4**(9).

Cooper, D.L. and Fair, J. (1978) Developing and testing flexibility. *The Physician and Sports Medicine*, **10**, 137–8.

Corbin, C.B. and Noble, L. (1980) Flexibility: a major component of physical fitness. *Journal of Physical Education and Recreation*, **6**, 23–60.

Denslow, J.S. (1947) The place of the osteopathic concept in the healing art.

Glick, J.M. (1980) Muscle strains: prevention and treatment. *The Physician and Sports Medicine*, **11**, 73–7.

Hellebrant, F. and Houtz, S. (1956) Mechanisms of muscle training in man: experimental demonstration of the overload principle. *Physical Therapy Review*, **36**, 371–83.

Klafs, C.E. and Arnheim, D.D. (1981) *Modern Principles of Training*, C.V. Mosby, St Louis.

Shelton, R.E. (1977) What is exercise? *Osteopathic Annals*, **9**, 48–54.

FURTHER READING

Marino, M., Nicholas, J.A., Gleim, G.W., Rosenthal, P. and Nicholas, S.J. (1982) The efficiency of manual assessment of muscle strength using a new device. *American Journal of Sports Medicine*, **10**(6), 360–4.

Williams, P.E., Catanese, T., Lucey, E.G. and Goldspink, G. (1988) The importance of stretch and contractile activity in the prevention of connective tissue accumulation in muscle. *Journal of Anatomy*, **158**, 109–14.

Index

Page numbers appearing in **bold** refer to figures and page numbers appearing in *italics* refer to tables.